# Movement Disorders in Neurologic Disease

## Effects on Communication and Swallowing

# Movement Disorders in Neurologic Disease

## Effects on Communication and Swallowing

Leonard L. LaPointe, PhD
Bruce E. Murdoch, PhD

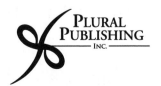

PLURAL
PUBLISHING
INC.

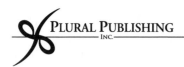

5521 Ruffin Road
San Diego, CA 92123

e-mail: info@pluralpublishing.com
Web site: http://www.pluralpublishing.com

Library of Congress Cataloging-in-Publication Data

LaPointe, Leonard L.
  Movement disorders in neurologic disease : effects on communication and
swallowing / Leonard L. LaPointe, Bruce E. Murdoch, authors.
     p. ; cm.
  Includes bibliographical references and index.
  ISBN-13: 978-1-59756-152-5 (alk. paper)
  ISBN-10: 1-59756-152-5 (alk. paper)
  I. Murdoch, B. E., 1950- II. Title.
  [DNLM: 1. Movement Disorders—complications. 2. Communication Disorders
—etiology. 3. Deglutition Disorders—etiology. 4. Speech Disorders—etiology.
WL 390]
  RC376.5
  616.8'3—dc23
                         2013015065

# Contents

# Contributors

**Leonard L. LaPointe, PhD**
Francis Eppes Distinguished Professor of Communication Science and Disorders
Faculty, Program in Neuroscience
Faculty, College of Medicine
Florida State University
Tallahassee, FL
Editor-in-Chief
Journal of Medical Speech-Language Pathology
*Chapters 1, 2, 3, 9, and 11*

**Bruce E. Murdoch, PhD, DSc**
Director
Center for Neurogenic Communication Disorders Research
 School of Health and Rehabilitation Sciences
The University of Queensland
Australia
*Chapters 4, 5, 6, 7, and 10*

**Julie A. G. Stierwalt, PhD**
Associate Professor
School of Communication Science and Disorders
Florida State University
Tallahassee, FL
*Chapter 8*

*This book is dedicated to Woody Guthrie and Slim Dusty, two iconic singer-songwriters who knew the perils of movement disorders and cancer. Each carved their indelible impressions on the cultures of their respective lands. We hum their songs and pass along their messages.*

# 1

# Introduction, Definitions, Foundations, and Scope

*LEONARD L. LAPOINTE*

*Executing a triple-twisting dismount from the parallel bars . . . playing a violin concerto . . . juggling a bowling ball, a machete, and a mango . . . driving a pickup truck . . . paddling a canoe . . . tying a knot . . . typing . . . walking . . . eating . . . zipping . . . sipping . . . scratching . . . washing . . . writing . . . hugging . . . humming . . . laughing . . . talking . . .*

Human movement can be a wonder and a curse. We take for granted not only the complex movement sequences that go into creative activity, but also the mundane moves of everyday life. When things are going along well, our preoccupations are elsewhere, and we give only a passing thought to the automatized programs of ordering and executing the muscles of the body into some sort of action. But all of these movements, many of which relate to activities that characterize us

as uniquely human, are the result of a finely coordinated neuromuscular system that is composed of, presided over, and regulated by a delicate balance of nervous system integrity.

Bad things, however, can happen to good people, and the thousands of little activities that we piece together in a day can be at once jeopardized by pathology to the nervous system. In seconds, or sometimes insidiously over a span of days or months, our ability to conduct ourselves in an efficient and dignified fashion can be lost or irrevocably impaired. The network of levels and systems that program and effect such simple movements as saying our name or picking up the phone or drinking a cup of coffee can be grossly affected. Sitting up, walking, writing, or putting speech sounds together into sentences can be so impaired as to make daily living a challenge for some

1

and a living nightmare for others. To humanize these conditions we include the thoughts, quotations, and impressions of the most important segment of people impacted by the movement disorders, those who have experienced them. Although we desire our work to be firmly grounded in scholarliness, objectivity, and sound science, we want also to never lose touch with the thoughts and feelings of those who are within the eye of the storm of movement disorders and have lost those things that make us most human: the gifts of communication and thinking.

The following account provides the impressions of a 60-year-old woman, originally from India, as she waited to see a physician in the Highgate Hill Surgery in Brisbane, Australia. The first author (LLL) observed and spoke with this woman during that interminable span of time both were waiting to see a physician. She was diagnosed with a unique pastiche of movement disorders: spasmodic torticollis or cervical dystonia, with accompanying blepharospasm and oromandibular focal dystonia. Her voice was weak. Her speech was imprecise and difficult to comprehend. She had trouble chewing and swallowing a piece of apple she retrieved from a small plastic bag. Her impressions reveal some of the genuine psychosocial impact on her self-esteem and her discomfort at having her condition so readily revealed and apparent within the confines of a general practitioner's waiting room:

> I can hardly make myself look at the other people in the doctor's office. My friend Jerry brought me to my appointment once again. He is a godsend. He usually sits outside and

smokes a cigarette while I wait. I love this doctor, but today she is backed up and running behind. The small office is full. There are two young women, one with a child who looks like he is perhaps half aboriginal. Nice little boy. About 3 years old. Yellow cotton shirt. He looks like he might have to go to the bathroom. Another woman with a cervical collar and elastic wraps around her ankle. She appears to be in great distress, very emaciated, and wan-looking. Two Yanks are seated next to me. Looks to be a man and wife. She's reading a picture book of Tasmania. He looks anxious, but interested in me in sort of a clinical way. I later got to know him and shared with him some of my thoughts. She keeps trying not to notice me, but I can see her noticing out of her peripheral vision. I cannot sit still. My cervical dystonia, or spasmodic torticollis, or whatever they're calling it now is really bad this week. This waiting room is small, and we're all cramped together, and I got one of the non-comfortable wooden chairs that keeps squeaking and making noise as I writhe and shift position to try to find some semblance of comfort or rest. Ha. Cramped together. Good choice of words. I'm the only one who is really cramped. My neck is full of spasms and twisting way over to the right today. I change my posture by sitting up as straight as I can and trying to forcibly extend my neck backwards. It is drawn, as if by some thick rubber band to the right, and contorts and pulls my neck inexorably to the right. I try straightening it with my hand, first by just stroking the side of my face, then by resting my chin in my hand and applying gradual pressure to try to get my head and face turned to the midline more. My mouth region seems particularly affected today, as well. My lips keep pursing and the round lip muscles draw up like a purse string. Sometimes a smacking or sucking noise is emitted by these movements, though I certainly try to stop them. My tongue is tense and moving around inside my mouth. I keep my mouth closed as best I can and hope that the tongue-stirring inside of it is not observable through my cheeks. My eye is worse today also. I have to keep changing positions and each time I do, this wooden chair squeaks or grates noisily. The little boy is wandering all around the waiting room. He has an apple, partly eaten and brown-stained, and a little cloth bunny that he is playing with. He looks up at me and stares at my twisting and chair-squeaking. He takes the apple over to a bronze statue of a young girl and tries to offer the statue a bite of his apple. It doesn't bite. He then places the cloth bunny on the leg of the statue as a gesture of sharing. I can't wait until my name is called and I can get in to see the doctor. These public displays in confined spaces are the worst. You'd think I'd be used to it by now. I've had this condition for years and still it is so exhausting to go out in public, especially in small, confined rooms like this. I twist my body to try to compensate for my twisted head position. This triggers more of the unwanted head and neck movement and writhing, and this chair seems to be getting louder. I can't sit still. I can't sit straight. Why can't I just relax? Why are they looking at me? I can't help it. Sometimes this is so humiliating I want to cry. But I have cried enough. I want to scream. Why can't they do something for me? Maybe acupuncture. Maybe nothing. Maybe I'll just have to get used to it. I'm much better at home. These are

the painful times. If only it didn't hurt so much. At least it's better when I sleep. I'll take a nap when I get home. To sleep perchance to rest easy, without my neck and head twisted in some abnormal, grotesque posture. To sleep perchance to steal some relief. To sleep perchance to dream of when I was a young woman in India. When I was popular and the pride of my village. When I was not twisted. When I was free of pain . . . Maybe this doctor will have some help for me. I've heard of a new treatment being used of a powerful injection to break the cramping muscles. I would like some relief. I would like to stop being the object of everyone's curiosity. I would like to be free of pain and be able to walk straight again, and sit quietly, without writhing and twisting and being the object of attention of everyone in this small waiting room at the top of the hill.

Numerous and variegated diseases and conditions fit under the umbrella of movement disorders. Some are common and easily recognizable. Some are rare and bizarre. When they affect human communication and swallowing, individuals are robbed of precious and vital aspects of living. The area of movement disorders focuses on a variety of conditions that are characterized by hypokinetic, hyperkinetic, or abnormally coordinated movements. These conditions include tremor, parkinsonism, dystonia, myoclonus, chorea, ballismus, ataxia, tic disorders, dyskinesia, akathisia, restless limbs, and others. The term "movement disorders" may be used to refer to either abnormal movements or to syndromes that cause these abnormal movements. The classification of movement disorders is based on phenomenology, individual syndromes, or etiology. In this book, we first review the terminology used to describe movement disorders, then discuss individual movement disorder syndromes. Appendix 1–A contains a brief description of some of the basic nomenclature used in movement disorders. It would be useful to study this list prior to reading further. A more extensive glossary can be found at the end of the book.

## Scope of the Problem: How Many and What Impact?

The scope and extent of movement disorders worldwide is mind-boggling. Unfortunately, completely accurate statistics do not exist on the incidence or prevalence of these myriad disorders. We have educated guesses and estimations based on such factors as number of diagnoses made in hospitals and health care facilities. This in no way accounts for the number of unreported cases and some estimations are that anywhere from 10% to 50% of living, breathing persons with these disorders go undiagnosed or unreported. Epidemiology is the medical term used for the study of diseases and disorders in a given population. It is important because it forms the basis for making intervention and public health decisions as well as providing evidence and logic to support allocation of resources to keep communities and populations healthy. Incidence and prevalence are two of the cornerstones of epidemiology. Prevalence refers to the actual number of cases or people in

a defined or given group or community at a point in time (e.g., 7 people with diagnosed Parkinson disease lived in Channing, Michigan in 2013; 81 individuals with ataxia were reported in Noosa, Queensland in 2010). Incidence is a related term but refers to a measure of the risk or probability of developing some new condition within a specified period of time. Although sometimes loosely expressed simply as the occurrence of new cases during some time period, it is more accurately expressed as a proportion or a rate with a denominator (e.g., out of 1,000 live births in Toowoomba during 2005 to 2010, 12 infants were born with cerebral palsy). These examples are illustrative only. Epidemiologic data help physicians and other health professionals understand the probability of certain diagnoses or conditions and is regularly used by epidemiologists, health care providers, government agencies, and insurers. It informs us as to whether certain conditions are rare or common. Epidemiology does not, however, measure the full scope of the problem of movement disorders. The amount of suffering, disability, lost income, shattered lives, mental anguish, blood, sweat, and lachrymal secretion are not captured in the cold, hard numbers.

The brain and nervous system are major players on the field of diseases and abnormal conditions. The brain is protected, to a degree, but nasty things happen to it every minute of every day. The scope of the global problem of nervous system disease is broad and getting broader. Major new epidemiologic analyses are focusing attention on disorders of the nervous system as important causes of death and disability around the world (Bergen & Silberberg, 2002; Neuroepidemiology, 2012). These authors characterize nervous system disease as a global epidemic.

On our big blue marble of a world, one in every nine individuals dies of a disorder of the nervous system. Stroke outweighs all other neurologic disorders combined as a cause of mortality. Most disorders of the nervous system occur in developing countries. Developmental disability due to malnutrition, and cognitive dysfunction associated with parasitic infections, are the most common neurologic disorders. As the world's population ages and the effects of infectious disease decline, the life-altering effects of many disorders of the nervous system, including stroke and dementia, are increasing. Bergen and Silberberg (2002) contend that the disorders of the nervous system causing the highest rates of death and disability are preventable and treatable. Not all, but many, of these brain-based conditions result in disorders of movement. As with all convincing epidemiologic studies, increased awareness of the global effects of neurologic disorders should help health care policymakers and health care workers generate and establish appropriate priorities in research, prevention, and management of these conditions.

The world is full of brain-based diseases and conditions, and the array of those that affect moving are daunting. Of the most common movement disorders, Parkinson disease and parkinsonism account for about 1% of the general population (Figure 1–1). In a country of approximately 310 million people (World Population Clock, 2010), that means that over 3 million people have Parkinson disease.

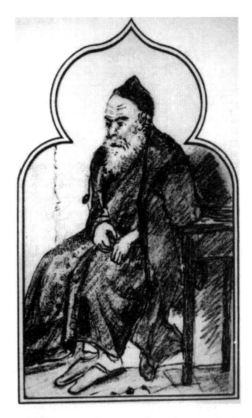

**FIGURE 1–1.** Famous French neurologist Jean-Martin Charcot's drawing of a patient with Parkinson disease in Morocco, 1889.

## References

Bergen, D. C., & Silberberg, D. (2002). Nervous system disorders: A global epidemic. *Archives of Neurology, 59,* 1194–1196.

Neuroepidemiology. (2012). 2012 Neuroepidemiology Annual Report. Retrieved January 24, 2013 from http://www.wfneurology.org/2012-neuroepidemiology-annual-report

WeMove (2010). Glossary. Retrieved January 24, 2013 from http://www.wemove.org/glossary/

World Population Clock. (2010). Retrieved February 3, 2010 from http://www.census.gov/main/www/popclock.html/

## Appendix 1–A
# Specialized Terms Related to Movement Disorders

**Action tremor:** A tremor that occurs during the performance of voluntary movements. Such tremors include postural, isometric, kinetic, and intention tremors.

**Agonist:** A muscle whose contraction executes an intended movement.

**Akinesia:** Absence of movement or loss of the ability to move such as temporary or prolonged paralysis or "freezing in place."

**Akinetic:** Referring to absence or poverty of voluntary movement; loss of the ability to move all or part of the body.

**Ambulation:** The act of walking.

**Antagonist:** (1) A muscle whose contraction opposes an intended movement. (2) A drug that blocks a receptor, preventing stimulation.

**Anticholinergic agents:** Anticholinergic medications are drugs that block the action of acetylcholine, a neurotransmitter with an effect opposite to that of dopamine. By blocking the action of acetylcholine, these drugs increase the ability of dopamine to control movement.

**Apraxia:** Loss of the ability to sequence, coordinate, and execute certain purposeful movements and gestures in the absence of motor weakness, paralysis, or sensory impairments. Apraxia may affect almost any pattern of voluntary movements, including those required for proper eye gaze, walking, speaking, writing, or handling a chicken.

**Ataxia:** A condition characterized by an impaired ability to coordinate voluntary movements. Ataxia may result from damage to the cerebellum, cerebellar pathways, or the spinal cord due to various underlying disorders, conditions, or other factors.

**Athetosis:** Involuntary, relatively slow, writhing movements that essentially flow into one another. Athetosis is often associated with chorea, a related condition characterized by involuntary, rapid, irregular, jerky movements. Although athetosis may be most prominent in the face, neck, tongue, and hands, the condition may affect any muscle group.

**Automatic behavior:** Automatic behaviors are those during which a person performs a routine task without any awareness of doing so.

**Ballismus:** An abnormal neuromuscular condition that is generally considered a severe form of chorea. Involvement of the upper muscles of the arms and legs results in uncontrolled, violent, flinging, or throwing actions.

**Basal ganglia:** Specialized nerve cell clusters of gray matter deep within each cerebral hemisphere and the upper brainstem, including the striate body (caudate and lentiform nuclei) and other cell groups such as the subthalamic nucleus and substantia nigra. The basal ganglia assist in initiating and regulating movement.

**Botulinum toxin (BTX):** Any of a group of toxins, designated as A through G, produced by *Clostridium botulinum* bacteria. Localized injection of minute amounts of commercially prepared BTX may help to relax an overactive muscle by blocking the release of acetylcholine, a neurotransmitter responsible for the activation of muscle contractions. BTX-A is currently the only form (i.e., serotype) of botulinum toxin approved for clinical use. (BTX-A [BOTOX®] is produced by Allergan, Inc., and used in the United

---

Adapted from and used with the permission of WE MOVE 2007. Retrieved January 24, 2013 from http://www.wemove.org/

States and many other countries. Outside the United States, it is available as Dysport® from Ipsen, Ltd.) It was originally introduced in the 1970s for the treatment of misalignment of the eyes (strabismus) and involuntary contraction of eyelid muscles (blepharospasm) associated with dystonia or facial nerve disorders. BTX-A is now increasingly being used as a therapeutic option for selected patients with other disorders characterized by severely increased muscle activity (hyperactivity), such as tremor, other focal dystonias, and spasticity.

**Brady Bunch:** An American television situation comedy based around a large blended family that aired in the 1970s. Ambulation by the cast members of the Brady Bunch has been referred to by some as bradykinesia.

**Bradykinesia:** Slowness of voluntary movements. The gradual loss of spontaneous movement.

**Caudate nuclei:** One of the three major substructures that, together with the globus pallidus and putamen, form the basal ganglia. The caudate nuclei and putamen, which are relatively similar structurally and functionally, are collectively known as the striatum. Specialized clusters of nerve cells or nuclei within the caudate receive input from certain regions of the cerebral cortex. This information is processed and then relayed (by way of the thalamus) to areas of the brain responsible for controlling complex motor functions. The caudate nuclei are specifically thought to process and transmit cognitive information that influences the initiation of complex motor activities.

**Cerebellum:** A two-lobed region of the brain located behind the brainstem. The cerebellum receives messages concerning balance, posture, muscle tone, and muscle contraction or extension. Working in coordination with the basal ganglia and thalamus, the cerebellum integrates, adjusts, and refines messages transmitted to muscle groups from the cerebral cortex (i.e., motor cortex). Thus, the cerebellum plays an essential role in producing smooth, coordinated, voluntary movements; maintaining proper posture; and sustaining balance.

**Chorea:** Jerky, irregular, relatively rapid involuntary movement that primarily involve muscles of the face or extremities. Choreic or choreaform movements are relatively simple and discrete or highly complex in nature. Although involuntary and purposeless, these movements are sometimes incorporated into deliberate movement patterns. When several choreic movements are present, they often appear relatively slow, writhing, or sinuous, resembling athetosis. Chorea may occur in association with certain neurodegenerative diseases, including Wilson disease and Huntington disease, or systemic disorders, such as lupus. In addition, chorea is a dominant feature in Sydenham chorea or may result from the use of certain medications, such as particular anticonvulsant or antipsychotic agents.

**Clonus:** Movements characterized by alternate contractions and relaxations of a muscle, occurring in rapid succession. Clonus is frequently observed in conditions such as spasticity and certain seizure disorders.

**Contractures:** Fixed resistance to passive stretching of certain muscles due to shortening or wasting (atrophy) of muscle fibers or the development of scar tissue (fibrosis) over joints.

**Corticobulbar:** Referring to or connecting the cerebral cortex with the nuclei or groups of cell bodies of the diencephalon (thalamus, hypothalamus, and other nuclei) or brainstem (bulb).

**Corticospinal:** Referring to or connecting the outer region of the brain (cerebral cortex) and the spinal cord.

**Cranial nerve nuclei:** Specialized groups of nerve cells (nuclei) that give rise to and convey or receive impulses from sensory and motor constituents of the cranial nerves, which are the 12 pairs of nerves that emerge from the brain. These nerve pairs convey sensory impulses for various functions including taste, smell, hearing, and vision; motor impulses involved in controlling eye movements, chewing, swallowing, facial expressions, etc.; and impulses for transmission to certain organs and glands for regulation of various involuntary or autonomic activities.

**Dopamine:** Dopamine is a chemical that is known as a neurotransmitter. Neurotransmitters help relay messages from one nerve cell to another. Dopamine is especially important in relaying messages about movement.

**Dopamine agonist (DA):** A drug that acts like dopamine. DAs combine with dopamine receptors to mimic dopamine actions. Such medications stimulate dopamine receptors and produce dopamine-like effects.

**Dysarthria(s):** A group of movement-based disorders of speech (respiration, phonation, resonance, articulation) due to disturbances of muscular control (range, velocity, or direction of movement) or muscular planning and coordination usually resulting from damage to the central or peripheral nervous system.

**Dyskinesias:** Abnormal neuromuscular conditions characterized by disorganized or excessive movement (also known as hyperkinesia). Forms of dyskinesia include sudden, brief, "shock-like" muscle contractions (myoclonus); involuntary, rhythmic, oscillatory movements of a body part (tremor); rapid involuntary jerky movements (chorea); relatively slow writhing motions (athetosis); or abrupt, purposeless, simple, or complex muscle movements or vocalizations (motor or vocal tics).

**Dysphagia:** Difficulty in swallowing. Dysphagia may be associated with structural etiologies as well as certain neurodegenerative or motor disorders involving the tongue, pharynx, or esophagus, and their innervation.

**Dyspraxia:** Partial loss of the ability to coordinate and perform certain purposeful movements and gestures that are not the result of paralysis, paresis, or sensory impairments. Dyspraxia is technically an impairment of function and apraxia a loss of function, but the term apraxia in North America is understood to refer to all levels of loss of purposeful movement. Dyspraxia is favored in Europe, Australia, and elsewhere.

**Dystonia:** A neurologic movement disorder characterized by sustained muscle contractions, resulting in repetitive, involuntary, twisting, or writhing movements and unusual postures or positioning. Dystonia may be limited to specific muscle groups (focal dystonia), such as dystonia affecting muscles of the neck (cervical dystonia or spasmodic torticollis) or the eyes, resulting in closure of the eyelids (blepharospasm).

**Essential tremor (ET):** A common, slowly, and variably progressive neurologic movement disorder characterized by involuntary, rhythmic, "back-and-forth" movements (i.e., tremor) of a body part or parts. In ET patients, tremor is primarily a "postural" or "kinetic" tremor or may be a combination of both types, that is, tremor while voluntarily maintaining a fixed position against gravity (postural tremor) and/or when conducting self-directed, targeted actions (kinetic intention tremor).

**Extrapyramidal system:** Refers to central nervous system structures (i.e., outside the cerebrospinal pyramidal tracts) that play a role in controlling motor functions. The extrapyramidal system includes substructures of the basal ganglia and the brainstem and interconnections with certain regions of the cerebellum, cerebrum, and other areas of the central nervous system. Extrapyramidal disturbances may result in postural and muscle tone abnormalities as well as the development of certain involuntary movements.

**Gait:** The style or manner of walking. Gait disturbances may be associated with certain neurologic or neuromuscular disorders, orthopedic conditions, inflammatory conditions of the joints (i.e., arthritic changes), or other abnormalities.

**Globus pallidus:** A major substructure of the basal ganglia deep within the brain. Specialized groups of nerve cells in the globus pallidus function as an "intermediate relay system." This system processes and transmits information from the basal ganglia by way of the thalamus to areas of the brain that regulate complex motor functions (e.g., motor cortex, premotor area of frontal lobe).

**Hoehn and Yahr Scale:** The Hoehn and Yahr Scale is a commonly used physician-administered rating of the global severity of the motor symptoms of Parkinson disease. Scores range from 0, no signs of disease, to 5, wheelchair bound or bedridden without assistance.

**Huntington disease (HD):** A hereditary, progressive, neurodegenerative disorder primarily characterized by the development of emotional, behavioral, and psychiatric abnormalities; gradual deterioration of thought processing and acquired intellectual abilities (dementia); and movement abnormalities, including involuntary, rapid, irregular jerky movements (chorea) of the face, arms, legs, or trunk.

**Hyperkinetic:** Characterized by excessive movement because of abnormally increased motor activity or function. Certain movement disorders are termed "hyperkinetic" such as tics or essential tremor.

**Hypokinetic:** Diminished movement and decreased motor function. Some movement disorders are hypokinetic, such as Parkinson disease.

**Levodopa:** Levodopa is a drug used to treat Parkinson disease. It is also called L-dopa and, in the United States, is sold as Sinemet®. Levodopa crosses the blood-brain barrier and is converted by the body to dopamine. A loss of dopamine-producing nerve cells in the part of the brain that controls movements leads to the symptoms of Parkinson disease.

**Motor fluctuations:** Motor fluctuations occur when levodopa is used to treat Parkinson disease. As the disease becomes worse, the number of cells in the brain that store dopamine decreases, the symptoms of Parkinson disease worsen, and levodopa is not as effective in controlling the symptoms. When this happens, a person is said to have "off" episodes.

**Motor signs and symptoms:** Signs or symptoms that affect movement. The motor symptoms of Parkinson disease include tremor, stiffness (called rigidity), slowness or absence of movement (called bradykinesia or akinesia, respectively), and difficulty maintaining balance or unstable posture.

**Multiple sclerosis (MS):** A progressive disease of the central nervous system characterized by destruction of myelin (demyelination), the fatty substance that forms a protective sheath around certain long nerve fibers (axons). Myelin serves as an electrical insulator, enabling the effective transmission of nerve signals. People with MS may develop paresthesias, such as numbness or tingling; muscle weakness and stiffness; impaired coordination; abnormal reflexes; an inability to control urination (urinary incontinence); hypokinetic dysarthria; visual disturbances; and/or other signs and symptoms.

**Myoclonus:** A neurologic movement disorder characterized by brief, involuntary, twitching or "shock-like" contractions of a muscle or muscle group. These jerk-like movements may be accompanied by periodic, unexpected interruptions in voluntary muscle contraction, leading to lapses of sustained posture (known as "negative myoclonus"). "Positive" and "negative" myoclonus is often seen in the same individuals and may affect the same muscle groups. Myoclonus is often a nonspecific finding, meaning that it may occur in the setting of additional neurologic abnormalities and be associated with any number of underlying conditions or disorders. In other patients, myoclonus appears as an isolated or a primary finding.

**Neurodegenerative:** Marked by or pertaining to neurologic degeneration; deterioration of the structure or function of tissue within the nervous system.

**Neurotransmitter:** A specialized substance (such as norepinephrine or acetylcholine) that transfers nerve impulses across spaces between nerve cells (synapses). Neurotransmitters are naturally produced chemicals by which nerve cells communicate.

**Off episodes:** This term refers to the times when people with Parkinson disease have a decrease in the ability to move (hypomobility) and other signs and symptoms that cause difficulty rising from a chair, speaking, walking, or performing their usual activities. Off episodes occur because the person's dose of levodopa has worn off too soon or has suddenly and unexpectedly stopped providing benefit.

**On time:** Motor fluctuations occur when levodopa is used to treat Parkinson disease. As the disease becomes worse, the number of cells in the brain that store dopamine decreases, the symptoms of Parkinson disease worsen, and levodopa is not as effective in controlling the symptoms. When this happens, a person is said to have "off" episodes. The times in which the levodopa is effective and the person with Parkinson disease is able to function normally is called "on time."

**Paresthesias:** Abnormal sensations occurring spontaneously or in response to stimulation. Paresthesias may include prickling, tingling, burning, or tickling feelings; numbness; "pins and needles"; or cramp-like sensations. Various neurologic movement disorders may be characterized by paresthesias, including restless legs syndrome (RLS), paroxysmal kinesigenic dyskinesia (PKD), and paroxysmal nonkinesigenic dyskinesia (PNKD).

**Parkinson disease (PD):** A slowly progressive degenerative disorder of the central nervous system characterized by slowness or poverty of movement (bradykinesia), rigidity, postural instability, and tremor primarily while at rest.

**Parkinsonism:** A constellation of the following symptoms: tremor, rigidity, bradykinesia (slow movements), and loss of postural reflexes. Although classically seen in Parkinson disease, parkinsonism may have other causes. In the elderly, parkinsonism may be caused by dopamine-blocking drugs, multiple system atrophy, striatonigral degeneration, Shy-Drager syndrome, cortico basal degeneration, diffuse Lewy body disease, and Alzheimer disease with parkinsonism. In younger people, parkinsonism may be caused by juvenile-onset dystonia/parkinsonism, Westphal variant of Huntington disease, Wilson disease, L-dopa-responsive dystonia, Hallervorden-Spatz disease, and progressive pallidal degeneration.

**Paroxysmal movement disorders:** Certain neurologic movement disorders characterized by abrupt, transient episodes of abnormal involuntary movement, such as chorea, athetosis, dystonia, and/or ballismus (i.e., the paroxysmal dyskinesias) or impaired coordination of voluntary actions and other associated findings (i.e., paroxysmal ataxias).

**Postural tremor:** Any tremor that is present while an individual voluntarily maintains a position against gravity, such as holding the arms outstretched.

**Progressive supranuclear palsy (PSP):** A progressive neurologic disorder characterized by neurodegenerative changes of certain brain regions, including particular areas of the basal ganglia and the brainstem. Symptom onset most often occurs in the sixth decade of life. Associated findings may include balance difficulties, sudden falls, stiffness (rigidity), slowness of movement (bradykinesia), an impaired ability to perform certain voluntary eye movements, and visual disturbances.

**Putamen:** One of the three major brain regions that, together with the caudate nuclei and the globus pallidus, comprise the basal ganglia. Relatively similar in function and structure, the putamen and the caudate nuclei are collectively referred to as the striatum. Specialized groups of nerve cells within the putamen receive input from various regions of the cerebral cortex. The messages are processed and relayed by way of the thalamus to the motor cortex, influencing voluntary movement.

**Range of motion (ROM):** The extent of a structure's free movement. The normal ROM of the elbow, for instance, carries the forearm through a half-circle. Passive ROM is tested while the limb is relaxed. Active ROM is movement controlled by the individual. Tongue range of motion is frequently related to types of dysarthria.

**Rhythmic myoclonus:** Involuntary, shock-like contractions or spasms of a muscle or muscle group that occur in a rhythmic pattern. This usually occurs as a result of a lesion in the central nervous system.

**Rigidity:** Stiffness and resistance to movement; may be a sign of a neurologic movement disorder such as Parkinson disease.

**Sialorrhea:** Excess production of saliva, or increased retention of saliva in the mouth, due to difficulty swallowing.

**Spasmodic dysphonia (SD):** A manifestation of dystonia. SD involves the muscles of the larynx and surrounding muscles and therefore involves phonation and the production of voice and speech. In individuals with SD, phonation is interrupted by intermittent spasms of the muscles of the larynx.

**Spasmodic torticollis (ST):** A form of dystonia involving the muscles of the neck, and therefore called "cervical dystonia." As a result of the abnormal involuntary contractions of the neck muscles, the head may be rotated, tilted, flexed, extended, or any combination of these postures. The movements may be quick, sustained, or patterned and, therefore, may be associated with tremor.

**Spasticity:** An abnormal increase in muscle tone that may be caused by certain types of damage to the nerve pathways regulating muscles. Spasticity is a common complication of cerebral palsy, brain injuries, spinal cord injuries, multiple sclerosis, and stroke. Spasticity can lead to incoordination, loss of function, pain, and permanent muscle shortening, or contracture.

**Stereotypic:** Inappropriate, persistent repetition of particular bodily postures, actions, or speech patterns. These are typically involuntary, rhythmic, coordinated, and purposeless movements, postures, or vocalizations that may appear ritualistic or purposeful in nature. Stereotypies may be associated with a variety of neurologic and behavioral disorders, such as Tourette syndrome, obsessive-compulsive disorders, Rett syndrome, restless legs syndrome, schizophrenia, and autism.

**Striatum:** An area of the brain that controls movement and balance. It is connected to and receives signals from the substantia nigra.

**Substantia nigra:** A dark band of gray matter (cell bodies) deep within the brain where cells manufacture the neurotransmitter dopamine for movement control.

Degeneration of cells in this region may lead to a neurologic movement disorder such as Parkinson disease.

**Substrate:** A chemical substance that is acted upon by an enzyme is called a substrate.

**Thalamus:** An area of the brain consisting of two relatively large masses of gray matter. The thalamus relays information from most sensory organs to the outer region of the cerebrum or cerebral cortex; receives and processes messages from the body concerning heat, cold, pain, pressure, and touch; and influences motor activity of the cerebral cortex.

**Tics:** Involuntary, compulsive, stereotypic muscle movements or vocalizations that abruptly interrupt normal motor activities. These repetitive, purposeless motions (motor tics) or utterances (vocal tics) may be simple or complex in nature; may be temporarily suppressed; and are often preceded by a "foreboding" sensation or urge that is temporarily relieved following their execution.

**Tremor:** Rhythmic, involuntary, oscillatory (or to-and-fro) movements of a body part.

**Unified Parkinson Disease Rating Scale (UPDRS):** The UPDRS is the most commonly used tool to rate the signs and symptoms of Parkinson disease.

**Upper motor neurons:** Nerve cells extending from the brain to the spinal cord that control movement.

**Ventral intermediate (VIM) nucleus:** A specific region of the thalamus. This area of the brain is involved in the control of movement and is the "target" area for thalamotomy and deep brain stimulation when treating patients with tremor.

**White matter:** Bundles of myelinated nerve fibers or axons. These nerve fibers have a creamy white appearance due to myelin, a whitish substance that primarily contains fats and proteins. Myelin forms a protective, insulating sheath around certain axons, functioning as an electrical insulator and ensuring efficient nerve conduction. The breakdown, destruction, or loss of myelin from a nerve or nerves (demyelination), such as seen in certain neurodegenerative diseases, results in impaired nerve impulse transmission.

# 2

# Etiologies of Movement Disorders

*LEONARD L. LAPOINTE*

## Introduction

Major new epidemiologic analyses are focusing attention on disorders of the nervous system as important causes of death and disability and mayhem around the world. This is true for Florida, Tasmania, Beijing, Cape Town, and Channing. This has been documented by Bergen and Silberberg (2002) and many other epidemiologists. One in every nine individuals dies of a disorder of the nervous system. Stroke outweighs all other neurologic disorders combined as a cause of mortality. Most disorders of the nervous system occur in developing countries. Not everyone gets enough to eat. The plethora of fast food restaurants and street food is not present in every land. The undernourished outnumber the obese. Skinny trumps fat. There are over 900 million people in the world today who are

undernourished and about 500 million who are obese (Stop the Hunger, 2012). An undernourished body can be the harbinger of poor nervous system disease and later problems with all things related to brain control of the body. Developmental disability due to malnutrition, and cognitive dysfunction associated with parasitic infections are the most common neurologic disorders. As the world's population ages and the effects of infectious disease decline, the relative effects of many disorders of the nervous system, including stroke and dementia, are increasing. The longer we live, the more susceptible to turmoil in an aging nervous system we become. Many of the disorders of the nervous system causing the highest rates of death and disability are preventable and treatable. Increased awareness of the worldwide effects of brain disorders will help health care planners and the neurologic community set appropriate priorities in research, prevention, and management of these conditions. So far, we are much more aware as a global society of the sparkle of celebrity and amusement than we appear to be of some of the manageable problems that affect how we walk and talk and swallow and think.

## Gestalt

The American Speech-Language-Hearing Association (ASHA) estimates that 49 million Americans have some type of communication disorder. Persons of all ages can be affected by a communication disorder that may result from a variety of causes (e.g., stroke, trauma, or other injury to the brain, injury to facial structure or muscles, neurodegenerative diseases, pediatric cancer, occult differences in neural development as in autism spectrum disorders). These communication disorders can occur in isolation (specific language impairment) or they may coexist with other developmental disorders such as intellectual handicap or cerebral palsy. In young children, communication disorders represent the most common developmental problem. As broadly defined by ASHA, it is estimated that between 15 and 25% of young children have some form of communication disorder (ASHA, 2012; LaPointe, Murdoch, & Stierwalt, 2010).

## General Causes of Communication Disorders

Frequently, the specific cause of a communication disorder is unknown. Some common problems that coexist with communication disorders include cerebral palsy and other nerve/muscle disorders, traumatic brain injury, stroke, viral diseases, mental retardation, effects of certain drugs, structural impairments such as cleft lip or palate, vocal abuse or misuse, or inadequate speech and language models (ASHA, 2012).

The specialty of movement disorders in neuroscience focuses on a large number of neurologic disorders that share the common clinical feature of either hypo- or hyperkinetic character. Too little or too much. The Golden Age of Greece in the fifth century BC taught us the valuable concept of "nothing in excess," and this notion of the great thinkers follows us through all aspects of life. This broad conceptualization dictates that there is the possibility of many causes. What jeopardizes the brain can create movement disorders, if the motor or movement scheme of the nervous system is vulnerable and affected. Classification systems in movement disorders abound. Movement disorders may be classified first behaviorally and experientially and then etiologically. Muscles, the great conveyors of movement, may be weak, hypo, or too little. Interestingly, the nervous system is composed of checks and balances and the inhibition of movement as well. If these inhibitions of movements are unleashed, the result may be involuntary, unchecked, sometimes bizarre patterns of involuntary movement. Involuntary movements generally occur in the absence of weakness, and therefore these disorders were originally termed extrapyramidal, although this term has been largely dropped from current nosology, despite that the side effects generated by certain drugs are frequently referred to as extrapyramidal signs or symptoms. People taking antipsychotic drugs are at risk of developing certain movement side effects. These signs and symptoms can include things such as repetitive, involuntary muscle movements (such as lip smacking) or an irresistible urge to be moving constantly.

## Extrapyramidal Signs and Symptoms

In human anatomy, the extrapyramidal system is a neural network that is part of the motor system that causes involuntary reflexes and movement, and modulation of movement (i.e., coordination). The system is called "extrapyramidal" to distinguish it from the tracts of the motor cortex that reach their targets by traveling through the "pyramids" of the medulla. The pyramidal pathways (corticospinal and some corticobulbar tracts) may directly innervate motor neurons of the spinal cord or brainstem (anterior, or ventral, horn cells or certain cranial nerve nuclei), whereas the extrapyramidal system centers around the modulation and regulation (indirect control) of anterior (ventral) horn cells (Reeves & Swenson, 2012).

Extrapyramidal tracts are chiefly found in the reticular formation of the pons and medulla, and target neurons in the spinal cord involved in reflexes, locomotion, complex movements, and postural control. These tracts are in turn tempered and modulated by various parts of the central nervous system, including the nigrostriatal pathway, the basal ganglia, the cerebellum, the vestibular nuclei, and different sensory areas of the cerebral cortex. All of these

regulatory components can be considered part of the extrapyramidal system, in that they modulate motor activity without directly innervating motor neurons (Reeves & Swenson, 2012).

## Idiopathic: An All Too Familiar Term

Idiopathic is an adjective used primarily in medicine meaning arising spontaneously or from a murky or unknown cause. From Greek ἴδιος, idios (one's own) + πάθος, pathos (suffering), it suggests a disorder that arises from "a disease of its own kind." It is technically a term from nosology, the branch of medicine concerned with the classification and description of known diseases. For some medical conditions, one or more causes are somewhat understood, but in a certain percentage of people with the condition, the cause may not be readily perceptible or apparent. In these cases, the origin of the condition is said to be idiopathic. We do not know. We are not exactly sure what is causing this constellation of signs and symptoms you have brought to us.

With some medical conditions, perhaps far too many, the medical community cannot establish a source cause for a large percentage of all cases. Some examples from a broad spectrum of medical disorders include coagulation disorders, cyclic vomiting syndrome, Fanconi syndrome (a rare condition that has touched the family of Jimbo and Candy Fisher, the head football coach family of the Florida State University Seminoles). Other idiopathic conditions include hirsutism, hyperhidrosis, idiopathic infiltrative lung diseases, proteinuric syndrome, idiopathic thrombocytopenic purpura (a disease characterized by purple or brownish-red spots on the skin or mucous membranes, caused by the extravasation of blood) or the very common juvenile arthritis, or Raynaud disease (a vascular disorder of unknown cause, characterized by recurrent episodes of blanching and numbness of the fingers and toes and sometimes the tip of the nose and ears, usually triggered by stress or exposure to cold). With some conditions, however, idiopathic cases account for a small percentage (for example, pulmonary fibrosis).

Humans are not the only animals prone to idiopathic diseases. Poodles and Australian Shepherds are prone to idiopathic epilepsy, a disease that can be distressing for both dog and owner—and sheep. If sheep are frightened by barking, think of how upset they would be by a dog seizure. Dog owners of the human sort are prone to Parkinson disease, in many cases labeled idiopathic as the exact cause may be unknown. Annoyingly for some people, no actual cause can be found for the runny-nose condition of idiopathic rhinitis that can be disconcerting for both a conversational partner as well as for the sufferer during the act of eating.

In his book, *The Human Body*, Isaac Asimov noted a comment about the term *idiopathic* made in the 20th edition of *Stedman's Medical Dictionary*: "A high-flown term to conceal ignorance." (Asimov, 1963, p. 179).

In the American television show *House*, the title character remarks that the word is "from the Latin, meaning: 'We're idiots because we can't figure out what's causing it.'" This popular television show, known for its sarcasm and candor, had a way of hitting the

nail on the head. Far too many conditions are designated idiopathic, and when this labeling diagnosis is proffered, disenchanted receivers of the label are likely to nod knowingly and respond, "Oh," as it sounds so official.

As medical and scientific advances are made with relation to a particular condition or disease, more root causes are, and likely will be, discovered, and the percentage of cases designated as idiopathic is destined to decrease. But this may turn out to be a zero sum balance as new diseases and disorders are discovered or thrust upon us. So the etiology of "idiopathic" remains firmly entrenched in medical practice and science and it unfailingly indicates that more research is necessary and we must carry on in the creation of new knowledge, which is exactly the aim of all research.

Not all movement disorders are idiopathic, however, and many of the etiologies of them are well documented and understood. A discussion of these causes and their relationship to neuroanatomy and neurophysiology follows, but not before an overview of neural anatomy and physiology are reviewed. For a more in-depth review of the neuroanatomy of human communication the reader is referred to the *Atlas of Neuroanatomy for Communication Science and Disorders* (LaPointe, 2012).

## Brain Foundations

The brain is an extraordinary organ, which may be one of the greatest understatements ever generated. It has been captured and celebrated in poem and song and called everything from an enchanted loom that weaves a never ending stream of dissolving patterns to an über computer on steroids. Though our species is a bit chauvinistic, we think our homo sapien brain has allowed the mostly human developments of art, theater, literature, music, religion, architecture, and cuisine. Paradoxically, it is also the source of prejudice, hatred, and war. Sophisticated and creative communication is another trait that some reserve only for humans, although animal communication models are undergoing a genuine re-examination. Many of us regard the human brain as an instrument of elegant and as yet unknown capacity, though surely there are limits. Listen to Macdonald Critchley (1979), the famous British neurologist, talk about the brain as a divine banquet: "We must admit that the divine banquet of the brain was, and still is, a feast with dishes that remain elusive in the blending, and with sauces whose ingredients are even now a secret."

Sometimes that three-pound ball of squish, that factory and seat of our dreams, ideas, and precise movements creates a nightmare. We are afforded some protection, but it is not complete protection from both intrinsic and extrinsic villains. As the eminent philosopher George Costanza (a character on the TV show "Seinfeld") has said: " . . . important things go in a case. You got a skull for your brain, a plastic sleeve for your comb, and a wallet for your money."

When the skull does not protect and brain goes bad, there is misery to pay. Although many diseases or conditions that affect the brain do not result in communication disorders, there is a vast array of disturbances of speech,

voice, and language that are a direct consequence of brain damage; thus, a communication disorder can be the consequence and is many times one of the very first signs of brain dysfunction.

Aphasia is a not infrequent accompanying condition in movement disorders. Many times movement disorders exist without language or cognitive involvement, but language impairment can coexist with motor speech disorders. Aphasia, that complicated disruption of language, is always caused by injury to the brain, most commonly from a stroke, particularly in older individuals. Even though stroke is the most common cause of brain injury resulting in aphasia, it also may occur from head trauma, brain tumors, or brain infections. Not every stroke or brain injury results in aphasia, but the condition of aphasia is never present without some sort of brain damage. The language system that overrules semantics (word meanings) and syntax (word order) and the cognitive system that is interwoven with the use of language (memory, attention, discrimination, categorization) are frequently implicated in aphasias and dementias, but are not the principal systems that are related to movement disorders and motor speech disorders.

## Movement and Motor Speech Disorders

By definition, these disruptions of speech are the result of underlying movement changes in range, direction, velocity, or coordination of movement. Body movement requires a series of intricate and imperceptible interactions among the brain, spinal cord, nerves, and muscles. Movement disorders are caused by abnormal function (damage or malfunction) in the brain components involved in movement, including the basal ganglia and cerebellum. The neural impulse that commands movement must be passed at lightning speed along the billions of brain cell connections that join with muscles. If some of these transmissions are off just a little, the precision is compromised and this results in either too much or too little movement.

The marvel of movement that results in speech is complex and fast. As Van der Merwe (1997) and Netsell (1982) have explained, speech is the incredible externalized expression of language and sensorimotor control. The Netsellian motor-afferent mechanisms that direct and regulate these behaviors are goal directed and guided by sensory information and feedback loops. It is performed with very precise accuracy, incredible speed, uses motor plans and programming, can be modified with practice, uses knowledge of results, demonstrates great motoric flexibility, and can relegate all of this precision to automatic control where consciousness is liberated from the details of the motoric action plans (Netsell, 1982).

Of course voluntary movement is dependent on the primary cortical motor strips found in each hemisphere of the brain. Brodmann's area 4, along with area 6 and other cortical and cerebellar areas, are the principal players in planning, programming, and initiating a movement ("Pick up that cup of Starbuck's venti caramel macchiato.") But another major player in the world of movement and movement disorders is the group of deep brain cells known as the basal ganglia.

One should have a basic knowledge of the anatomy of the basal ganglia and how it relates to certain disorders in order to understand movement disorders and how these disorders can demolish speech production.

## Basal Ganglia 101

The basal ganglia are groups of neural cell bodies found on both sides of the thalamus, outside and above the limbic system but below the cingulate gyrus and within the temporal lobes of the cerebrum. Boeree (2006) presents a good summary of the basal ganglia. The term *ganglia* is used generally in neuroanatomy to refer to a collection of neural cell bodies that reside outside the central nervous system (brain and spinal cord). *Nucleus* or *nuclei* (plural) designate cell body collections that are found inside the central nervous system. In the case of the basal ganglia, however, this rule is violated. Why this misnomer has been allowed to continue and be perpetuated is lost in the dim recesses of brain history. The basal ganglia are definitely found within the central nervous system, in a deep area of the brain within the cerebrum.

Glutamate is the most common neurotransmitter here as everywhere in the brain, but the inhibitory neurotransmitter GABA plays the most important role in the basal ganglia. This explains why so many of the functions of basal ganglia are based on a lack of adequate inhibition of function. The disorders of the basal ganglia are characterized by not only loss of movement function (negative or decreased movement characteristics) but also by too much or uncontrolled movement (positive behaviors) such as tremor, hyperkinesias, tics, writhing, and a mixture of movements gone wild. The basal ganglia along with the cerebellum are responsible for smoothing, controlling, fine-tuning, and inhibiting movements after they have been planned, programmed, and initiated. The online feedback and amendment functions of movement allow lightning-like corrections in direction, velocity, range, and coordination to be implemented, but when the basal ganglia or cerebellum are compromised we observe a stew of movement impairment. This does not bode well for movements that require fine motor coordination such as playing the piano, walking down stairs, or human speech.

The largest group of these nuclei are called the corpus striatum ("striped body"), made up of the caudate nucleus ("tail"), the putamen ("shell"), the globus pallidus ("pale globe"), and the nucleus accumbens ("leaning"). All of these structures are bilateral, one set on each side of the central septum. Figure 2–1 presents a simplified overview of these groups of cell bodies that are so important for movement.

The caudate begins just behind the frontal lobes and curves in a posterior direction towards the occipital lobes. These groups of cell bodies are bilaterally located as are other groups of cell bodies in the basal ganglia. These cell groups are paired and that explains why some lesions cause unilateral as opposed to bilateral effects. The caudate nucleus is highly innervated by dopamine neurons.

## Dopamine

Dopamine is a powerful neurotransmitter that is very involved in movement and its disorders. Without dopamine

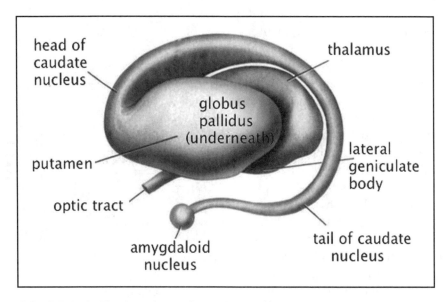

**FIGURE 2–1.** The basal ganglia is shown. (Adapted from Boeree, 2006)

or with a reduction of it, we would not only have trouble moving but also have difficulty learning the alphabet or how to shoot a free throw, getting a good night's rest, balancing our checking account, learning from experience, or enjoying our honeymoon.

Dopamine has many functions in the brain, including important roles in behavior and cognition, voluntary movement, motivation, punishment and reward, inhibition of prolactin production (involved in lactation and sexual gratification), sleep, mood, attention, working memory, and learning. Dopaminergic neurons (i.e., neurons whose main neurotransmitter is dopamine) are present mainly in the ventral tegmental area (VTA) of the midbrain, the substantia nigra pars compacta, and the arcuate nucleus of the hypothalamus (Benes, 2001; Stollerman, 2010).

Insufficient dopamine biosynthesis in the dopaminergic neurons is intricately related to the loss of neurons in the substantia nigra of the midbrain and can cause Parkinson disease, the condition in which one loses the ability to execute smooth, controlled movements. In the frontal lobes, dopamine serves a floodgate function and controls the flow of information from other areas of the brain. Dopamine disorders in this region of the brain can cause a weakening in neurocognitive functions, especially memory, attention, and problem solving. Reduced dopamine concentrations in the prefrontal cortex are thought to contribute to attention deficit disorder (Biederman, 1998). Many other movement disorders are related to inadequate dopamine production. Dopamine, amazingly, also has a role in the browning of fresh fruits and vegetables when they are cut or bruised.

That brown spot on your banana may be associated with dopamine.

The caudate system sends its messages to the frontal lobe (especially the orbital cortex, just above the eyes) and appears to be responsible for informing us that something is not right and we should do something about it. Sometimes this checking behavior gets a little out of control and the dopamine basal ganglia usual suspects are implicated. Check to see if the door is locked! Check the burners on the stove! Arrange all the papers on your desk in a straight line! Bite the corner of your bed nightstand seven times! Wash your hands until they're scrubbed raw! Drive around for hours to make sure that the bump you heard while driving wasn't a person you ran over! Compulsively twist your hair until it falls out or is broken off (trichotillomania) or engage in obsessive skin or scab picking! Figure 2–2 depicts a case of trichotillomania.

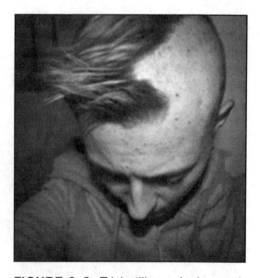

**FIGURE 2–2.** Trichotillomania (compulsive hair twisting/pulling) associated with dopamine-related obsessive-compulsive disorder.

These examples may be the awful offspring of obsessive-compulsive disorder (OCD) and many times involves an overactive caudate. An underactive caudate may be implicated in a variety of disorders as well, such as depression, aspects of schizophrenia, and lethargy. It is also involved in PAP syndrome, a dramatic loss of motivation only recently reported (see below).

The putamen lies just below and behind the front of the caudate. It appears to be involved in coordinating automatic behaviors such as tying your shoes, riding a bike, driving a car, or working on an assembly line and screwing widgets onto bolts. Problems with the putamen may be associated with some of the signs and symptoms of Tourette syndrome as well. The globus pallidus is located just within the putamen, with an outer part and an inner part. It receives inputs from the caudate and putamen and provides outputs to the substantia nigra. The nucleus accumbens is a nucleus just below the previous nuclei. In fact, most members of the basal ganglia community are richly interconnected. The nucleus accumbens receives signals from the prefrontal cortex (via the ventral tegmental area) and sends other signals back by way of the globus pallidus. The nucleus accumbens is the little Las Vegas or Disney World of the brain, the "pleasure center." It has traditionally been studied for its role in addiction, and it plays an important role in processing many rewards such as food and sex. Interestingly, the nucleus accumbens is selectively activated during the perception of pleasant, emotionally arousing pictures and during mental imagery of pleasant, emotional scenes. A 2005 study found

that it is involved in the regulation of emotions induced by music, perhaps consequent to its role in mediating dopamine release (Menon & Levitin, 2005). Daniel J. Levitin has contributed much on the neuroscience of music, and his book, *This Is Your Brain on Music: The Science of Human Obsession* (2006), is required reading for anyone interested in the marvelous and intricate alliance of brain, pleasure, movement, and music. The nucleus accumbens plays a role in rhythmic timing and is considered to be of central importance to the limbic–motor interface. Many drugs, including dopamine, are known to greatly increase these messages to the nucleus accumbens. Overall, this area of the basal ganglia, particularly the special little pleasure center of the nucleus accumbens, is thought to play an important role in reward, pleasure, laughter, addiction, aggression, fear, and the placebo effect. Where would we be without it? What a pity that it sometimes goes a bit over the top. It is implicated in sexual arousal and activity as well as gambling addiction. People who gamble and play cards *during* sex are thought by some to signal problems with the nucleus accumbens.

Another nucleus of the basal ganglia is the substantia nigra ("black substance") which is associated with Parkinson disease. Located in the upper portions of the midbrain, below the thalamus, it gets its color from neuromelanin, a close relative of the skin pigment. One part (the pars compacta) uses dopamine neurons to send signals up to the striatum. The exact function is not known but is believed to involve reward circuits and movements, as is its little party-all-night neighbor the nucleus accumbens. Parkinson disease is due to the death of dopamine-producing neurons there, and when about 70% of these neurons in the substantia nigra are impaired or lost, the signs and symptoms of Parkinsonism become evident. Another part of the substantia nigra (the pars reticulata) is mostly associated with GABA neurons. GABAergic neurons are those which secrete GABA (gamma-aminobutyric-acid) as their primary neurotransmitter. Basically, GABA is an inhibitory neurotransmitter that inhibits whichever neurons to which it binds. It is the primary inhibitory neurotransmitter in the brain. Its opposite is glutamate, which is the primary excitatory neurotransmitter in the brain. It is easy to conceive that GABA neurons might be the culprits involved in those positive, involuntary, uncontrollable movements that are seen so frequently in movement disorders. This part of the substantia nigra is involved in controlling eye movements and has a role as well in Parkinson disease as well as epilepsy (Boeree, 2006).

The following material on the basal ganglia is adapted from LaPointe (2012). For a broader and more detailed treatment of the topic of neural control of movements the reader may wish to consult the publication *Atlas of Neuroanatomy for Communication Science and Disorders* (LaPointe, 2012). Figure 2–3 presents images and text on the complexity and feedback loops of the basal ganglia.

There is no definitive and uncontested consensus of the precise structures and connections included in the extrapyramidal or pyramidal (arising from pyramidal shaped motor cells) motor systems, but all lists would include the basal ganglia (caudate, putamen, and globus pallidus), and

the subthalamic nucleus. The substantia nigra is an associated structure with important basal ganglia interconnections and plays a major role in Parkinsonism. The cerebellum and perhaps the red nucleus are involved in some abnormalities associated with basal ganglia disorders (Reeves & Swenson, 2012). The brain is such a complex network of structures and systems and interconnections (100 billion neurons; trillions of interconnections) that the basics are modestly well understood but the precision of specifics continue to be revealed by new and important advances in neuroimaging and neuroscience innovations.

The normal functions of the human basal ganglia have largely been deduced from study of functional problems associated with destructive or irritative lesions. To a large degree, many brain anomalies result in deficits in motor function, and therefore the extrapyramidal system and basal ganglia have been associated with a rich garden of movement disorders. Ironically, movement disorders have enlightened us about basic functions of the motor systems. For the most part, these clinical perceptions have been supported and expanded by basic science investigations, although it is becoming increasingly evident that these brain regions are involved in a greater array of functions than was obvious during the infant years of our understanding of human movement. Although far from complete, this understanding has permitted development of some effective therapies for movement disorders (Reeves & Swenson, 2012). For every yin there may be a yang, and sadly, some of these therapies have created additional problems and side effects that create movement disorders.

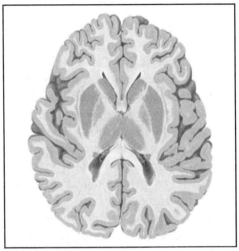 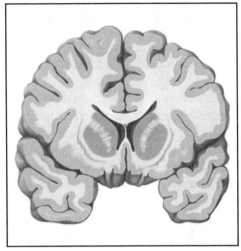

**A**                                    **B**

**FIGURE 2–3. A** and **B.** The basal ganglia are shown. **A.** Transverse section through the cerebrum at the level of the corpus striatum, viewed from above. In a strict anatomic sense, the basal ganglia consist of the caudate nucleus, putamen, and globus pallidus. Developmentally, the globus pallidus is a part of the diencephalon that has migrated into the telencephalon, but it is still counted among the basal ganglia. The basal ganglia are an essential component of the extrapyramidal motor system. The extrapyramidal system is composed of motor fibers that do not pass through the pyramidal tracts of the medulla but that nevertheless exert a measure of control over bodily movements. The system is composed of complex pathways and feedback loops. Nevertheless, the extrapyramidal system can be divided into three controlling systems: the cortically originating indirect pathways, the feedback loops, and the auditory-visual-vestibular descending pathways. The basal ganglia and extrapyramidal system are important in fine-tuning and coordinating movements and in neurologic movement disorders, such as Parkinson disease and dystonia, and can greatly affect motor control of speech and other movements. The claustrum ("barrier") is a strip of gray matter lateral to the putamen. It is not part of the basal ganglia but instead has reciprocal connections with sensory areas of the cerebral cortex. **B.** Coronal section through the cerebrum at the level of the olfactory tract, anterior view. This section demonstrates how the caudate nucleus and putamen are separated from each other by the fibrous white matter of the internal capsule. The caudate nucleus and putamen together constitute the corpus striatum (often shortened to "striatum"). The globus pallidus is not visible because it is occipital to this plane of section.

In primates and other neomammalian species, the basal ganglia appear to be important in the process of initiation of movement and the maintenance of stereotyped movements once these rivers and tributaries of movement are initiated. Postural control, resting muscle tone, automatic associated movements (e.g., swinging the arms while walking), and possibly emotional motor expression (e.g., smiling, frowning, laughing, crying, etc.) appear to be important functions of the basal ganglia (Reeves & Swenson, 2012).

## Speech Production: An Enigmatic and Highly Complex Motor Task

Pascal Perrier has worked and commented upon, along with many other researchers in speech motor control, the blinding complexity of motor control of the human speech process. Compared with many other human motor tasks classically studied in motor control research, speech production has a number of idiosyncrasies that make it particularly knotty (Perrier, 2006). This complexity has been frequently discussed in the speech motor control literature and is a recurring topic of debate, heat, and occasional enlightenment at the biennial motor speech control conferences in Europe and the United States. As Perrier (2006) reflects, this complexity and uniqueness of speech motor control, as opposed to limb control for such functions as reaching or grasping, is founded in the following premises:

- Because of its semiotic nature (based on signs, signals, sounds, words, and meanings of symbol systems), the goal of speech production is actually defined in an abstract domain; hence, its physical characterization is not straightforward, and this has two consequences. First, there is no unique physical correlate for a given elementary speech sound, and a large variability of patterns can be observed in the neurophysiologic, articulatory, and acoustic domains. Second, the issue of the physical space in which the motor task is planned becomes particularly complex, since the distal space can be defined either by articulatory posi-

tions (e.g., tip of the tongue touches the alveolar ridge and valves or interrupts an airstream) or by spectral properties of the speech signal, or by perceptual characteristics of this signal or a multimodal space associating orosensory, auditory and even visual characterizations.

- Speech production has a large number of degrees of freedom that confer a many-to-one characteristic on the relationships between motor commands, articulatory positions, and acoustic or auditory properties. This characteristic, together with the above mentioned intrinsic variability of the physical correlates of the production of a given sound, has the consequence that a large set of motor equivalence strategies can be used to implement a range of coarticulation strategies. These real-time manipulations and minute, quick-as-a wink adjustments can deal with artificial perturbations (such as talking with a Meerschaum pipe or a small Italian meatball in the mouth). These features of immediate adjustment in the face of conditions that alter the oral mechanism during speech contribute to the head-scratching complexity of the speech motor control system that innervates the hundred or so muscles that must be temporally adjusted among the seven articulators. These flashing space–time coordinate requirements are necessary for accurately perceived speech and may in fact play into explanation of some of the disorders of speech planning, programming, and production.

- Compared with other skilled human motor activities, speech movements in normal conditions can be very short, since vowels have a mean duration of approximately 80 ms and conso-nants have mean durations around 40 ms. These characteristics seem to exclude any potential on-line con-tribution of long-latency orosensory feedback that would be processed by the cortex, and to limit the role of auditory feedback to a supraseg-mental level and to an a posteriori monitoring used to correct segmen-tal aspects of speech after it is pro-duced. The absence of online use of auditory feedback to control speech at a segmental level is supported by experimental work showing that speakers can produce intelligible speech even after hearing loss. Like-wise, work with people who stut-ter and normal speakers shows that delaying auditory feedback in the range of 50 to 200 ms affects prosodic (speaking rate, fluency, rhythm, into-nation, and emphatic stress) rather than segmental or speech phoneme features. At the same time, speech gestures have to be accurate enough in order to ensure that the associated acoustic signal can be correctly per-ceived by a listener. How accuracy can be obtained without the use of long-latency feedback that would be processed by the cortex is a key issue for speech production research, but not for other human motor tasks except for eye saccades (Perrier, 2006).

To deal with the complexity and the multimodality of speech task rep-resentations, with the numerous motor or auditory equivalence strategies, and with the accuracy requirements in the absence of long-latency feedback going through the cortex, the large majority of speech motor control models published in the literature assumes the existence of internal representations of the speech apparatus, called internal models. I am indebted to the excellent review by Per-rier (2006) for this summary that high-lights, but only hints at, the remarkable complexity of the speech motor control system. It is no wonder that it is dif-ficult to both understand and generate treatment strategies for motor speech disorders. The paradox of bedazzling complexity superimposed on the ironic flexibility and adaptability of speech production coordination poses immense challenges to the clinician who would both understand and treat people with disrupted speech control.

## Etiologies: Background of Brain-Based Disorders

The river of movement disorders flows from many sources. The basis of all neuropathology is the interruption of function of the peripheral, central, or autonomic nervous systems. In the case of movement disorders we ignore damage to the other myriad functional systems and concentrate on just those causes of interruption of the sensori-motor system. As intricate feedback loops exist in our complex motor sys-tems, that means that planning, pro-gramming, and unavailability of sen-sory feedback also can wreak havoc on accomplished and precise movement patterns. Even without implication of the motor nerves, a visit to the dentist that involves the lovely injection of an anesthetic (articaine, in most contempo-rary clinical practice) can produce inter-esting results that impair speech move-ments (Wynn, 2003). Many of us have experienced the temporary dysarthria and difficulty producing precise speech articulation caused by nerve block during dental procedures. This emphasizes the role of oral sensation and perception in the sensory feedback loop model that is involved in motor control. If we cannot feel or appreciate position of the articulators, we have less probability of precisely controlling and correcting their movements. My colleague, William N. Williams, and I spent a good deal of our research time during the 1970s and 1980s investigating methods of measurement and effects of disruption of mechanisms of oral sensation and perception (Jensen, Sheehan, Williams, & LaPointe, 1975; LaPointe, Williams, & Hepler, 1973; Williams, LaPointe, Blanton, 1984; Williams, LaPointe, Mahan, & Cornell, 1984, 1985; Williams, Levin, LaPointe, Cornell, 1985). Despite the models of speech motor control that emphasize internal models, there yet may be a role of oral sensation and perception important to understanding and setting up motor-control-based models of intervention. Currently, the role of oral sensation and perception and its role in speech movements is experiencing a bit of a renaissance of research interest particularly as it relates to motor-guided learning theory and swallowing disorders (de Wijk, 2012; Schmidt & Bjork, 1992).

## Specific Causes of Movement Disorders

In general, the causes of movement disorders can be organized into several general categories with no perfect consensus across the movement disorder literature. The etiologic classification of disorders includes neurodegenerative, genetic, infectious, metabolic, nutritional, traumatic, toxicologic, and vascular. As such, movement disorders may be considered *primary* when they occur as an isolated neurologic syndrome or *secondary* when they occur as a part of a larger process of known cause. To appreciate the diversity of these categories of causes, the health care professional must become familiar with the characteristics and descriptions of the clinical manifestations such as Parkinsonism, tremors, chorea, dystonia, tics, stereotypies, and myoclonus. (The Glossary provides definitions of these clinical expressions.) With increased familiarity of these disorders and their clinical features, the health practitioner will be able to distinguish the characteristics and separate disorders into primary and secondary ones. These clinical syndromes are sometimes labeled in confusing and inconsistent fashion. They are based sometimes on etiology, sometimes on clinical description of principal signs and symptoms, sometimes on the researcher or physician who first described the condition, and sometimes in seemingly arbitrary fashion. Try to discern the reason for the following:

- Parkinson disease
- Parkinsonian syndromes
- Progressive supranuclear palsy
- Multiple system atrophy
- Corticobasoganglionic degeneration
- Huntington disease
- Tourette syndrome
- Idiopathic dystonia
- Essential tremor
- Wilson disease

- Tardive dyskinesia
- Restless leg syndrome.

The impact of these terms and their contribution to the understanding of movement disorders is considered in more detail in the next chapter. Figure 2–4 illustrates a neural image of the effects of traumatic brain injury (arrow) and how such an injury can disrupt the basal ganglia and centers and pathways of movement in the brain.

## Movement Disorder Society

This is a good place to introduce the Movement Disorder Society with the wealth of material assembled on their website. This site is ever expanding and is a wellspring of clinical and basic information about the salad bar of movement disorders. This website can be accessed at http://www.movement disorders.org/membership/. An overview of the clinical and professional business of the society as articulated on this website is as follows (Movement Disorders Society, 2012):

The Movement Disorder Society is an international professional society of clinicians, scientists, health care professionals, and persons with movement disorders who are interested in Parkinson disease, related neurodegenerative and neurodevelopmental disorders, hyperkinetic movement disorders, and abnormalities in muscle tone and motor control. The spectrum of clinical disorders represented by the Society includes but is not limited to:

- Parkinson disease and parkinsonism
- Dystonia
- Chorea, Huntington disease
- Ataxia
- Tremor, essential tremor
- Myoclonus and startle
- Tics and Tourette syndrome
- Restless legs syndrome
- Gait disorders
- Stiff person syndrome.

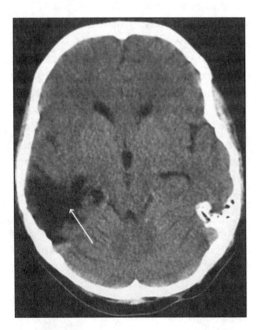

**FIGURE 2–4.** Neural image of traumatic brain injury.

## Summary of Etiologies

Movement, and especially movement for precise and complex activities such as human speech, requires an astonishing amount of control of synergistic and coordinated integration of the nervous system and muscles. This accounts for why so many parts of the motor control system are implicated in movement disorders. These disorders that rear their ugly influence on smooth, coordinated movement sequences deprive us of the ability to make purposeful movements and interact effectively with our environment. Ballet is out of the question. Hitting a curve ball is questionable. Descending stairs is perilous. Eating can be sloppy. Playing the violin, piano, dobro, or accordion is difficult beyond expectation. To rip off a chorus of the polka "Just Because You Think You're So Pretty" on the 120 bass accordion is a complex feat of its own with the requirements of smoothly pulling the bellows and sending air through the little beeswax reeds while coordinating the bass buttons of the left hand with the piano keyboard of the right side. Imagine trying to pull off this coordination against the backdrop of hand tremors and explosive involuntary jerks. Now multiply that feat by 10 or so to effect the precise space–time coordinates necessary for saying "I think I just lost my pants!" or swallowing a Krispy Kreme donut.

What is lost in all of these movement-necessary activities are some of the most basic abilities that have contributed to the success of the human species. This not only includes a lot of functions that are shared with other species, such as locomotion, drinking water, or jumping on the back of a mate for a brief pony ride, but also includes functions that make us uniquely human such as making a speech at the Rotary club or asking our mate for a little sugar. Not only is speech vulnerable, but skilled use of the hands for using a toothbrush or a Black and Decker drill is rendered difficult as is trying to get from a D 7th to G chord on your Martin guitar.

The brain controls skeletal muscles for all these activities through specialized nerve cells, that is, lower and upper motoneurons. Lower motoneurons are located in the spinal cord and brainstem and send axons, the cable-like extensions, to muscles where they make specialized contacts called neuromuscular junctions. Not only are the muscles necessary for these precise movements, but the neurotransmitter juice that facilitates passing along the nerve signals are also a vital part of the movement equation. During movement of a body part, signals are sent from the upper motor neurons located in the cerebral cortex of the brain to the lower motoneurons located in the brainstem (for head and facial muscles) and spinal cord (for limb and trunk muscles). Lower motoneurons then send signals to muscles to cause contraction. In between, complex feedback circuits fine-tune and purify these signals.

Injury and dysfunction at any point in this network can result in disorders of movement and muscle contraction. Not unexpectedly, these disorders include a large number of highly capricious conditions depending on what part of the network is injured or dysfunctional; however, what all of these conditions have in common is that they affect some aspect of motor function. Signs and symptoms may include weakness, muscle wasting, pain, spasticity (exaggerated reflexes and muscle spasms), rigidity (muscle stiffness), tremor, involuntary movements, slow movements, inability to initiate voluntary movements, inaccurate movements, and unstable gait.

The root causes of these disorders include genetic mutations, viral infections, autoimmune disorders, hormonal disorders, metabolic disorders, drugs, toxins, and trauma. Add to these the vascular system upheaval of embolisms, thromboses, and hemorrhage, as well as the vast number of idiosyncratic diseases of nerve and muscle. For many of these disorders the causes can be pinpointed, but for far too many, the etiologies are a mystery and fall into the previously mentioned waste category of idiopathic. Health care professionals who deal with movement disorders can appreciate from the foregoing discussion not only the complexity of the speech motor control system but also the abundant array of etiologies that can affect it and cause movement to go off track. Figure 2–5 illustrates an early health care provider with his tools for neurologic intervention.

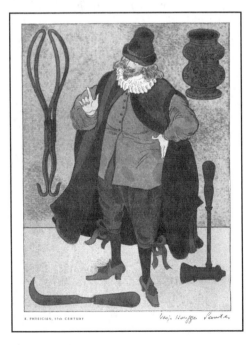

**FIGURE 2–5.** A seventeenth century healer with tools of the trade.

## References

American Speech-Language-Hearing Association (ASHA). (2012). Communication Disorders Statistics. Retrieved September 13, 2012 from http://www.asha.org/default.htm/

Asimov, Isaac. (1963). *The human body: Its structure and operation* (p. 179). New York, NY: Houghton Mifflin.

Benes, F. M. (2001). Carlsson and the discovery of dopamine. *Trends in Pharmacological Sciences, 22(1)*, 46–47.

Bergen, D. C., & Silberberg, D. (2002). Nervous system disorders: A global epidemic. *Archives of Neurology, 59*, 1194–1196.

Biederman, J. (1998). Attention-deficit/hyperactivity disorder: A life-span perspective. *Journal of Clinical Psychiatry, 59*(Suppl. 7), 4–16.

Boeree, C. G. (2006). Basal ganglia. Retrieved May 6, 2011 from http://webspace.ship.edu/cgboer/basalganglia.html/

Critchley, M. (1979). *The divine banquet of the brain*. London, UK: Raven Press.

de Wijk, R. A., Janssen A. M., & Prinz, J. F. (2012). Oral movements and the perception of semi-solid foods. *Physiology and Behavior*. 2011 May 3 [Epub ahead of print].

Jensen, P. J., Sheehan, J. G., Williams, W. N., & LaPointe, L. L. (1975). Oral sensory-perceptual integrity of stutterers. *Folia Phoniatrica, 27*, 38–45.

LaPointe, L. L. (2012). *Atlas of neuroanatomy for communication science and disorders*. New York, NY: Thieme.

LaPointe, L. L., Murdoch, D. E., & Stierwalt, J. A. G. (2010). *Brain-based communication disorders*. San Diego, CA: Plural.

LaPointe, L. L., Williams, W. N., & Hepler, E. L. (1973). Illusion in size perception of intra-orally presented holes. *Perceptual and Motor Skills, 36*, 1047–1050.

Levitin, D. J. (2006). *This is your brain on music: The science of human obsession*. New York, NY: Dutton (a division of Penguin).

Menon, V., & Levitin, D. J. (2005). The rewards of music listening: Response and physiological connectivity of the meso-limbic system. *NeuroImage, 28*(1), 175–184.

Movement Disorders Society. (2012). Retrieved October 3, 2012 from http://www.movementdisorders.org/

Netsell, R. (1982). Speech motor control and selected neurological disorders. In S. Grillner, B. Lindblom, J. Lubker, & A. Persson (Eds.), *Speech motor control* (pp. 247–261). Oxford, UK: Pergamon Press.

Perrier, P. (2006). About speech motor control complexity. In J. Harrington, & M. Tabain (Eds.), *Speech production: Models, phonetic processes, and techniques* (pp. 13–26). New York, NY: Psychology Press.

Reeves, A. G., & Swenson, R. S. (2012). Disorders of the nervous system. Retrieved September 10, 2012 from http://www.dartmouth.edu/~dons/index.html/

Schmidt, R. A., & Bjork, R. A. (1992). New conceptualizations of practice: Common principles in three paradigms suggest new concepts for training. *Psychological Science, 3,* 207–217.

Stolerman, I. P. (2010). *Encyclopedia of psychopharmacology* (Vol. 2). New York, NY: Springer.

Stop the Hunger. (2012). Skinny and fat. Retrieved October 26, 2012 from http://www.stopthehunger.com/

Van der Merwe, A. (1997). A theoretical framework for the characterization of pathological speech sensorimotor control. In M. R. McNeil (Ed.), *Clinical management of sensorimotor speech disorders* (pp. 1–25). New York, NY: Thieme.

Williams, W. N., LaPointe, L. L., & Blanton, R. S. (1984). Human discrimination of different bite forces. *Journal of Oral Rehabilitation, 11,* 407–413.

Williams, W. N., LaPointe, L. L., Mahan, P. E., & Cornell, C. E. (1984). The influence of TMJ and central incisor sensory impairment on bite force discrimination. *Journal of Craniomandibular Practice, 2*(2), 120–124.

Williams, W. N., LaPointe, L. L., Mahan, P. E., & Cornell, C. E. (1985). Bite force discrimination with mandibular movement. *Journal of Craniomandibular Practice, 3,* 133–137.

Williams, W. N., Levin, A. C., LaPointe, L. L., & Cornell, C. E. (1985). Bite force discrimination by individuals with complete dentures. *Journal of Prosthetic Dentistry, 54*(1), 146–150.

Wynn, R. L. (2003). Paresthesia associated with local anesthetics: A perspective on articaine. *Journal of the Academy of General Dentistry, 51* (6), 498–501.

# 3

# Characteristics of Movement Disorders

*LEONARD L. LAPOINTE*

The year 1861 has a good deal of prominence in the history of neuroscience and especially in behavioral neurology. This year is forever bonded to the work of Pierre Paul Broca, the prodigious anatomist, surgeon, anthropologist, neurologist, French senator, and horn player who revolutionized the history of neuroscience and human communication by publishing the first clinicopathologic evidence for a connection between the parts of the the brain that are intimately related to speech and language. In *Paul Broca and the Origins of Language in the Brain* (2013), LaPointe traces these nineteenth century developments that still impact current thinking about the delicate connections between our neurons and our words.

As it turns out, 1861 was important for our understanding of movement disorders and speech as well. The great British neuroscience historian J. M. S. Pearce has called attention to the role of his predecessor British neurologists Russel Reynolds and Hughlings Jackson in attempting to clarify the nature of positive and negative signs and symptoms in brain disease (Pearce, 2004). These signs and symptoms are particularly relevant to movement disorders that portray a rich and puzzling array of not enough movement and too much movement. All of this can interfere with speech and swallowing. As Pearce reports, these two early observers and neurologists were prominent in characterizing positive and negative signs of brain disease. Pearce highlights some of Russel Reynolds contributions to epilepsy but comments that perhaps of greater consequence was his 1861 paper in which he championed the concept of positive and negative neurologic signs and symptoms as being the excess or negation of vital properties. Positive symptoms were abnormal "superimposed" and no doubt unintentional and unwanted behaviors that included not only clonic jerking and abnormal movements but also hallucinations and paranoid delusions. Negative signs and symptoms included loss of sensation, paralysis, and coma. This introduced the theme of too much and too little, especially of movement, and set the stage for Hughlings Jackson to elaborate. As Pearce explains, the roots of positive and negative neurologic signs and symptoms are inextricably intertwined with Herbert Spencer's dissolution and evolution of the nervous system. Hughlings Jackson stretched Spencer's idea to positive and negative aspects of other diseases. Jackson trusted that negative symptoms related to suspension or reduction of neural function, whereas positive symptoms resulted from excitation or the release of lower levels from higher inhibitory control. If neural circuits are incapable of exercising their inhibitory function or cannot rein in unbridled movements, then an overabundance of movement will result and tics and tremor may be the result.

## Basics of Movement Disorder Characteristics

To thoroughly understand the complexities of the human neuromotor system requires a strong foundation of neuroanatomy and neurophysiology. The structures and functions of this system are interrelated and intricate. We encounter terms such as upper motor neuron, lower motor neuron, pyramidal, extrapyramidal, reflex and feedback circuits, and initiation and inhibition circuits. Overriding these terms are the concepts of etiology, specifics of each disease process, and type and extent of damage to a nervous system that is scattered all over the body. No wonder determining the significance of observed characteristics is such a riddle and mystery to all but the most neurologically sophisticated. All of these factors play out in determining which characteristics will be evident when the neuromotor system is visited by devils and disease.

As most texts and papers on characteristics of brain disease mention, the most obvious motor deficits result from serious brain damage and are hard to miss. The Dana Foundation (http://www.dana.org/) is a rich source of information on the brain and its disorders, as is the accurate and dependable We Move (2012) website, the worldwide education website for movement disorders (http://www.wemove.org/).

Indeed, we move and are an ambulatory and nonstationary species. We use our arms and our legs and our tongues; when these stop working everyone takes notice. As reviewed in Chapter 2, strokes result in paralysis and spasticity of the arm and leg on one side (hemiplegia) due to damage of the precious tracts and nerves that carry the signal to move, that is, the tract connecting the motor cortical outflow to the brainstem, cerebellum, and spinal cord. Other influences on movement are not so obvious. Damage in certain areas in the parietal or frontal cortex can affect motor functions more slowly and be subtly harmful or destructive.

## Apraxias

Some of these lesions may result in apraxias of various kinds, meaning difficulty in planning and programming the motor skills a person has already learned (for example, how to dress, strike a match, say the phrase "red velvet cupcake"). If we attempt or are asked to copy shapes from a template or from memory, assemble objects from component parts, or imitate common gestures, these complex moves can also be affected and disorders of these abilities cross into the netherworld of perceptual and motor disorders. Many of these planning and programming disorders are not evident for automatic, reflexive movements but show themselves during volitional movement requests. Such difficulties will not become apparent until the person is asked to volitionally perform these actions. "Stick out your tongue." "Draw a clock." "Imitate a wallaby about to do the mating dance." This multiplex of disorders, known as apraxia, is the result of damage to both motor, supplementary motor, and association areas of the cortex, and perhaps circuits that connect to the cerebellum as well.

## Coordination Disorders

Disorders of coordination and balance are more commonly the result of cerebellar damage. Motor coordination is the combination of body movements created with the kinematic (such as spatial direction) and kinetic (force) factors that result in intended actions. Motor coordination is achieved when sub-sequent parts of the same movement, or the movements of several limbs or body parts, are combined in a manner that is well timed, smooth, and efficient with respect to the intended goal. This involves the incorporation of proprioceptive information detailing the position and movement of the musculoskeletal system or the tongue or the vocal folds with the neural processes in the brain and spinal cord which control, plan, and relay motor commands. The cerebellum plays a critical role in this neural control of movement, and damage to this part of the brain or its connecting structures and pathways results in impairment of coordination, known as ataxia. These diseases can interfere with the fine-tuning of muscular movement and result in coarse, uncoordinated movement. This type of condition is easily seen in a person's jerky to-and-fro motion of the trunk and unsteady gait (Dana Foundation, 2012; Latash & Anson, 2006).

The word ataxia is derived from Greek and means "without order." In a medical sense, it refers to lack of coordination. The first sign of the condition is usually walking with poor balance and a slow and unsteady gait. That is often followed by impaired hand coordination, including deteriorating handwriting and difficulty with complex hand motions. Later a person may have imprecise and inarticulate speech and in fact represent a type of motor speech disorder within the category of the dysarthrias called ataxic dysarthria. Ataxia can also be associated with the positive signs of shaking or tremors, especially when a person tries to use his or her hands. This is the classic sign called intention tremor, and my personal experience with a bit of intention tremor occurred when I first attempted to access the tiny keyboard on an early-version Blackberry. Sometimes ataxia reveals itself as altered eye movements, producing distorted vision and impaired perception of movement. Disrupted movement can be pervasive and impinge itself into the wonderful world of perception as well. *Sensorimotor* is not a bad concept to keep in mind when dealing with movement disorders and is featured in a book on speech production disorders by M. R. McNeil entitled *Clinical Management of Sensorimotor Speech Disorders* (Dana Foundation, 2012; McNeil, 2008).

To outsiders, a person suffering from ataxia may seem drunk: reeling totteringly, slurring his or her speech, and making clumsy and awkward hand gestures. But people with the condition, their family, and their friends know that too many margaritas is not the cause. Usually, the person's obvious difficulty in walking causes the kinfolk to seek medical attention promptly. They are often concerned that the signs and symptoms are due to stroke, brain tumor, multiple sclerosis, or other serious neurologic disorders, and indeed in some cases ataxia might be the first sign of those problems (Dana Foundation, 2012). Diagnosing ataxia and its cause as swiftly as possible is critical to prevent further losses of dexterity and to obtain the best chance for full recuperation.

The types of disorders and subsequent movement disorder characteristics that result from damage or disease to different parts of the motor system are complex and sometimes puzzling. How do the different components of the motor system work together to produce the fluid, effortless body movements that we take for granted? The motor system can appear to be a riddle wrapped inside an enigma when one observes the salad bar of positive and negative signs and symptoms that can result from damage.

## Levels of Damage and Differences in Characteristics

Motor system dysfunction can result from damage or disease at any level of the motor system hierarchy and side loops (Knierim, 2012). Differences in the strange array of aberrant movements that result from damage at different levels allow the neuroscientist or neuroclinician to understand and localize where in the hierarchy of nervous system organization the damage is likely to be.

### Lower Motor Characteristics

Damage to alpha motor neurons results in a distinctive set of signs sometimes called the *lower motor neuron syndrome* (recall that the lower motor neurons refer to alpha motor neurons in the spinal cord and brainstem; all motor system neurons higher in the hierarchy are referred to as upper motor neurons) (Knierim, 2012). This damage usually results from certain diseases that selectively affect alpha motor neurons (such as polio) or from localized lesions such as traumatic dissection of the neuron groups, nerves, or tracts of the spinal cord by, say, a cutlass slash to the spine by a drunken pirate. Lower motor neuron syndrome is characterized by a cluster of characteristic signs:

1. The effects can be *limited to small groups of muscles*. Remember that a motor neuron pool is a nucleus of alpha motor neurons that innervate a single muscle. Furthermore, nearby motor neuron pools control nearby muscles; thus, restricted damage to lower motor neurons, either within the spinal cord or at the ventral roots of the spinal cord, affect only a restricted group of muscles and damage may be easily localized (Knierim, 2012).

2. *Muscle atrophy.* When alpha motor neurons call it a day and fade into the great beyond, the muscle fibers that they innervate become deprived of necessary nutritional factors (blood, glucose, hamburgers, and other nutritional favorites) and eventually the muscle itself atrophies or wastes away.

3. *Weakness.* Because of damage to alpha motor neurons and the wasting away of muscles, weakness is profound in lower motor neuron disorders. We cannot lift, run as fast, punch with much force, or even walk up stairs.

4. *Fasciculation.* Damaged alpha motor neurons can produce spontaneous action potentials or neuron firings. These spikes cause the muscle strings that are part of that neuron's motor unit to fire, resulting in a visible twitch (called a fasciculation) of the affected muscle.

5. *Fibrillation.* With further worsening or collapse of the alpha motor neuron, only fragments and leftovers of the axons near the muscle fibers remain. These individual axon fibers also can spawn spontaneous action potentials; however, these action potentials will only cause singular muscle fibers to contract. This spontaneous twitching of individual muscle fibers is called a fibrillation. Fibrillations are too tiny to be seen as a visible muscle contraction. They can only be noticed with electrophysiologic recordings of the muscle activity (an electromyogram) (Knierim, 2012).

6. *Hypotonia.* Because alpha motor neurons are the only way to stimulate extrafusal muscle fibers, the loss of these neurons causes a decrease in muscle tone. Muscle tone (the backdrop state of slight muscle contraction) can be caused by neurologic disease but is also a product of aging. As people reach middle age and go headlong into the great swamp of aging, the struggle to keep muscle tone increases even more. This is due to a condition known as *sarcopenia*, which is a degenerative process of muscles associated with aging. What arthritis is to cartilage or osteoporosis is to bone, sarcopenia is to muscle: a plodding journey to the wearing away of extrafusal muscle fibers, steering its way to low muscle tone. Sarcopenia coupled with alpha motor neuron disease equals weakness and negative movement characteristics.

7. *Hyporeflexia.* The myotatic (stretch) reflex is weak or absent with lower motor neuron disorders, because the alpha motor neurons that cause muscle contraction are damaged. Weak reflexes are signs of motor disorders.

## Upper Motor Neuron Syndrome

Damage to any part of the motor system hierarchy above the level of alpha motor neurons (not including the side loops and circuits) results in a set of signs termed the *upper motor neuron syndrome*. Some of these signs and symptoms are just the opposite of those of lower motor neuron disorders. Consequently, one of the critical decisions a clinician must understand is whether a person presenting with movement disorder has an upper motor neuron disorder or a lower motor neuron disorder (Knierim, 2012).

Upper motor neuron disorders typically arise from the garden of cruel etiologies such as stroke, tumors, and blunt or penetrating trauma. For example, cerebrovascular accidents (CVA) to the middle cerebral artery, lateral striate artery, or the medial striate artery can cause damage to the lateral surface of cortex or to the internal capsule, where the descending axons of the corticospinal tract collect. The internal capsule is a particularly unfortunate site for a CVA as a very small lesion can pick of many important and compressed tracts of descending axons carrying vital motoric signals. As Knierim (2012) instructs us, the primary signs and characteristics of upper motor neuron syndrome include the following considerations:

1. *Large groups of muscles.* As we remember from textbooks and atlases of neuroanatomy (LaPointe, 2012), our familiar friend, the little homunculus man, portrays that muscles from different body parts are activated by stimulation of parts of motor cortex (and that body parts that require fine motor control and dexterity are represented with big hands, fingers, lips, and tongue). All of this is in harmony as well with the concept that the motor cortex represents some movements that are controlled by many joints and muscles, rather than individual muscles; thus, a stroke in a particular part of the motor cortex may affect the initiation of many muscles in the body. Likewise, a stroke that affects the internal capsule or crus cerebri (two symmetric tracts of nerve fibers at the base of the midbrain, linking the pons and the cerebral hemispheres) could involve muscles on the entire contralateral side of the body (Knierim, 2012).

2. *Atrophy is rare.* Because alpha motor neurons are present, muscles will continue to receive nourishing material necessary for their survival. A mild amount of atrophy may result from disuse, but it will not be as distinct as that resulting from a lower motor neuron disorder.

3. *Weakness.* This is the characteristic of disordered movement that is most apparent across many etiologies of motoric impairment and is the chief negative sign and symptom of poorly innervated muscle groups. Weakness is the result of muscles not functioning optimally. We cannot lift or move our arms as well as before. We cannot even elevate our tongue with enough speed and range of movement to make /l/, /n/, /t/, or /d/ sounds. An adequately strong tongue must elevate to the alveolar ridge to produce these sounds clearly. A weakened tongue may produce an imprecise attempt to say "ladder" or "Nadine" or "tanning salon," and the results may be poorly understood. Weakness can have a significant effect on the muscles (includ-

ing the tongue) to initiate the process of swallowing a mouthful of a deliciously vanilla pudding-filled Dunkin' Donuts mound of pleasure or a chunk of lamb flank as well. When Mary has a little lamb she might end up aspirating it and getting pneumonia—all because of weak muscles in the motor system innervated by the corticobulbar system. All of the parameters of movement, such as velocity, range, and even direction, can be affected by weakness and produce both speech and swallowing disruption. Upper motor neuron disorders produce a graded weakness of movement (paresis), which differs from the complete loss of muscle activity caused by paralysis (plegia). Of course, hemiparesis and hemiplegia refer to half of the body or structure being affected.

4. *Absence of fasciculations.* Because alpha motor neurons themselves are spared in upper motor neuron conditions, fasciculations do not occur. No twitching of muscle groups is visible.

5. *Absence of fibrillations.* Just as with fasciculations, the junior version of rapid twitching, fibrillations, do not occur in upper motor disease or disorder.

6. *Hypertonia.* Upper motor neuron disorders may cause an increase in muscle tone. Remember, there are numerous and rich circuits from the cerebellum and basal ganglia that can work their magic on descending motor pathways and can modulate the intrinsic circuitry that is existent in the spinal cord. This modulatory input can be either inhibitory or excitatory and can be a benefit or get in the way and create new and unwanted signs and symptoms. Although all of these processes and mechanisms are not well understood, the loss of descending inputs tends to result in an increased firing rate

of alpha and/or gamma motor neurons (Knierim, 2012). The higher firing rate in upper motor neuron disruption can cause an increase in the resting level of muscle activity, resulting in hypertonia. This abnormal increase in the steady-state background contraction of muscle groups can appear as stiffness and impede movement by slowing or weakening range of motion. Doctor Frankenstein's monster was portrayed as walking with serious stiffness or hypertonia.

7. *Hyperreflexia.* Because of the loss of inhibitory modulation from descending pathways and the circuits of the basal ganglia and cerebellum, the myostatic (stretch) reflex is exaggerated in upper motor neuron disorders. The stretch reflex is a major clinical diagnostic test of whether a motor disorder is caused by damage to upper or lower motor neurons. This is why physicians use the little rubber hammer (I have heard it called many things) to observe the knee-jerk stretch reflex. Hyperreflexia is defined in many sources as overactive or overresponsive reflexes. Examples of this can include twitching or spastic (hypercontractive) tendencies, which are suggestive of upper motor neuron disease as well as the dwindling or loss of control ordinarily exerted by higher brain centers of lower neural pathways (disinhibition). Checking reflexes is the part of the clinical neurologic exam conducted by neurologists and other physicians to help solve the puzzle of "Lesion, lesion, where is the lesion? Where is the damage and what is the reason?" The neurologist or family practitioner must be careful, however, since hyperreflexia can be the result of many other causes, including medication and stimulant side effects, hyperthyroidism,

electrolyte imbalance, serotonin syndrome, and severe widespread brain trauma. One significant variant of hyperreflexia, especially seen in some instances of spinal cord injuries above the thoracic zone (T1), is *autonomic hyperreflexia*. Autonomic hyperreflexia is a potentially life-threatening condition that can be considered a medical emergency requiring immediate attention. It occurs when the blood pressure in a person with a spinal cord injury (SCI) above T5–T6 becomes excessively high due to the overactivity of the autonomic nervous system, which is so intimately involved in the secretion of hormones and regulation of homeostasis of the body (Streeten, 2012).

The autonomic nervous system is an intricate and sometimes poorly explored system that helps regulate emotions, stress, and especially our "fight or flight" reactions to external stimuli and happenings. It conveys sensory impulses from the blood vessels, the heart, and all of the organs in the chest, abdomen, and pelvis through nerves to other parts of the brain (mainly the medulla, pons, and hypothalamus). These signals often do not reach our full levels of consciousness, but frequently are mostly automatic or reflex responses through the efferent autonomic nerves, thereby triggering appropriate reactions of the heart, the vascular system, and all the organs of the body to variations in environmental temperature ("I'm freezing!"), posture ("I'm falling!), food intake ("I'm choking!"), stressful experiences ("There's a badger in my toilet!"), and other changes to which all individuals are exposed ("I'm alive and everything is after me!"). The sympathetic nervous system is one section of the autonomic

nervous system that is largely responsible for organizing responses such as emotional excitement, fear, apprehension, psychic distress, panic reactions, the opportunity of immediate sexual activity when at the bakery, or a wide variety of other emotion-based, fight-or-flight stimuli. These activate many parts of the sympathetic nervous system, including the adrenal glands, that organize the special neurotransmitters such as acetycholine, adrenaline, and dopamine. Interestingly, many anxiety disorders are associated with dysregulation or a high set point of the sympathetic nervous system. The parasympathetic nervous system is the other main part of the autonomic nervous system and functions to calm things back down and set the emotions and involuntary body functions back to a balanced level (Streeten, 2012). Pupils dilate, heart rate returns to normal, sweating stops, goose bumps disappear, and skin color of the face returns to normal, all the result of the modulating parasympathetic nervous system which changes the alarmist sympathetic response of "I've got to get the heck out of here right away" to "Maybe this isn't such a major threat after all."

The most common signs and symptoms of this most severe condition of *autonomic dysreflexia* are sweating, pounding headache, tingling sensation on the face and neck, blotchy skin around the neck, and goose bumps, or piloerection. In untreated and extreme cases of autonomic dysreflexia, it can lead to stroke and death (Streeten, 2012).

8. *Clonus.* Sometimes the stretch reflex is so strong that muscles contract a number of times in a 5- to 7-Hz little oscillation dance when the muscle is rapidly stretched and then held at a con-

stant length. This abnormal oscillation, called clonus, can be observed visually or felt if it is too subtle to be seen.

9. *Initial contralateral flaccid paralysis.* In the initial stages after damage to the motor cortex, the contralateral side of the body shows a flaccid paralysis. The arm is limp and swings during ambulation, or the leg is dragged. Gradually, over the course of a few weeks, motor function returns to the contralateral side of the body. This continuing and sometimes way too gradual recovery of function results from the ability of other motor pathways so they can take over some of the lost or impaired operations of movement. Once again, we must remember that in the wonderful layout of the motor system, there are multiple descending motor pathways by which high-order information can reach the spinal cord; therefore, and with thanks to the redundancy of the systems that we appreciate in airplanes and our motor system, descending pathways such as the rubrospinal and the reticulospinal tracts, which receive direct or indirect cortical input, can take over the function lost by the damage to the corticospinal tract. Additionally, the primary motor cortex itself, that little homunculous land on the motor strip just anterior to the central sulcus or fissure of Rolando is capable of regrouping and reorganizing itself to recover some vanished function; thus, if the part of motor cortex that controls a certain body movement is damaged, neighboring parts of the motor cortex that are undamaged can, to some extent, alter their function to help compensate for the damaged areas. The one major exception to the recovery of function is that fine control of the distal musculature will not be regained after a lesion to the corticospinal tract. This is due to the motor system characteristic that there are direct connections from primary motor cortex neurons to alpha motor neurons controlling the fingers. These connections ostensibly underlie our abilities to manipulate objects with great precision and to do such tasks as playing "Just Because You Think You're So Pretty" on the accordion or performing the delicate surgery of removing the testicles from a cat. None of the other descending pathways have direct connections onto spinal motor neurons, and none of them can offset the loss of fine motor control of the hands and fingers after damage to the corticospinal tract (Knierim, 2012).

10. *Spasticity.* A clinical sign of upper motor neuron disorder is a velocity-dependent resistance to passive movement of the limb. If the neurologist moves a person's limb slowly, there may be little resistance to the movement. As the passive movement becomes quicker, however, at a certain point the muscle will sharply resist the movement. This is referred to as a "spastic catch." The mechanism for this spasticity is not entirely understood, but altered firing rate of gamma motor neurons and their regulating interneurons may be involved, as well as an increase in alpha motor neuron activity, causing an inappropriately powerful stretch reflex to a fast stretch of the muscle. Sometimes, the resistance becomes so great that the autogenic inhibition reflex is initiated, causing a sudden drop in the resistance; this is referred to as the *clasp-knife reflex* (Knierim, 2012; Streeten, 2012)

11. *Babinski sign.* A classic neurologic test for corticospinal tract damage is the Babinski test. In this test, the physi-

cian strokes the sole of the foot firmly with the thumb, finger, or a blunt instrument. This elicits a normal *plantar response* in normal individuals, as the toes curl inward. In individuals with an upper motor neuron disorder, however, an abnormal *extensor* plantar response is elicited, as the big toe extends upward and the remaining toes fan out. This is called a positive Babinski sign. Interestingly, the positive Babinski sign is normal in infants for the first 2 years of life. During development, however, the reflex changes to the normal adult pattern, presumably as corticospinal circuits become established over time (Knierim, 2012).

## Paralysis

Dissection or crushing of the spinal cord results in paralysis of all parts of the body below the damaged region. Even though such an injury occurs in the spinal cord, it is not considered a lower motor neuron disorder, as the alpha motor neurons themselves are not directly damaged. If the damage occurs at the cervical level, as in the unfortunate circumstance of the late American actor Christopher Reeve, then all four limbs will be paralyzed (quadriplegia). If the damage occurs below the cervical enlargement, then only the legs are paralyzed (paraplegia). The cervical enlargement corresponds with the attachments of the large nerves which supply the upper limbs. The cervical enlargement extends from about the third cervical to the second thoracic vertebra, and its maximum circumference (about 38 mm) is at about the level with the attachment of the sixth pair of cervical nerves. The explanation behind the enlargement of the cervical region is that it is related to the increased neural input and output to the upper limbs (some call them *arms*). An equivalent region in the lower limbs occurs at the lumbar enlargement. Other terms used to describe patterns of paralysis are hemiplegia (paralysis to one side of the body) and monoplegia (paralysis of a single limb).

## Basal Ganglia

The basal ganglia have traditionally been considered part of the motor system because of the variety of motor deficits that occur when they are damaged, and these disorders represent all of the motoric disinhibition known as positive signs and symptoms. These types of disorders that result from basal ganglia disorders are classified and typed in several different ways. In some texts they are divided into two classes: dyskinesias, which are abnormal, involuntary movements; and akinesias, which are abnormal, involuntary postures. An example of a dyskinesia would be the involuntary, rhythmic tremors that are seen in many neurologic diseases. An akinesia example would be the abnormal head and neck posture seen in what has been called cervical dystonia or spasmodic torticollis. Because the basal ganglia were once considered to form a separate, "extrapyramidal" motor system, these symptoms are sometimes called extrapyramidal disorders, but this term is losing favor in the contemporary literature.

## Dyskinesias

Resting tremors are most often associated with Parkinson disease (PD) or the variety of movement disorders increasingly known as parkinsonism. When a person with PD is at rest, certain body parts display a characteristic and very observable and almost countable 4- to 7-Hz tremor. The thumb and forefingers move back and forth against each other in a characteristic tremor called by some "pill-rolling tremor." The tremor stops when the body part engages in active movement. As mentioned, as the nature of the tremor can be diagnostic of which part of the nervous system is affected, these positive signs can be very diagnostic (Knierim, 2012; LaPointe, 2012; Streeten, 2012).

*Athetosis* is another classic dyskinesia and is characterized by involuntary, writhing movements, especially of the hands and face. Athetosis can vary from mild to severe motor dysfunction; it is generally characterized by unbalanced, involuntary movements of muscle tone and a difficulty maintaining a symmetric posture. The associated motor dysfunction can be restricted to a part of the body or present throughout the body, depending on the individual and the severity of the symptoms. One of the pronounced signs can be observed in the extremities in particular, as the writhing, convoluted movement of the digits (Morris et al., 2002). Athetosis can appear as early as 18 months from birth with first signs including difficulty feeding, hypotonia, spasm, and involuntary writhing movements of the hands, feet, and face, which progressively worsen through adolescence and at times of emotional distress. Readers will recognize these signs and symptoms as the cluster of characteristics that has been described traditionally as one of the types of cerebral palsy (CP). "Cerebral palsy" is now considered by some a rather outmoded term

that encompasses the characteristics of movement disorders; and the types of CP relate to different levels and structures of disruption of the motor control system. Cerebral palsy has been, and to an extent still is, a group of non-progressive, non-contagious motor conditions that cause physical disability in human development, primarily in the various areas of body movement. Cerebral palsy is caused by damage to the motor control centers of the developing brain and can occur during pregnancy, during childbirth, or after birth up to about age 3 years. The resulting limitations of movement and posture cause activity limitation and are often accompanied by disturbances of sensation, depth perception, and other sight-based perceptual problems. Communication and cognitive impairments are not uncommon, and epilepsy is found in about one-third of cases. Cerebral palsy, no matter what the type, is often accompanied by secondary musculoskeletal problems that arise as a result of the underlying disorder, one of which is occasionally still referred to as "athetoid" CP, but as is understood from the previous discussion, athetosis can occur as a complex of movement disorders that is acquired at any age.

Athetosis may be caused by lesions in more than a few brain areas, such as the hippocampus and the motor thalamus, as well as the corpus striatum; therefore, children with athetosis may show rather widespread signs and symptoms as they develop and could present cognitive deficits, speech impairment, hearing loss, and slow acquisition of sitting balance (Morris, 2002).

*Chorea*, another descriptor of movement gone wrong, is a term derived from the Greek word for "dance," and is characterized by continuous, writhing movements of the entire body. It is viewed by some as an intense form of athetosis, though choreiform movements can be either slow and writhing or quick and jerky. Chorea is associated with Huntington disease, the genetic, progressive, degenerative condition that can rob movement and cognition.

*Ballismus* is characterized by involuntary, ballistic movements of the extremities. This author is reminded of a young survivor of the Vietnam War who presented for evaluation of shrapnel wounds to the head and subsequent motor speech disorder. Part way through the evaluation in a cramped, tiny office at Fitzsimons Army Hospital, the examiner/author was treated to a sudden, flailing back-of-the-hand slap on the side of the face, the result of the condition of *hemiballismus*. This young veteran had no control over his sudden, involuntary flailing arm movement and provided for a first-hand (no pun intended) experience with the hyperkinetic condition of ballismus.

*Tardive dyskinesia* (TD) can result from the long-term use of antipsychotic drugs that target the dopamine system. It is characterized by involuntary movements of the tongue, face, arms, lips, and other body parts. The classic form of TD refers to stereotypic movements of the mouth, where patients look as though they are chewing gum; however, TD can take the form of other involuntary movements such as chorea, dystonia (slow hypercontractions), or tics.

## Akinesias

*Rigidity* is a resistance to passive movement of the limb. When one attempts to raise or move a limb, a rigid resistance is felt. Unlike spasticity, rigidity does not depend on the speed of the passive movement. In some persons, this resistance is so great that it is referred to as lead-pipe rigidity, because moving the person's limb is reported to feel like bending a lead pipe, though it is safe to say that most of us have had little experience bending lead pipes. In some individuals, this rigidity is combined with tremors and is called *cogwheel rigidity*, as moving the limb feels to the clinician like the catching and release of gears. As with spasticity, the mechanism is not totally understood but may result from unremitting firing of alpha motor neurons causing a continual contraction of the muscle (Morris, 2002).

*Dystonia* is the involuntary slow hypercontraction of muscle groups that results in abnormal movements and postures, as agonist and antagonist muscles both contract and become so rigid that the patient cannot maintain normal posture. Dystonia is the third most common movement disorder, after essential tremor and Parkinson disease. It is characterized by sustained co-contractions of opposing muscle groups that cause twisting or repetitive movements and abnormal postures. Dystonia is categorized according to the number of muscle groups affected. It may be focal and limited to one area (such as the face, neck, larynx/vocal cords, or limbs), or it may be generalized and affect the whole body.

One of the most common types of focal dystonia is called *cervical dystonia* or *spasmodic torticollis* (ST) and is recognized by its abnormal posture of the head. The most detailed study of speech in people with ST is that of LaPointe, Case, and Duane (1994). Our group of people with ST, most of whom were filmed and evaluated by the late James Case at Arizona State University, exhibited reduced reading rate, reduced speech alternate movement rates, reduced sequential movement rates, reduced maximum duration of /s/ and /z/ sounds, and prolonged vowels. They also presented with reduced phonation reaction time; and, in women, reduced habitual pitch, reduced highest pitch, and reduced pitch range. This study of speech and voice effects in cervical dystonia was "functional and intelligible, even if it was subtly different along some parameters."

Dystonia can be both painful and debilitating. Aside from medications, dystonias are frequently treated with Botox injections. Individuals with regional and generalized dystonias and normal MRI scans may benefit from deep brain stimulation (DBS) therapy. The following are examples of the variety of focal dystonias:

*Blepharospasm* is marked by involuntary contraction of the eyelid muscles. Symptoms may range from intermittent, increased frequency of blinking to constant, painful eye closure leading to practical blindness.

*Oromandibular* dystonia is characterized by mighty contractions of the lower face causing the mouth to open or close. Chewing and unusual tongue movements also may be part of the complex. This focal dystonia, of course, has the potential to wreak havoc on speech articulation and tongue movements required for motor speech production.

*Laryngeal dystonia* or *spasmodic dysphonia* (SD) is the result of abnormal contraction of intrinsic muscles in the larynx producing changes in the voice. Patients may have a strained/strangled quality to their voice or in some cases a whispering/breathy quality. Phonatory interruption is particularly noticeable on vowel sounds. For years, this disorder was thought to be laryngeal or even psychosomatic, but these days it is increasingly viewed as a neurologically based movement disorder. Spasmodic dysphonia is formally classified as a movement disorder, one of the focal dystonias, and is also known as laryngeal dystonia (Merati et al., 2005). Supporting evidence that SD is a neurologic disorder includes:

- SD may co-occur with other neurologic movement disorders such as blepharospasm (excessive eye blinking and involuntary forced eye closure), tardive dyskinesia (involuntary and repetitious movement of muscles of the face, tongue, body, arms, and legs), oromandibular dystonia (involuntary movements of the jaw muscles, lips, and tongue), torticollis (involuntary movements of the neck muscles), or tremor (rhythmic, quivering muscle movements).
- SD runs in some families and is thought to be inherited. Research has identified a possible gene on chromosome 9 that may contribute to the SD that is common to certain families.
- Histologic examination of the nerve to the vocal folds in patients with SD demonstrates that the percentage of abnormally thin nerve fibers was higher than in normal controls.
- Functional MRI signal is reduced in sensorimotor cortices associated with movement of the affected body part in laryngeal dystonia, supporting a dystonic basis for this voice disorder (Merati et al., 2005).

Spasmodic dysphonia or laryngeal dystonia is not as unknown as it was for many years, and many notable persons have struggled with the condition including Diane Rehm, host of the Diane Rehm Show on National Public Radio (NPR) in the United States. Others include Linda Robinson, British folk-rock musician, Scott Adams, creator of the comic strip *Dilbert*, Robert F. Kennedy, Jr., and Darryl McDaniels, of the rap group Run DMC.

*Writer's cramp and musician's cramp* is a task-specific dystonia, meaning that it only occurs when performing certain tasks. Writer's cramp is a contraction of hand and/or arm muscles that happens only when a person is writing. What could be worse for an author than to have writer's block and writer's cramp? It does not occur in other situations, such as when a person is using a keyboard or when eating. *Musician's cramp* occurs only when a musician plays his or her instrument. For example, pianists may experience cramping of their hands when playing, while brass players may have cramping or contractions of their mouth muscles. The Arizona Dystonia Institute, where we studied focal dystonias with neurologist Drake Duane, treated several cases of musician's cramp including a cello player for the Phoenix Symphony.

*Bradykinesia* refers to a slowness or insufficiency of movement. Bradykinesia ("slow movement") is characterized by slowness of movement and has been linked to Parkinson disease and other ailments of the basal ganglia. Rather than being a slowness in initiation (akinesia), bradykinesia designates a slowness in the execution of movement. It is one of the three key symptoms of parkinsonism ("the triad of signs") which are bradykinesia, tremor, and rigidity.

Bradykinesia and rigidity are also the underlying explanations for what is normally referred to as "the mask-like face" (expressionless face) noticed in those with Parkinson disease.

## Tics

Tics are involuntary, usually quick movements that are stereotyped, meaning that they tend to recur with the same or a very similar pattern in the same muscles. They most commonly involve the face, mouth, eyes, head, neck, or shoulder muscles. Tics can be motor (pertaining to movement) or vocal (pertaining to speech). Tics usually vary in relentlessness and severity over time and worsen in times of stress.

## Tourette Syndrome

When both motor and vocal tics are present and persist for more than one year, a diagnosis of Tourette syndrome (TS) is likely. Tourette syndrome is an inherited neurobehavioral disorder characterized by both motor and vocal tics. Some individuals with TS may develop obsessions, compulsions, inattention, and hyperactivity, and obsessive-compulsive disorder (OCD) is not infrequently a comorbid condition with TS. Tourette syndrome usually starts in childhood. In contrast to the abnormal movements of other movement disorders (for example, choreas, dystonias, myoclonus, and dyskinesias), the tics of TS are temporarily suppressible, nonrhythmic, and often preceded by an unwanted premonitory urge (Jankovic, 2001). Immediately preceding tic onset, many people with TS are aware of an urge, described as similar to the need to sneeze or scratch an itch. The crave to tic is characterized as a buildup of tension, pressure, or energy which they consciously choose to release, as if they "had to do it" to relieve the sensation or until it feels "just right." Examples of this baffling and unrelenting premonitory urge by those who have commented on their tics include the feeling of having something in the throat ("a lump of food; a medium-sized hawker"), or a localized discomfort in the shoulders ("a little hamster or something") leading to the need to clear one's throat or shrug the shoulders. The actual tic may be felt as relieving this tension or sensation, similar to scrabbling an itch. Another example is blinking to relieve an uncomfortable sensation in the eye ("seems like I had a fleck, or a small booger in my eye.").

In 1885, Gilles de la Tourette published an account of nine patients, *Study of a Nervous Affliction,* concluding that a new clinical category should be defined (Gille de la Tourette, Goetz, & Llawans, 1982). The eponym was later bestowed by one of the most famous in a long line of famous French neurologists, Charcot, on behalf of Gilles de la Tourette. Charcot, Gilles de la Tourette, Bouillaud, Aubertin, Dejerine, Dupuytren, and many others labored in the hospitals of Paris and contributed much of what we know about contemporary neurology and nervous system afflictions (LaPointe, 2013).

Only about 10 to 20% of people with TS exhibit copralalia (the reports vary, come from different cultures and languages, and methodologic differences are difficult to reconcile), the utterance of naughty words. Coprolalia refers to the involuntary swearing or utterance of obscene words or socially inappropriate and derogatory remarks. Cop-

rolalia comes from the Greek (kopros) meaning "feces" and (lalia) from lalein, "to talk." So quite literally, coprolalia means to "talk shit." Related terms are copropraxia, performing obscene or forbidden gestures, and coprographia, making obscene writings or drawings (Singer, 1997).

Coprolalia encompasses words and phrases that are culturally taboo or generally unsuitable for acceptable social use when used out of context. The term is not used to describe contextual swearing; or the polysyllabic 14-carat nasty words that flow trippingly off the tongue when we bang our thumb with a hammer. Genuine coprolalic utterances are usually expressed out of social or emotional context, and may be spoken in a louder tone or different cadence or pitch than normal conversation. It can be a single word or a complex phrase replete with adjectives considered to be socially unacceptable, such as offensive words regarding race, weight, body parts, or ethnicity.

A person with coprolalia may repeat the word mentally rather than saying it out loud, and even these subvocalizations can be very distressing. Imagine how socially penalizing and isolating this condition can be. Barks, grunts, and screamed obscenities are not fit behaviors for church, movie theaters, office jobs, or school, and the people who exhibit these uncontrollable behaviors soon find themselves better off by self-imposed social isolation.

Although coprolalia is an occasional characteristic of TS in a minority of those with the disorder, it is not required for a diagnosis of TS. In TS, compulsive swearing can be uncontrollable and undesired by the person uttering the phrases. Involuntary outbursts, such as racial or ethnic slurs in the company of those most offended by such remarks, can be particularly embarrassing. The phrases uttered by a person with coprolalia do not necessarily reflect the thoughts or opinions of the person, and that is what makes it dually embarrassing. A young girl with TS with a YouTube video posting discusses how utterly embarrassed she is for her uncontrollable utterance of a racial slur in the presence of her best friend, who is a member of the ethnic group which the girl disparages. Interestingly, cases of deaf persons with TS swearing in sign language have been described, showing that coprolalia is not just a corollary of the short and sudden sound pattern of many swear words.

Coprolalia is not unique to tic disorders. It has been described as well as a rare symptom of other neurologic disorders. Swearing in aphasia after stroke is not uncommon. It may occur after other injuries to the brain, such as encephalitis, and in other neurologic conditions, such as choreoacanthocytosis (an autosomal-recessive syndrome characterized by tics, chorea, and personality changes, with acanthocytes in the blood), seizure disorder, and sometimes in persons with dementia or OCD in the absence of tics.

## Communication Disorders Embedded in Movement Disorders

The speech, language, and swallowing impairment and disability in movement disorders are complex and varied. The characteristics of motor speech disorders are treated in depth in a number of excellent texts on the topic. One of the premier and lasting works on this topic that covers the neurologic substrates, differential diagnosis, and management of motor speech disorders is *Motor Speech Disorders* by Joseph R. Duffy (2013). This book is based on the rich foundation of clinical research that has been going on for decades at the Mayo Clinic (Rochester, Minnesota). It has a footing in the classic research conducted by Darley, Aronson, and Brown (1975) and has incorporated all of the necessary updates and revisions to contemporary understanding of the speech disorders that are born of movement impairment (Kent, 2008). Lowit and Kent (2010) also have produced a useful summary of assessment of the communication disorders embedded in movement disorders. Their book brings together a wide range of researchers who present an updated summary of assessment and evaluation techniques for disordered speech, with both a clinical and a research emphasis. This resource examines research evidence pertaining to best practice in the clinical assessment of established areas such as intelligibility and physiological functioning. It also introduces recently developed topics, such as conversational analysis, participation measures, and the burgeoning area of telehealth, which is on the horizon of more and more programs that find they must supplement in-clinic assessment with increasingly sophisticated methods of remote measurement. Lowit and Kent (2010) concoct a rich omelet of motor speech ingredients including the eggs of phonetics, kinematics, imaging, and neural modeling. Understanding disarranged speech in movement disorders requires consideration of all of these components.

## Harvesting the Internet

Motor speech disorders are typically categorized into two predominant types: dysarthria (or more precisely dysarthrias (since several identifiable subtypes exist) and apraxia of speech. Summations of speech motor control and subsequent motor speech disorders are available from many sources, including the textbooks listed above by Duffy (2013), Freed (2011), McNeil (2008), Murdoch (1998), Weismer (2006), Yorkston and Beukleman (2010), and others. The Internet is also a viable source of information on motor speech disorders, though, as with most Internet information, one can expect to find trash and treasures. For the most part, sites endorsed or generated by learned societies or professional organizations are the most dependable, although considerable variance exists among these sites as well.

Some of the information below has been garnered from the fertile collections of sources available on the Internet. Included among these are those of the American Speech-Language-Hearing Association's website (http://www.asha.org/SLP/clinical/Dysarthria/); the website of the Academy of Neurologic Communication Disorders and Sciences (ANCDS); (http://www.ancds.org/); The Movement Disorders Society (http://www.movementdisorders.org/); and the collection of material on movement disorders and speech difficulties from Parkinson disease societies across the globe such as the following:

http://www.parkinsons.org.uk/

http://www.parkinson.org/

http://www.parkinson.ca/site/c.kgLNIWODKpF/b.5842619/k.C7EB/Welcome/apps/s/custom.asp

https://www.michaeljfox.org/

Much information is available and can be gathered from academic, hospital, and research websites as well. The following list is representative but certainly not exhaustive of reputable sites that are instructive on movement disorders and motor speech disorders:

http://www.d.umn.edu/~mmizuko/2230/msd.htm

http://www.asu.edu/clas/shs/liss/Motor_Speech_DIsorders_Lab/Home.html

http://www.utdallas.edu/calliercenter/

http://www.cmds.canterbury.ac.nz/research/motorspeechdisorders.shtml

http://www.shrs.uq.edu.au/centre-for-neurogenic-communication-disorders-research

http://commdisorders.cci.fsu.edu/

http://www.waisman.wisc.edu/HOME.HTML

http://mdc.mbi.ufl.edu/

http://www.mayoclinic.org/movement-disorders/

http://www.mayoclinic.com/health/dysarthria/DS01175

http://my.clevelandclinic.org/Documents/Head_Neck/2010-face-sheet-final.pdf

http://www.ganeurosurg.org/
specialties/movementdisorders
.htm

http://www.hopkinsmedicine.org/
neurology_neurosurgery/specialty_
areas/movement_disorders/

http://www.thebarrow.org/
Neurological_Services/Muhammad
_Ali_Parkinson_Center/Movement
_Disorders_Clinic/index.htm

http://www.uihealthcare.org/
MovementDisorders/

http://swpadrecc.neurology.ucla
.edu/mdisorder/home.html

http://www.rush.edu/rumc/
page-1099611538174.html

http://www.chp.edu/CHP/
Movement+Disorders+Clinic

http://www.swedish.org/
Services/Neuroscience-Institute/
Neuroscience-Services/Movement-
Disorders#axzz2GwhUPa1v

## Motor Speech Disorders Primer

Contemporary textbooks and reputable websites are replete with some of the primer basics about motor speech disorders characteristics. This foundation for understanding the speech disorders accompanying movement disorders usually includes attention to definitions, motor processes of speech production, neuroanatomic and neurophysiologic substrates, classification systems, and perceptual characteristics. These bricks and mortar in the foundation of understanding motor speech disorders are reviewed and synthesized below:

## Definitions

Motor speech disorders are group of speech production disorders resulting from disturbances in muscular control (weakness, slowness, or incoordination) of the speech production muscle groups and systems that are due to damage or impairment to the central or peripheral nervous system or both. As discussed earlier, the central nervous system (CNS) includes the brain, brainstem, cerebellum, and spinal cord. The peripheral nervous system refers to parts of the nervous system outside the brain and spinal cord. It includes the vital connections of the cranial nerves, spinal nerves, and their roots and branches, peripheral nerves, and neuromuscular junctions. The anterior horn cells, although technically part of the CNS, are sometimes discussed with the peripheral nervous system because they are part of the motor unit. In the peripheral nervous system (PNS), bales, wads, cables, wires, filaments, and myriad assemblies of nerve fibers or axons conduct information to and from the CNS. The most simplistic metaphor of these intricate assemblies is the electrical cord or cable, but that is far short of the intricacy and complexity of these networks of conductivity to the muscles. The autonomic nervous system is the part of the nervous system concerned with the innervation of involuntary structures, such as the heart, smooth muscle, and glands within the body. The autonomic nervous system with its family of glands, hormones, and neurotransmitters, including the most important functions of the sympathetic and parasympathetic nervous subsystems, are frequently overlooked in the study of nervous system diseases, but they should not be. Bad glands and hormonal influences can result in diabetes, renal failure, huge goiters, hyper- or hypothyroidism, polycystic ovaries, and cancer. These are some of the diseases caused due to the failure of the glands in the human body. Dwarfism, gigantism, outbursts of acne, infertility, miscarriage, skin disorders, early or late puberty, and excessive weight are some of the upshots of hormonal imbalances in the body. The malfunctioning of one or more glands in the body can lead to mental disturbances, mood swings, depression, and high/low blood pressure. Movement disorders can be the result of faulty autonomic nervous system function and have either direct or indirect insinuation on the cousin systems that control and regulate movements. The wonder of the hypothalamus, for example, is ever so close to basal ganglia systems involved in movement, and is known as the "control and relay center of the endocrine system." The autonomic nervous system is reined over by the hypothalamus. It plays an important role in many metabolic processes and body functions, and in basic neuroanatomy courses we get great delight in generating and assigning associated sounds to the functions of the hypothalamus to aid in remembering its vital functions. Located near the pituitary gland at the basal part of the skull (deep within the cerebrum), the hypothalamus controls many secretions that relate to hunger, thirst, sleep, emotional behavior and sexual activity, body temperature, blood pressure, function of the car-

diovascular system (heart rate), and abdominal visceral regulation. So the central, peripheral, and autonomic systems are far reaching and impose their influence on everything that is human.

The definitional implications of the term dysarthria or the dysarthrias encompass coexisting neurogenic disorders of several or all of the basic processes of speech: respiration, phonation, resonance, articulation, and prosody and these definitional distinctions are largely the result of the clinically based research and writing of the Mayo Clinic influence by Darley et al. (1975) followed by Duffy (2013). Some of these distinctions include the following observations:

1. The medical dictionary definitions: "imperfect articulation" in speech is simplistic, reductionist, and fails to acknowledge the importance of the other speech production processes. The dysarthrias result from disruption of muscular control due to damage of the CNS or PNS, or both. This implies involvement of the basic motor processes used in the production and control of speech and is the consequence of a movement disorder. The dysarthrias include possible disruption of all basic motor processes of speech. Involvement of several motor speech control processes may contribute more to overall severity than just disrupted articulation. These processes include:
   a. Respiration: Slow, restricted, weak, or uncoordinated muscle activity used in breathing for speech.
   b. Phonation: Producing sound and regulating the airstream

and vibratory sound stream by the larynx.

   c. Resonance: Selectively amplifying sound by changing the size, shape, and number of cavities through which the sound or airstream must pass.

   d. Articulation: Valving and modifying the airstream or voice stream by the movement of speech structures (vocal folds, velum, tongue, jaw, lips) employed in producing the sounds of speech.

   e. Prosody: Varying intonation, stress, rhythm, and rate of speech.

2. As highlighted earlier, dysarthria refers to a group of disorders rather than a single disorder. It is more appropriate to refer to the plural form "dysarthrias" rather than the singular form "dysarthria."

3. Dysarthrias are neurogenic speech disorders. They should not be confused with language disorders such as aphasia, the language of confusion, disorientation, psychosis, or language of generalized intellectual impairment or dementia, or speech disorders due to developmental or structural problems (although these conditions can and sometimes do coexist).

4. The clinical relevance of this distinction is in assessment, intervention, and management. Treatments for the dysarthrias differ from those employed for language disorders, or developmental or structurally based disorders.

5. Localization: The neuroanatomic areas or systems involved are many and can be correlated with deviant speech dimensions and perceptual characteristics. The dysarthrias, depending on the type, can result from impairment of many levels and systems of the motor systems of the nervous systems including the upper motor neuron system, the lower motor neuron system, the cerebellum, the basal ganglia and extrapyramidal systems, or combinations of these areas.

6. Classification and taxonomy systems used with dysarthrias are grounded on the site of lesion and common clusters of speech perceptual characteristics. Dysarthrias are neuromuscular speech disorders that can arise from motor pathway damage at singular or multiple sites from the cortex to muscle. The type of dysarthria demonstrated depends on the site of lesion within the motor pathway.

7. Perceptual characteristics. Darley, Aronson, and Brown (1975) developed the widely used perceptual classification system of dysarthrias. Their seminal work has been updated and refined, and these changes are highlighted in the work of Duffy (2013). This breakthrough clinical research has come to be associated with the Mayo Clinic and marked a paradigm shift in understanding and managing motor speech disorders. The history of this innovative clinical research is chronicled in many sources, including the Mayo Clinic website (Mayo Clinic, 2013): http://mayoresearch.mayo .edu/mayo/research/neurology/ speech_pathology.cfm/.

In the late 1960s, several seminal publications by speech-language pathologists Fredrick L. Darley, Arnold

E. Aronson, and neurologist Joe R. Brown described the distinctive speech characteristics associated with motor speech disorders resulting from neurologic diseases affecting various components of the motor system. This work established a system for classifying the dysarthrias now used throughout the world. Darley, Aronson, and Brown, in collaboration with numerous speech pathology fellows and other Mayo Clinic neurologists, subsequently published numerous papers that contributed importantly to our understanding of apraxia of speech and the speech characteristics associated with dysarthrias associated with a variety of neurologic diseases (e.g., stroke, multiple sclerosis, motor neuron disease, Wilson disease, Shy-Drager syndrome, Parkinson disease).

In recent years, Joseph R. Duffy and Edythe Strand (speech-language pathologists), in collaboration with speech-language pathology fellows and neurology consultants, have published numerous additional papers addressing the speech deficits associated with a variety of other disorders (e.g., progressive supranuclear palsy, corticobasal degeneration, paraneoplastic cerebellar degeneration, primary progressive aphasia, progressive apraxia of speech, and childhood apraxia of speech). This work, conducted over many decades, continues and has had a strong influence on the classification and understanding of neurologic motor speech disorders.

Today, the system used for classifying the dysarthrias in many parts of the world is often referred to as the "Mayo classification system."

The original researchers collected speech samples from 2,000 persons diagnosed with motor speech disorders from the vast caseloads and vaults of the Mayo Clinic and associated them with diagnosed neurologic lesions or disease. They concluded that dysarthrias resulting from damage in different parts of the nervous system sound different and can be differentiated according to specific perceptual dimensions. A summary is reproduced below.

Speech dimensions:

- Pitch
- Loudness
- Voice quality
- Respiration
- Prosody
- Articulation

Classification type and neuroanatomic areas involved:

1. *Flaccid dysarthria*
   - Site of lesion
     - Peripheral nervous system or lower motor neuron system
   - Neuromuscular symptoms
     - Weakness
     - Lack of normal muscle tone
   - Perceptual characteristics
     - Hypernasality
     - Imprecise consonant productions
     - Breathiness of voice
     - Nasal emission

2. *Spastic dysarthria*
   - Site of lesion
     - Pyramidal and extrapyramidal systems
   - Neuromuscular symptoms
     - Muscular weakness
     - Greater than normal muscular tone

- Perceptual characteristics
  - Imprecise consonants
  - Harsh voice quality
  - Hypernasality
  - Strained/strangled voice quality

3. *Ataxic dysarthria*
   - Site of lesion
     - Cerebellum
   - Neuromuscular symptoms
     - Inaccuracy of movement and slowness of movement
   - Perceptual characteristics
     - Imprecise consonants
     - Irregular articulatory breakdowns
     - Prolonged phonemes
     - Prolonged intervals
     - Slow rate

4. *Hypokinetic dysarthria*
   - Site of lesion
     - Subcortical structures involving basal ganglia
   - Neuromuscular symptoms
     - Slow movements
     - Movements limited (limited range of movement)
   - Perceptual characteristics
     - Articulatory mechanism—impaired because of reduced range of motion involving the lips, tongue, and jaw; disturbance may range from mildly imprecise to total unintelligibility
     - Monopitch; monoloudness

5. *Hyperkinetic dysarthrias*
   - Site of lesion
     - Subcortical structures involving basal ganglia
   - Neuromuscular symptoms
     - Quick, unsustained, involuntary movements

- Slow hypercontraction of muscle groups
- Perceptual characteristics associated with TS
  - Emission of grunts as a result spontaneous contractions of the respiratory and phonatory muscles
  - Barking noises
  - Echolalia
  - Coprolalia: shocking, obscene, or socially inappropriate language without provocation or reason.

6. *Mixed dysarthrias*
   - Amyotrophic lateral sclerosis and other multisystem pathologies
   - Site of lesion
     - Progressive degeneration of the upper and lower neuron systems.
   - Neuromuscular symptom
     - Impairs the function (weakness and paralysis) of all the muscles used in speech production
   - Perceptual characteristics
     - Slow rate
     - Shortness of phrases
     - Imprecise of consonants
     - Hypernasality
     - Phonatory harshness

7. *Apraxia of speech*
   As revealed earlier, apraxia is a problem in planning, selecting, and assembling the appropriate sequence of movements. When the task involves these assemblies for speech production or executing the appropriate serial ordering of sounds for speech, the condition is called *apraxia of speech*. The primary disorder is a difficulty with

programming articulatory movements. Since these problems cannot be explained by significant slowness, weakness, restricted range of movement, or incoordination of the articulators, apraxia is not one of the dysarthrias and no significant muscle involvement exists. Prosodic alterations may be associated with the articulatory problem, perhaps in compensation for it, and Darley has referred to this as "tiptoeing through speech." (Darley, Aronson, & Brown, 1975).

- Localization—Apraxia results from a unilateral, left hemisphere lesion involving the third frontal convolution, Broca's area. There is a possibility of apraxia following more posterior, probably parietal lesions. Lesions in many areas have been associated with apraxia of speech. The cortical insula, subcortical structures, and even the cerebellum has been suggested by some research as being implicated.
- Speech characteristics
  - Articulation and prosodic processes
    - Distortions, sound substitutions, intrusive schwa sounds, islands of error-free production, sound cluster creation, sound cluster reduction, inconsistency in repeated utterances of polysyllabic words
    - Articulatory errors vary greatly with severity but have been described as primarily substitutions, additions, repetitions, and

prolongations (essentially complications of the act of articulation). Articulation errors are inconsistent and highly variable, not referable to specific muscle dysfunction

- Common characteristic is the patient's groping to find the correct articulatory postures and sequences
  - Facial grimaces, articulatory groping, moments of silence, and phonated movements of articulators
- Consonant phonemes are involved more often than vowel phonemes
- Prosody process
  - Durational relationships of vowels and consonants are distorted
  - Rate of production is slow
  - Alterations of the intonation

## Diagnosis and Management Principles

Just as the Mayo Clinic approach has brought a semblance of order from the seeming chaos of motor speech disorders, the work of Duffy (2013), McNeil (2008), Murdoch (1998), Freed (2011), and researchers in Europe (Maassen, Kent, Peters, van Lieshout, & Hulstijn, 2004; Maassen & van Lieshout, 2010) and elsewhere, has crystalized some principles to diagnosis and management. The ongoing bienniel conferences of the Motor Speech Disorders Conference in the United States (http://www.madonna.org/clinical_education/conferences/motorspeechconference

.html) and of international conferences in the Netherlands (http://
www.slp-nijmegen.nl/smc2011/index
.php?part=home) have honed both the-
oretic and clinical thinking and practice
about diagnosis and management of
movement-based motor speech control
and disorders. Detailed contours of the
issues involved in differential diagnosis
and management are available in many
of the sources cited in this chapter, but
the reader may benefit from an outline
of the basic principles involved. No one
does this as well as Duffy (2013), and
I am indebted to his work and the many
discussions we have generated during
the pre-Clinical Aphasiology Conference Boyz Week meetings for the conceptualization of these processes. As
Duffy explains, to arrive in the land of
adequately thought-through diagnosis
and management principles, one must
first pose and attempt to answer a number of salient questions:

- Is a speech disorder present? Dialects, speech in the non-native language, horribly sloppy diction, and
  unfortunate speech habits may
  intrude and may or may not be
  discounted.
- Is the speech disorder neurogenic?
  Many disorders of speech are structural, developmental, or the result
  of factors not causually related to
  the nervous system. One consulta-
  tion request I answered at bedside
  revealed not the "possible dysarthria" on the request, but rather an
  intrusive wad of chewing tobacco
  the size of a small bird that was
  impeding articulation. This country
  gentleman had conveniently hid-
  den his necessary Styrofoam "spit

cup" to allow him to continue his
nicotine-driven habit while he was
in the hospital.
- What does the pattern of impaired
  speech imply about possible location
  of neurologic lesion? Many motor
  speech disorders are already well
  associated with lesion site, but occasionally the appearance of aberrant
  speech is the first sign on nonstatic
  neuropathology such as neoplasms
  and tumor growth.

The guidelines posed by Duffy
(2013) for differential diagnosis are
imperative to create the proper path
of discovering the diagnostic nature of
the disorder. These days, we can avail
the increasingly sophisticated strategies of instrumental supplementation
to our diagnostic dilemmas. Murdoch's
work (1998) on a physiologic approach
to managing dysarthrias and the continuing research and publications of
the Centre for Neurogenic Communication Disorders Research (http://www
.shrs.uq.edu.au/centre-for-neurogenic-
communication-disorders-research) are
testaments to the application of innovative instrumental analysis to the clinical
problems of motor speech disorders.

Differential diagnosis of motor speech
disorders is no task for a neophyte, and
considerable study and clinical experience must be logged before one can
accurately and reliably toil in these
fields. As Duffy (2013) has dauntingly
outlined, the astute clinician must be
able to understand and distinguish
dysarthrias from apraxia of speech,
aphasia, neurogenic stuttering, palilalia, echolalia, abulia (cognitive and
affective disturbances), aprosodia, and
a variety of psychogenic disorders (e.g.,

depression, schizophrenia, conversion disorders). The scope of our practice in the diagnosis and management of clinical speech, language, and swallowing disorders is wide indeed, and there is ample evidence that refinement and specialization is an evolutionary reality. Few clinicians can be generalists these days, even within the more restricted realm of brain-based disorders.

As pointed out in many writings with depressing frequency, the management of many medically based disorders lags behind description and diagnosis of them. This is certainly true with movement disorders and motor speech disorders, though there are enough innovative developments and an occasional breakthrough to give us expectation. Medical, surgical, pharmacological, and technological advances may continue to impress us, but behavioral management is still the foundation of intervention. Duffy (2013) reminds us in his summary of managing motor speech disorders:

■ Communication is key. The goal of all management may include attempts to manipulate improvement in speech intelligibility and speech naturalness, but in many it may focus on developing and implementing augmentative or alternative means of communication.

■ In addition to efforts to restore or compensate for motor speech disorders, we may have to assist in adjustment and acceptance of things that are unlikely to change. LaPointe's (2011) chapter on "aristos" and making the best of a bad situation may guide facilitating acceptance of unchangeable conditions.

■ Not everyone is a candidate for therapy. Many factors enter into this decision of treat or do not treat. These factors include medical diagnosis and prognosis, societal and environmental support factors, extent of cognitive limitations, availability of services, motivation and need for communication, and of course access to health care resources.

■ Criteria for termination of treatment is still a quandary. Termination must be based on ethical, cost-effective assessment of the individual's needs, and the achievement of realistic goals. In the best possible world, termination of treatment should not be based solely on the availability of reimbursement or insurance, but we all are aware that this is not the best possible "health care world." In many societies, and certainly in the United States, availability and provision of treatment is an economic, bottom-line decision rather than one based on the needs of the individual.

■ Management of motor speech disorders may be medical, prosthetic, or behavioral. Computer-based interfaces, prosthetic palatal lifts, and perhaps transcranial magnetic stimulation may enter the picture, but for most patients, rather traditional behavioral treatment will be used.

■ Management includes counseling, family support, and the vast palette of supportive services that may be necessary.

■ Treatment most likely will occur frequently with sessions that are designed to move from easy to difficult tasks. Sessions should be constructed and implemented to minimize fatigue. Patients who nod off after a rigorous session of physical therapy probably are not benefiting maximally.

■ Treatment should adhere to principles of science and evidence, and not chase the pseudoscientific rainbows of copper bracelets, and cell salts (claimed effective against a wide variety of diseases, including appendicitis, baldness, deafness, insomnia, and worms). Quackery is still rampant, and pseudoscience leads people to believe weird things, especially if they are desperate or vulnerable. (See the website of Quackwatch for insightful contemporary examples: http://quackwatch.org/.) Efficacy data and evidence-based practice for motor speech disorders come mostly from case studies, case reports, and a small number of group studies, but guidelines for treatment exist and have been published in the *Journal of Medical Speech-Language Pathology* and among the practice guidelines on the website of the Academy of Neurologic Communication Disorders and Sciences (ANCDS) (http://www.ancds.org/index.php?option=com_content&view=article&id=9&Itemid=9).

## References

Dana Foundation. (2013). Brain and brain research. Retrieved May 4, 2013 from https://www.dana.org/

Darley, F. L., Aronson, A. E., & Brown, J. E. (1975). *Motor speech disorders*. Philadelphia, PA: W. B. Saunders.

Duffy, J. R. (2013). *Motor speech disorders: Substrates, differential diagnosis, and management* (3rd ed.). St. Louis, MO: Elsevier Mosby.

Freed, D. (2011). *Motor speech disorders: Diagnosis and treatment*. Albany, NY: Delmar Cengage Learning.

Gilles de la Tourette, G., Goetz, C. G., & Llawans, H. L. (1982). Étude sur une affection nerveuse caractérisée par de l'incoordination motrice accompagnée d'echolalie et de coprolalie. In A. J. Friedhoff, & T. N. Chase (Eds.), *Advances in neurology* (Vol. 35, pp. 1–16). New York, NY: Raven Press.

Jankovic, J. (2001). Differential diagnosis and etiology of tics. *Advances in Neurology, 85*, 15–29.

Kent, R. D. (2008). Perceptual sensorimotor speech examination for motor speech disorders. In M. R. McNeil (Ed.), *Clinical management of sensorimotor speech disorders* (2nd ed.). New York, NY: Thieme.

Knierim, J. (2012). Disorders of the motor system. Retrieved October 29, 2012 from http://neuroscience.uth.tmc.edu/s3/chapter06.html/

LaPointe, L. L. (2011). *Aphasia and related neurogenic language disorders*. New York, NY: Thieme.

LaPointe, L. L. (2012). *Atlas of neuroanatomy for communication science and disorders*. New York, NY: Thieme.

LaPointe, L. L. (2013). *Paul Broca and the origins of language in the brain*. San Diego, CA: Plural.

LaPointe, L. L., Case, J. L., & Duane, D. D. (1994). Perceptual–acoustic speech and voice characteristics of subjects with spasmodic torticollis. In J. A. Till, K. M. Yorkston, & D. R. Beukelman (Eds.), *Motor speech disorders: Advances in assessment and treatment* (pp. 57–64). Baltimore, MD: Paul H. Brookes.

Latash, M. L., & Anson, J. G. (2006). Synergies in health and disease: Relations to adaptive changes in motor coordination. *Physical Therapy, 86*(8), 1151–1156.

Lowit, A. & Kent, R. D. (2010). *Assessment of motor speech disorders*. San Diego, CA: Plural.

Maassen, B., Kent, R., Peters, H. F. M., van Lieshout, P. H. H. M., & Hulstijn, W.

(Eds.). (2004). *Speech motor control in normal and disordered speech*. Oxford, UK: Oxford University Press.

Maassen, B., & van Lieshout, P. H. H. M. (Eds.). (2010). *Speech motor control: New developments in basic and applied research*. Oxford, UK: Oxford University Press.

Mayo Clinic. (2013). Neurology: Speech pathology research. Retrieved May 4, 2013 from http://mayoresearch.mayo.edu/mayo/research/neurology/speech_pathology.cfm

McNeil, M. R. (2008). *Clinical management of sensorimotor speech disorders*. New York, NY: Thieme.

Merati, A. L., Heman-Ackah, Y. D., Abaza, M., Altman, K. W., Sulica, L., & Belamowicz, S. (2005). Common movement disorders affecting the larynx: A report from the neurolaryngology committee of the AAO-HNS. *Otolaryngology-Head and Neck Surgery, 133*(5), 654–665.

Morris, J. G., Jankelowitz, S. K., Fung, V. S., Clouston, P. D., Hayes, M. W., & Grattan-Smith, P. (2002). Athetosis I: Historical considerations. *Movement Disorders, 17*(6), 1278–1280.

Murdoch, B. E. (1998). *Dysarthria: A physiological approach to assessment and treatment*. London, UK: Nelson Thornes.

Pearce, J. M. S. (2004). Positive and negative cerebral symptoms: the roles of Russell Reynolds and Hughlings Jackson. *Journal of Neurology, Neurosurgery and Psychiatry, 75*, 1148.

We Move. (2012). Movement disorders. Retrieved October 29, 2012 from http://www.wemove.org/

Singer, C. (1997). Tourette syndrome. Coprolalia and other coprophenomena. *Neurologic Clinics, 15*(2), 299–308.

Streeten, D. (2012). The autonomic nervous system. Retrieved November 3, 2012 from http://www.ndrf.org/ans.html/

Weismer, G. (2006). *Motor speech disorders: Essays for Ray Kent*. San Diego, CA: Plural.

Yorkston, K., & Beukleman, D. (2010). *Management of motor speech disorders in children and adults*. Austin, TX: Pro-Ed.

# 4

# Differential Effects of Contemporary Treatments for Movement Disorders on Limb and Speech Function

## BRUCE E. MURDOCH

## Introduction

Movement disorders in most instances manifest as impaired performance in both limb and orofacial muscles, including the muscles of the speech production mechanism. Unfortunately, although many of the contemporary treatments (including both pharmacologic and neurosurgical) for movement disorders have been reported to be successful in relieving many of the motor signs in the limb muscles, their effect on the muscles involved in speech production is much less consistent. These findings are suggestive of the need to reconsider our current thinking in relation to the neurology of speech and possibly to differentiate it from limb neurology. The differential effects of treatments for movement disorders on limb and speech function are most extensively documented in relation to idiopathic Parkinson disease (PD); therefore, this chapter reviews and evaluates reports in the literature on the effects of pharmacologic and neurosurgical interventions for PD on speech.

As described in Chapter 3, the cardinal signs manifest in the limbs of persons with PD arising from the loss of the neurotransmitter dopamine include muscle rigidity (muscles resistant to movement), akinesia (inability to initiate movement), bradykinesia (slowness of movement), and rest tremor. Furthermore, as many as 50 to 90% of individuals with idiopathic PD develop speech and voice disorders in the form of a hypokinetic dysarthria, the most common perceptual features of which include reduced loudness (hypophonia), breathy voice, abnormal prosody (hypoprosodia or monotone speech), variability in speech rate, and imprecise movements of the articulators. In addition, individuals with PD frequently have reduced facial animation and limited mobility of their oral musculature. Although clearly the functioning of both limb and speech production muscles are affected in PD, the various treatments applied in an attempt to stop or slow the progress of PD (see Chapter 10) have primarily targeted the cardinal signs of PD, with any effects on speech only being regarded as a secondary outcome. Consequently, although pharmacologic treatments, such as levodopa therapy, have been effective, at least in the short term, in reducing limb akinesia, rigidity, and tremor, parallel improvements in speech production do not appear to occur. Likewise, the results of studies documenting the effects of contemporary neurosurgical interventions for PD on speech are equivocal.

## Effect of Pharmacologic Treatments for Parkinson Disease on Speech

Striatal dopamine denervation as a consequence of degeneration of the substantia nigra in the mesencephalon represents the neurochemical hallmark of PD. Therefore, pharmacologic treatment of PD is based on supplementation of the depleted dopamine levels in the brain through the use of dopamine precursors (e.g., levodopa) and dopamine receptor agonists or compounds that inhibit the metabolization of dopamine or levodopa such as monoamine oxidase-B (MAO-B) or catechol-O-methyltransferase (COMT). More than 40 years after its introduction in 1968, levodopa remains the gold standard in the pharmacologic treatment of PD. The initial effect of levodopa administration typically involves a consistent reduction in symptoms associated with PD, including akinesia and rigidity, and to a lesser extent, tremor. Subsequent to this initial "levodopa honeymoon" period (lasting 2 to 5 years), individuals treated with levodopa may experience motor side effects (e.g., dyskinetic and involuntary movements) as well as fluctuations in motor performance. One common type of fluctuation is the "ON–OFF" effect, characterized by unpredictable fluctuations in response to levodopa. There can be a sudden loss of the effectiveness of levodopa (OFF state) unrelated to any change in treatment schedule, which can then improve suddenly (to the ON state) without another levodopa dose (Djaldetti & Melamed, 1998). Many individuals become akinetic and experience postural instability during the OFF period. Although subtle at first, these complications of levodopa therapy progress to a level where they result in a significant impairment in quality of life. After years of levodopa therapy, the motoric improvements of the ON period begin to wane and become shorter in duration, and the person with PD becomes "disabled" due to prolonged reappearance of parkinsonian symptoms during the OFF period.

Investigations of the side effects and fluctuations in motor performance resulting from levodopa therapy have primarily examined these features with regard to limb control and other gross motor movements such as gait (Blin, Ferrandez, Pailhous & Serratrice, 1991; O'Sullivan, Said, Dillon, Hoffman, & Hughes, 1998). O'Sullivan et al. (1998) reported that measures of gait changed significantly and predictably along with levodopa fluctuations. In contrast, the effects of levodopa on speech are far less consistent. Indeed, the effect of levodopa on speech motor control has only rarely been objectively examined and the existing literature remains inconclusive. Although some studies report positive effects on speech characteristics such as fundamental frequency (Sanabria et al., 2001), articulation, loudness, and persistence of phonation (Critchley, 1981; Wolfe, Garvin, Bacon, & Waldrop, 1975), others did not find significant changes on oral function (Gentil, Tournier, Pollak, & Benabid, 1999) or general speech performance (Poluha, Teulings, & Brookshire, 1998). Louis, Winfield, Fahn, and Ford (2001) even reported worsening of speech with exacerbation of dysfluencies due to levodopa treatment. Although not supported by any quantitative speech data, Critchley (1981) proposed that alterations in speech may accompany levodopa fluctuations. Improvements in overall speech adequacy, clarity of articulation, normalcy of nasal resonance, and temporal aspects of speech (rate, pauses, and rhythm) were reported based on subjective assessments of spontaneous speech and oral reading following levodopa

therapy (Rigrodsky & Morrison, 1970); however, the authors noted that the improvements were not as dramatic as observed in limb symptoms. Mawdsley and Gamsu (1971) observed improved intelligibility in the majority of their cases with PD subsequent to levodopa treatment primarily stemming from improved vocal loudness and more regular distribution of both speech time and pauses. Two further subjective studies conducted in the 1970s also documented the effects of levodopa on intelligibility in PD. Nakano, Zubick, and Tyler (1973) used a multiple-choice speech intelligibility test to compare speech intelligibility in three conditions including levodopa, placebo, and procyclidine hydrochloride administration in 18 individuals with PD. Intelligibility ratings conducted by a group of 10 untrained listeners demonstrated levodopa administration to improve intelligibility to a greater extent than placebo or procyclidine. Likewise, Adelman, Hoel, and Lassman (1970) noted higher speech intelligibility ratings after levodopa therapy compared with a no-drug condition in a group of 25 individuals with PD. The findings of Nakano et al. (1973) and Adelman et al. (1970) were confirmed by De Letter, Santens, and Van Borsel (2005) who examined the effects of levodopa on word intelligibility in 10 individuals with PD via the Yorkston and Beukelman Intelligibility Test (1980). On the basis of ratings provided by a panel of speech-language pathologists, De Letter et al. (2005) reported improved word intelligibility in the ON versus OFF condition, although no correlation was found between intelligibility and overall severity of the disease or severity of the motor problems. Improved word intelligibility in a group of 25 individuals with idiopathic PD treated with levodopa was also observed by De Letter, Santens, De Bodt, Van Maele, Van Borsel, and Boon (2007a) on the basis of performance on the word subtest protocol of the Assessment of Intelligibility of Dysarthric Speech (Yorkston & Beukelman, 1980).

Reports in the literature relating to the effects of levodopa on tongue strength and endurance vary. Solomon, Robin, and Luschei (2000) reported a reduction in tongue strength and endurance in individuals with PD subsequent to levodopa administration. In contrast, De Letter, Santens, and Van Borsel (2003) reported a positive effect of levodopa on tongue strength and endurance. Comparison of maximum tongue force and contraction duration in the ON and OFF conditions in 10 individuals with PD showed that the integrated measure of both (area under the curve) was significantly larger in the ON state; however, no significant improvement or reduction could be found on maximum tongue protrusion force or sustaining of tongue protrusion following levodopa administration when these two parameters were examined in isolation leading De Letter et al. (2003) to conclude that reported improvements in speech intelligibility after levodopa do not appear to be related to alterations in tongue force or sustaining of tongue force.

Individuals with PD treated with levodopa have been reported to show a shorter period of time between the initiation of labial movement and speech as well as increased speech and symmetry of labial activity compared with procyclidine and placebo (Nakano et al., 1973). Consistent with this finding,

Cahill, Murdoch, Theodoros, Triggs, Charles, and Yao (1998) reported that lip force improves/decreases with increasing/decreasing plasma levodopa levels; however, Gentil, Tournier, Pollak, and Benabid (1999) reported no significant effect of levodopa on upper lip, lower lip, and tongue force production. Although the findings in relation to lip force are equivocal, electromyographic recordings of labial muscles of individuals with PD have revealed a decrease in tonic activity (indicative of reduced rigidity) in labial muscles after taking levodopa (Leanderson, Meyerson, & Persson, 1971) suggesting that the drug normalized the neuromotor control of labial muscular activity which in turn may contribute to observed subjective improvements in speech. Counter to this suggestion is the finding of Caligiuri and Abbs (1986) that movements of the lips do not change in parallel to a decrease in lip rigidity across the levodopa drug cycle. Consequently, although lip rigidity may decrease following administration of levodopa, improvement in labial movement may still be prevented by reduced motor drive to the labial muscles; hence, a reduction in rigidity of articulatory muscles does not necessarily imply improvements in articulatory movements. Consistent with this latter suggestion, Kompoliti, Wang, Goetz, Leurgans, and Raman (2000) found no significant improvement in articulatory function following central dopaminergic stimulation via apomorphine treatment.

Studies of the effects of levodopa on respiration have also yielded equivocal results. Gardner, Langdon, and Parkes (1987) reported improvements in respiratory function in persons with PD treated with levodopa. In contrast, Solomon and Hixon (1993) failed to find significant differences in speech breathing measures as a function of the levodopa drug cycle. Furthermore, several researchers have noted the occurrence of irregularities in respiration leading to deficient control of speech breathing in individuals with PD receiving levodopa therapy (Murdoch, Chenery, Bowler, & Ingram, 1989; Rice, Antic, & Thompson, 2002). Despite these inconsistencies, evidence is available to suggest that levodopa improves but does not normalize the rigidity of the chest wall and diaphragm in PD (De Letter et al., 2007a; Solomon & Hixon, 1993).

Several studies have failed to identify significant improvements in laryngeal function across the levodopa drug cycle (Daniels, Oates, Phyland, Feiglin, & Hughes, 1996; Larson, Ramig & Scherer, 1994; Poluha et al., 1998), nor following central dopaminergic stimulation (Kompoliti et al., 2000). Larson et al. (1994) examined phonatory characteristics during prolonged vowel production in two individuals across levodopa cycles. They found no consistent relationship between acoustic/electroglottographic measures (mean F0, intensity, jitter, shimmer abduction quotient) in the ON or OFF states. Likewise, Daniels et al. (1996) reported that individuals with PD had lower intensity, lower variability of Fo and intensity, and greater degrees of "whisperiness" and harshness in both the ON and OFF states as compared with healthy control subjects with no changes in these measures between the ON and OFF conditions.

Disturbances in speech prosody are well-documented features of hypokinetic dysarthria in PD. Recent studies suggest an absence of levodopa-induced effects on speech rate (De Letter, Santens, De Bodt, Boon, & Van Borsel, 2006; Goberman & McMillan, 2005). Individuals treated with levodopa, however, appear to demonstrate a reduction in the variation of pitch (De Letter, Santens, Estercam, Van Maele, De Bodt, Boon, & Van Borsel, 2007b; Goberman & McMillan, 2005; Wolfe et al., 1975).

In summary, it is apparent that while some aspects of speech production are changed by levodopa administration, others are not (De Letter et al., 2003; De Letter et al., 2006; Ho, Bradshaw, & Iansek, 2008). Based on an investigation of sequential changes in respiratory, articulatory, and phonatory speech characteristics across a levodopa drug cycle, De Letter, Van Borsel, Boon, De Bodt, Dhooge, and Santens (2010) confirmed that although a number of speech characteristics demonstrate sequential changes in response to levodopa, a consistent pattern across all speech characteristics was not evident. These findings have important implications. The use of fixed timing after medication intake, as has been used in most previous research, as well as the definition of a time of maximum ON based on motor performance, may not allow an estimation of all levodopa-induced changes in speech and possibly explains some of the inconsistencies between the studies outlined above. Furthermore, the moment during the drug cycle of maximum speech performance may not coincide with time of maximum overall motor improvement leading De Letter et al. (2010) to suggest that the determination of speech treatment programs in PD be based on individual assessments of changes in speech features across an entire levodopa cycle.

## Effects of Neurosurgical Treatments for Parkinson Disease on Speech

In recent years, renewed interest in the use of stereotactic neurosurgical procedures for the treatment of PD and other basal ganglia disorders has provided the opportunity for examining the effects of discrete circumscribed lesions in the globus pallidus and thalamus, and electrical stimulation of the subthalamic nucleus (STN) and thalamus on motor speech function. The most commonly utilized neurosurgical treatments include ablative procedures such as pallidotomy and thalamotomy and deep brain stimulation (DBS) applied to the subthalamic nucleus (STN-DBS). (For a detailed description of the various neurosurgical procedures used in the treatment of PD the reader is referred to Chapter 10.) Ablative techniques typically involve the generation of lesions within the internal segment of the globus pallidus (GPi) (i.e., pallidotomy) and thalamus (thalamotomy) by means of radiofrequency-mediated electrocoagulation, which aims to permanently disrupt or inactivate the relevant target. Pallidotomy has been found to alleviate akinesia, rigidity, and drug-induced dyskinesia while thalamotomy has been reported to ameliorate tremor (Goetz, DeLong, Penn, & Bakay, 1993). The DBS procedure involves the implantation of an electrode into a specific brain target (most commonly the STN) which is connected to a pacemaker placed subcutaneously over the chest wall. It is postulated that DBS suppresses the neuronal firing pattern in the target via neural jamming, depolarization blockade, or by induc-

ing the release of inhibitory transmitters. The DBS procedure has several advantages over ablative techniques including the fact that it is reversible and does not necessitate the creation of a destructive permanent lesion.

Although the beneficial effects of thalamotomy, pallidotomy, and DBS on general motor function in individuals with PD have been well documented (Benabid, Pollak, & Gross, 1994; Iacono, Shima, Lonser, Kuniyoshi, Maeda, Yamada, 1995; Kelly, 1995; Limousin et al., 1995), specific clinical evaluation of the effects of these surgical procedures on speech motor function has been limited. Of the studies that have reported the effects of pallidotomy, thalamotomy, and DBS on speech, the majority of the data collected has been subjective, unsophisticated, and perceptually based. Furthermore, the results of those studies that have investigated the effects of these procedures on speech are equivocal, with some studies reporting improvements in speech and/or voice (Iacono et al., 1995; Legg & Sonnenberg, 1998) and others reporting either no changes or a worsening of speech (Schneider, Duffy, & Uitti, 1999; Scott et al., 1998) after procedures such as pallidotomy.

### Effect of Pallidotomy on Speech

Although limb symptoms have been noted to improve dramatically following pallidotomy, the impact on speech function has been less striking. Indeed, the current literature is equivocal with respect to the effects of pallidotomy on speech function. On the one hand, several research groups have reported marked improvements in speech function following pallidotomy (Iacono et al., 1995; Laitinen, Bergenheim, & Hariz, 1992). On the other hand, other research groups have alluded to negative changes in speech function for some PD participants following pallidotomy (Ghika et al., 1999; Schrag et al., 1999; Scott et al., 1998; Theodoros, Ward, Murdoch, Silburn, & Lethlean, 2000; Uitti et al., 2000). In addition, other researchers have found that speech improved minimally or in only a minority of patients after unilateral pallidotomy (Baron et al., 1996; Schulz, Greer, & Friedman, 2000; Schulz, Peterson, Sapienza, Greer, & Friedman, 1999).

Overall, the majority of previous reports of speech change following pallidotomy have relied on nonspecific subjective ratings of speech function and failed to provide objective speech data. For example, Iacono et al. (1995) reported a significant improvement in speech function following pallidotomy based on a significant postoperative decline in the Unified Parkinson's Disease Rating Scale (UPDRS) speech rating. Although significant improvements were observed in UPDRS speech ratings, no information was provided about the type of speech disturbance the PD participants exhibited postoperatively. In contrast, other studies have reported that PD participants did not experience improvements in speech function following pallidotomy as measured by the UPDRS (Johansson, Malm, Nordh, & Hariz, 1997; Lang, Lozano, Montgomery, Duff, Tasker, & Hutchinson, 1997; Samuel et al., 1998).

In addition to studies of general ratings of speech function, several studies have examined more objective speech parameters in PD participants fol-lowing pallidotomy (Barlow, Iacono, Paseman, Biswas, & D'Antonio, 1998; Legg & Sonnenberg, 1998; Schulz et al., 1999; Schulz et al., 2000; Theodoros et al., 2000; Uitti et al., 2000). For example, Barlow et al. (1998) observed improved orofacial motor control and speech aerodynamics after bilateral pallidotomy in many of their 11 participants with PD, all of whom exhibited normal speech intelligibility. Based on their findings, Barlow et al. (1998) postulated that bilateral pallidotomy resulted in a rescaling of neural inputs or concomitant adjustments in muscle stiffness among muscle subsystems of the vocal tract.

One methodological limitation of the study by Barlow et al. (1998) was the timing of post-pallidotomy assessments, as testing was conducted 48 to 144 hrs following surgery. The relatively brief interval between surgery and postoperative speech testing was a concern, due to the possibility that the neurological system may not have stabilized and perilesional edema may have been present. Indeed, it is well documented that the perilesional edema that may accompany ablative lesions may last up to 4 weeks postoperatively (Samuel et al., 1998); therefore, the effects of pallidotomy on orofacial control and laryngeal aerodynamics noted by Barlow et al. (1998) may reflect the effects of perilesional edema and may not represent an accurate indication of the long-term effects of pallidotomy on speech production.

Similarly, Legg and Sonnenberg (1998) reported improved speech function in a single case as measured on the Frenchay Dysarthria Assessment (FDA) 1 to 4 weeks postoperatively. Specifically, the PD participant demonstrated increased laryngeal modulation (evident in fewer audible pitch breaks) as well as improved intonation, loudness, and tongue function postoperatively. The PD participant continued to exhibit dysarthric speech and impaired lip and jaw function postoperatively. One limitation of Legg and Sonneberg's (1998) study was the omission of qualitative information pertaining to the severity and perceptual features of the subject's dysarthria pre- and post-pallidotomy.

Other studies have reported mixed changes in speech function following pallidotomy. For example, Schulz et al. (1999) indicated that four of six PD participants demonstrated positive changes in either phonatory or both phonatory and articulatory acoustic parameters following unilateral pallidotomy. In particular, several PD participants demonstrated greater intensity, more syllables per second, and longer extended vowel duration at 3 months post-surgery. There was not, however, a consistent pattern of postoperative voice improvements across participants.

A further study of vocal intensity in 25 PD participants undergoing unilateral pallidotomy showed a mixed pattern of speech changes following surgery and high levels of inter-subject variability with respect to the effects of surgery on vocal intensity (Schulz et al., 2000). In particular, postoperative improvements in vocal intensity were noted for many participants with mild speech impairment, but negative changes were noted for most of the moderately to severely dysarthric speakers. This finding suggests that pallidotomy may pose a particular risk for speech for persons with

PD who also have marked dysarthria pre-operatively.

Other studies have found a substantial risk for persisting speech impairments, usually of mild severity after unilateral pallidotomy (Kumar, Lozano, Montgomery & Lang, 1998; Lozano et al., 1995), and even greater risk after bilateral pallidotomy (Scott et al., 1998). In particular, Scott et al. (1998) reported that 8 participants of a group of 20 PD participants recorded a significant deterioration in speech articulation rates following bilateral pallidotomy. The investigators reported that these negative changes in speech articulation rates were not judged to be functionally significant.

In addition, Theodoros et al. (2000) noted similar negative changes in speech function following bilateral pallidotomy as evidenced in the reduction in speech intelligibility in 10 of 12 PD participants following surgery. Similarly, Uitti et al. (2000) recorded a mild decline of speech intelligibility in one-third of a cohort of 57 PD participants following unilateral pallidotomy. Specifically, ratings of intelligibility were unchanged in 60% of patients, 33% demonstrated reduced intelligibility (usually mild), and 7% recorded mild improvements.

In summary, the current literature suggests that the effects of pallidotomy on motor speech function remain equivocal. Indeed, the current research has revealed that while pallidotomy results in consistent, significant improvements in nonspeech motor control (especially in the limbs), there are positive, neutral, and even negative outcomes recorded for speech. Clearly, there is a compelling case for further research that comprehensively examines the effects of pallidotomy on the motor speech mechanism of individuals with PD.

## Effect of Thalamotomy on Speech

Studies from the early stereotactic era reported that negative speech outcomes occurred in some individuals following thalamotomy. For example, several early studies noted the occurrence of postoperative impairments in respiratory support for speech, pitch, volume, and articulation following thalamotomy (Allan, Turner, & Gadea-Ciria, 1966; Bell, 1968; Canter & van Lancker, 1985; Jenkins, 1968; Petrovici, 1980; Samara et al., 1969). Moreover, several investigators suggested that unilateral thalamotomy in the PD individual's dominant hemisphere was more likely to produce negative speech changes than operations in the nondominant hemisphere (Allan et al., 1966; Jenkins, 1968).

In addition, investigations conducted in the early stereotactic era suggested that bilateral thalamotomy was more likely to result in negative speech outcomes than unilateral procedures (Allan et al., 1966; Matsumoto, Asano, Baba, Miyamoto, & Ohmoto, 1976; Selby, 1967). For example, Selby (1967) investigated 169 PD participants following thalamotomy and noted speech deterioration in 8.9% of participants following unilateral thalamotomy and in 23.8% of participants following bilateral thalamotomy. His study used nonspecific ratings, with speech impairments graded as absent, moderate, or severe; and postoperative speech was judged as improved, unchanged, or worse.

Interestingly, this investigator postulated that the presence of pre-operative speech impairments posed a higher risk for deleterious speech changes following bilateral thalamotomy.

Similar to the early stereotactic-era studies, more recent studies have reported speech deteriorations following contemporary bilateral thalamotomy (Countryman & Ramig, 1993; Tasker, DeCarvalho, Li, & Kestle, 1996). For example, a detailed case study indicated that no speech or voice deficits were present in a PD participant following a left thalamotomy; however, following a right-sided thalamotomy 4 years later, this participant showed a significant deterioration in speech and voice quality (Countryman & Ramig, 1993). Furthermore, Tasker et al. (1996) rated speech on a five-point perceptual scale and reported that 27% of the 43 PD participants experienced persistent worsening of dysarthria following bilateral thalamotomy. Interestingly, Tasker et al. (1996) noted that it was difficult to discern whether speech deterioration in some individuals resulted from thalamotomy or the progressive degenerative changes associated with PD.

In contrast to reports of deleterious speech change, several investigations of contemporary unilateral thalamotomy have suggested that speech remained largely unchanged in most PD participants following surgery (Fox, Ahlskog, & Kelly, 1991; Linhares & Tasker, 2000; Schuurman et al., 2000). For example, Fox et al. (1991) revealed that only 5% of 36 participants recorded persistent speech deterioration following left thalamotomy, whereas Schuurman et al. (2000) found only 14% of 34 participants demonstrated persistent speech change following unilateral thalamotomy. Furthermore, Linhares and Tasker (2000) reported neutral outcomes for speech and gait for 40 PD participants following thalamotomy.

Given that the majority of previous studies have used nonspecific speech rating scales, it is difficult to discern the exact nature of the speech changes that may or may not have occurred following thalamotomy. Clearly, there is a need for a more detailed examination of the effects of contemporary unilateral thalamotomy procedures on motor speech function in individuals with PD.

## Effect of Deep Brain Stimulation on Speech

Although the effects of DBS on the motor disturbances associated with PD have been well documented, there is a relative paucity of evidence detailing the effects of DBS on speech function in individuals with PD. Although effective in reducing nonspeech motor symptoms, this form of treatment has been reported to have no effect, minor improvements, or even a negative effect on speech (Frost, Tripoliti, Hariz, Pring, & Limousin, 2010; Klostermann et al., 2008; Tripoliti et al., 2008; Wang, Verhagen Metman, Bakay, Arzbaecher, & Bernard, 2003). To date, research has generally comprised single case and small group studies involving GPi and STN stimulation, and studies are equivocal as to the outcome for speech function. For example, wide variation in the effects of GPi stimulation on speech function was reported in a study of three PD participants with mild to moderate dysarthria (Solomon et al.,

2000). For example, GPi stimulation resulted in improved overall speech characteristics in one participant, while for another participant, marked hypophonia became apparent.

Other studies have reported that speech function was relatively unaffected following STN-DBS. In particular, a longitudinal study of 49 participants with advanced PD found that speech deficits appeared resistant to the effects of STN-DBS (Krack et al., 2003). Similarly, Bejjani et al. (2000) found that speech, swallowing, and neck rigidity were less likely to improve from STN stimulation than other axial signs. Benabid, Ni, Chabardes, Benazzouz, and Pollak (2001) postulated that the lack of change in voice deficits following STN-DBS was related to the location of stimulation targets. They speculated that stimulation targets made on the basis of limb symptoms may not be optimal for relieving orofacial deficits, and therefore, the correct target for speech might be located in another area.

In contrast to findings of no change in speech function, other studies have documented significant improvements in parameters of oral control and voice in participants with PD following STN stimulation (Gentil, Chauvin, Pinto, Pollak & Benabid, 2001; Gentil, Garcia-Ruiz, Pollak & Benabid, 1999; Gentil et al., 1999; Hoffman-Ruddy, Schulz, Vitek, & Evatt, 2001). Interestingly, Gentil et al. (1999) postulated that STN stimulation affected articulatory structures in an alternate manner to the dopaminergic pathways and hypothesized that articulatory system impairments may result mainly from non-dopaminergic lesions. Furthermore, Gentil, Pinto, Pollak, and Benabid (2003) reported that bilateral STN stimulation produced improvements in maximal force and reaction time of articulators as well as sustained vowel duration and fundamental frequency stability in a group of 16 participants with moderate dysarthria.

Additional studies have documented that, although changes occurred in a few speech parameters following DBS of the STN, these changes did not represent functional changes in speech function. In particular, Dromey, Kumar, Lang, and Lozano (2000) examined the effects of bilateral STN stimulation in 7 PD participants with mild–moderate dysarthria. Results revealed significant improvements in limb motor performance and small but significant increases in sound pressure level and fundamental frequency variability following bilateral STN stimulation. Overall, Dromey et al. (2000) concluded that speech measures did not change uniformly following DBS and that none of the speech changes were of a magnitude that would have a clinically relevant impact on functional communications.

Similarly, other studies have reported that bilateral STN-DBS did not result in clinically relevant speech changes (Santens, De Letter, Van Borsel, De Reuck, & Caemaert, 2003). Specifically, Santens et al. (2003) investigated the effects of left, right, and bilateral STN stimulation on perceptual ratings of prosody, articulation, speech intelligibility, voice quality, loudness, and speech rate. Results revealed no significant differences in participants' perceptual speech characteristics between ON and OFF bilateral STN stimulation conditions. Although there was no significant change in perceptual speech parameters following bilateral and right STN stimulation, left STN stimulation culminated in a significant deterioration in ratings of articulation, prosody, and speech intelligibility. Rousseaux, Krystkowiak, Kozlowski, Ozsancak, Blond, and Destée (2004) reported worsened speech following STN-DBS, particularly for spontaneous speech production.

As indicated above, stimulation parameters are often altered in STN-DBS to find optimal settings for the patient. Although increasing stimulation amplitude has been reported to provide better relief of motor symptoms in the limbs, simultaneously such an increase also leads to greater voice difficulties and reduced speech intelligibility (Krack, Fraix, Mendes, Benabid & Pollak, 2002; Tripoliti et al., 2008). Tornqvist, Schalen, and Rehncrona (2005) investigated the effects of different stimulation parameter settings on the intelligibility of speech in ten patients with bilateral STN-DBS. Under DBS ON and OFF conditions, five of the ten patients did not exhibit a change in intelligibility between the two conditions, while four exhibited decreased intelligibility while on stimulation. Increases in the amplitude and frequency of stimulation were reported to cause significant impairments in intelligibility.

Based on the above reports, it is apparent that STN-DBS can have a variable influence on speech function. Although the findings of a number of studies suggest that bilateral STN-DBS may be associated with improvements in speech on nonspeech oromotor measures, these benefits may not be clinically significant. Furthermore, negative speech changes with STN-DBS have also been reported. Given that negative side effects from STN-DBS may be controlled through adjustment of the parameters of stimulation, it has been suggested that negative speech changes associated with STN-DBS may be due to spread of electrical stimulation to the corticobulbar tracts in the internal capsule (Klostermann et al., 2008). More recently it has been demonstrated that dysarthria in STN-DBS is more likely to be caused by electrodes placed more medially in proximity to the anterior zona incerta (Åström et al., 2010; Tripoliti et al., 2011), and in the anterior zona incerta itself (Plaha, Ben-Shlomo, Patel, & Gill, 2006), the stimulation-induced dysarthria in these cases probably caused by the spread of the electrical stimulation to cerebellothalamic fibers in the area. It has been suggested that similar compromise of fibers passing into the ventral intermediate thalamus (VIM) may also be responsible for many cases of stimulation-induced dysarthria following VIM-DBS (Åström et al., 2010). Narayana et al. (2009) provided evidence that impaired speech production accompanying STN-DBS may result from unintended activation of the left dorsal premotor cortex.

Although the STN is the DBS target of choice for the treatment of motor symptoms in PD, a report by Plaha et al. (2006) indicated that stimulation of another target, the caudal zona incerta (cZi), may result in even better limb motor outcomes. The authors also reported that stimulation of this region avoided the speech deterioration often reported in association with STN-DBS suggesting that the caudal zona incerta be considered a promising target for DBS in terms of speech outcomes. Unfortunately, the findings of a recent study of seven participants with cZi-DBS suggest that cZi-DBS is more detrimental for extended articula-

tory movements than STN-DBS (Karlsson et al., 2011). More specifically the individuals with PD receiving cZi-DBS decreased in articulation rate in the stimulus ON condition and showed further reduction in their production quality. In a parallel study, Lundgren et al. (2011) reported that eight participants with PD fitted with cZi-DBS reported that vocal intensity decreased in the stimulator ON condition. Further studies based on larger participant numbers are required to further clarify the effects of cZi-DBS on speech; however, the early reports are not supportive of this target for DBS with regard to positive speech outcomes.

Overall there are several conclusions that can be drawn regarding the effects of neurosurgery procedures on speech in PD. First, surgery to any of the commonly utilized sites (VIM, GPi, STN) has greater therapeutic effects on limb than on bulbar performance, which raises questions regarding the relationships between speech and non-speech motor control in PD. In particular, the differential outcomes of neurosurgical procedures on limb, trunk, and orofacial systems suggests that distinct basal ganglia/neurotransmitter systems subserve limb, trunk, and orofacial control. Second, neurosurgical effects on speech are highly variable between patients. Third, the effects of neurosurgery on speech may vary at the individual patient level, with some aspects of speech showing deterioration while others remain unchanged. Finally, the best neuroanatomical site for surgery to relieve the symptoms of PD with the best outcome for speech has yet to be determined, although STN is currently the preferred surgical target.

## Implications of Speech Versus Limb Contrasts

Although the beneficial effects of pharmacologic and neurosurgical treatments for PD on general motor function are well documented, the effects of these procedures on speech motor control is far less consistent and beneficial. Based on the evidence available to date, it would appear that both pharmacologic (e.g., levodopa) and neurosurgical (e.g., STN-DBS) procedures do not always have the positive effects on speech production as seen in the muscles of other parts of the body such as the limbs. A number of possible explanations have been posed as the basis of these speech-versus-limb contrasts including neuroanatomic, neuropharmacologic, and research methodologic explanations. At a neuroanatomical level these differences may, at least in part, be the outcome of the segregated nature of the neuronal circuits that connect the cerebral cortex, basal ganglia, and thalamus with specific independent neural circuits subserving specific anatomic structures such as the orofacial structures versus the limb muscles (Alexander, Crutcher, & DeLong, 1990). Small inconsistencies in the site and volume of the lesions induced by stereotactic neurosurgery, therefore, could variably affect the functioning of the skeletal muscles in different regions of the body consistent with the case-to-case variability noted by several authors in their participants treated by neurosurgery.

From a neuropharmacologic perspective, another possible reason underlying the reported disparity between limb musculature and speech musculature is that subcortical modulation of the speech production muscles involves primarily nondopaminergic subcortical pathways (Agid, 1998; Steiger, Thompson, & Marsden, 1996). Among these pathways are neuronal systems originating in subcortical areas such as the cholinergic, serotoninergic, and noradrenergic systems. This suggestion is based on the observation that although treatment of PD with levodopa results in improvements in symptoms such as bradykinesia, rigidity, and tremors which arise from degradation of the nigrostriatal system, other symptoms, such as abnormal gait/postural instability, dysarthria, and cognitive impairment considered to be produced by non-dopaminergic systems, do not (Agid, 1998). This hypothesis is supported by the knowledge that the effect of levodopa therapy on speech production is less effective than on limb function in persons with PD (Kompoliti et al., 2000; Wolfe et al., 1975). Kompoliti et al. (2000) examined the effect of central dopaminergic stimulation with apomorphine on speech in individuals with PD and reported that no measure of laryngeal or articulatory function improved significantly after apomorphic stimulation. They concluded that laryngeal function and articulation are not under predominant dopaminergic control in PD, leading them to suggest that treatment for dysarthria in PD should focus on non-dopaminergic pharmacology and other therapies. Bonnet, Loria, Saint-Hilaire, Lhermitte, and Agid (1987) suggested that aggravation of PD following chronic levodopa therapy (e.g., increased involuntary abnormal movements, gait disorders, and dysarthria) mainly results from increasing severity of cerebral non-dopaminergic lesions.

Braak, Del Tredici, Rüb, de Vos, Jansen Steur, and Braak (2003) provided evidence in PD of an evolution of lewy body pathology starting in the lower brainstem and gradually evolving upwards to the mesencephalon. These findings may explain the presence of non-motor symptoms in many people with PD before motor signs arise as a consequence of degeneration of the substantia nigra in the mesencephalon. In support of this suggestion, vocal alterations have been reported in some pre-symptomatic persons with PD (Harel, Cannizzaro, & Snyder, 2004). There is evidence, therefore, that at least in some persons with PD, primary lewy body pathology and neurodegeneration in the brainstem instead of dopaminergic denervation may be responsible for disruption of some speech subsystems (Braak et al., 2003; Harel et al., 2004).

The variability in the results reported in studies that have investigated the effects of contemporary treatments for PD on speech, at least in part, may be the product of methodologic shortcomings in the research. For instance, participant-related differences across studies, such as varying age, gender, stage of disease, severity of dysarthria, time of assessment post-drug administration, time of day of assessment, as well as level of fatigue and anxiety, may all influence outcomes in PD making it difficult to compare results of one study with another (De Letter et al., 2010; Schulz & Grant, 2000). Furthermore, inter- and intraindividual variations in drug absorption rate are common leading to variations in clinical response during a drug cycle (Olanow, Gauger,

& Cedarbaum, 1991). Although most studies of the effects of levodopa on speech have utilized a standard protocol in which speech assessment is conducted approximately 1 hour post-drug administration and compared with the OFF medication state, this practice has been questioned (De Letter et al., 2010). As indicated earlier, long-term treatment with levodopa is complicated by ON and OFF fluctuations making predictions of these periods difficult in some cases; hence, studies based on standardized protocols may not be representative of an entire drug cycle. De Letter et al. (2010) concluded that individualized evaluation of speech during an entire drug cycle is warranted prior to initiation of a speech-language pathology program in advanced PD.

## References

Adelman, J. U., Hoel, R. L., & Lassman, M. E. (1970). The effect of L-DOPA treatment on speech of patients with Parkinson's disease. *Neurology, 20*, 410–411.

Agid, Y. (1998). Levodopa: Is toxicology a myth? *Neurology, 50*, 858–863.

Alexander, G. E., Crutcher, M. D., & DeLong, M. R. (1990). Basal ganglia-thalamocortical circuits: Parallel substrates for motor, oculomotor, prefrontal and limbic functions. *Progress in Brain Research, 85*, 119–146.

Allan, C. M., Turner, J. W., & Gadea-Ciria, M. (1966). Investigations into speech disturbances following stereotaxic surgery for parkinsonism. *British Journal of Disorders of Communication, 1*, 55–59.

Åström, M., Tripoliti, E., Hariz, M. I., Zrinzo, L. U., Martinez-Torres, I., Limousin, P., . . . Wårdell, K. (2010). Patient-specific model-based investigation of speech intelligibility and movement during deep brain stimulation. *Stereotactic and Functional Neurosurgery, 88,* 224–233.

Barlow, S. M., Iacono, R. P., Paseman, L. A., Biswas, A., & D'Antonio, L. (1998). The effects of postventral pallidotomy of force and speech aerodynamics in Parkinson's disease. In M. P. Cannito, K. M. Yorkston, & D. R. Beukelman (Eds.), *Neuromotor speech disorders* (pp. 117–156). Baltimore, MD: Paul H. Brookes.

Baron, M. S., Vitek, J. L., Bakay, R. A., Green, J., Kanoeke, Y., Hashimoto, T., . . . DeLong, M. R. (1996). Treatment of advanced Parkinson's disease by posterior GPi pallidotomy: One-year results of a pilot study. *Annals of Neurology, 40,* 335–366.

Bejjani, B. P., Gervais, D., Arnulf, I., Papadopoulos, S., Demeret, S., Bonnet, A. M., & Agid, Y. (2000). Axial parkinsonian symptoms can be improved: The role of levodopa and bilateral subthalamic stimulation. *Journal of Neurology, Neurosurgery and Psychiatry, 68,* 595–600.

Bell, D. S. (1968). Speech functions of the thalamus inferred from the effects of thalamotomy. *Brain, 91,* 619–638.

Benabid, A. L., Ni, Z., Chabardes, S., Benazzouz, A., & Pollak, P. (2001). How are we inhibiting functional targets with high frequency stimulation? In K. Kultas-Ilinsky & I. Ilinsky (Eds.), *Basal ganglia and thalamus in health and movement disorders* (pp. 309–315). New York, NY: Kluwer Academic/Plenum.

Benabid, A. L., Pollak, P., & Gross, C. (1994). Acute and long term effects of subthalamic nucleus stimulation in Parkinson's disease. *Stereotactic and Functional Neurosurgery, 62,* 76–84.

Blin, O., Ferrandez, A., Pailhous, J., & Serratrice, G. (1991). Dopa-sensitive and dopa-resistant gait parameters in Parkinson's disease. *Journal of Neurological Sciences, 103,* 51–54.

Bonnet, A. M., Loria, Y., Saint-Hilaire, M. H., Lhermitte, F., & Agid, Y. (1987). Does long term aggravation of Parkinson's disease result from non-dopaminergic lesions? *Neurology, 37,* 1539–1542.

Braak, H., Del Tredici, K., Rüb, U., de Vos, R. A., Jansen Steur, E. N., & Braak, E. (2003). Staging of brain pathology related to sporadic Parkinson's disease. *Neurobiological Aging, 24,* 197–211.

Cahill, L. M., Murdoch, B. E., Theodoros, D. G., Triggs, E. J., Charles, B. G., & Yao, A. A. (1998). Effect of oral levodopa treatment on articulatory function in Parkinson's disease: Preliminary results. *Motor Control, 2,* 161–172.

Caligiuri, M. P., & Abbs, J. H. (1986). *The influence of drug cycle on measures of labial kinematics in dysarthria associated with Parkinson's disease.* Paper presented at the Clinical Dysarthria Conference, Tucson, Arizona.

Canter, G. J., & van Lancker, D. (1985). Disturbances of the temporal organization of speech following bilateral thalamic surgery in a patient with Parkinson's disease. *Journal of Communication Disorders, 18,* 329–349.

Countryman, S., & Ramig, L. O. (1993). Effects of intensive voice therapy on voice deficits associated with bilateral thalamotomy in Parkinson's disease: A case study. *Journal of Medical Speech-Language Pathology, 1,* 233–250.

Critchley, E. (1981). Speech disorders of Parkinsonism: A review. *Journal of Neurology, Neurosurgery and Psychiatry, 44,* 751–758.

Daniels, N., Oates, J., Phyland, D., Feiglin, A., & Hughes, A. (1996). Vocal characteristics and response to levodopa in Parkinson's disease. *Movement Disorders, 11*(Suppl. 1), 117.

De Letter, M., Santens, P., De Bodt, M., Boon, P., & Van Borsel, J. (2006). Levodopa-induced alterations in speech rate in advanced Parkinson's disease. *Acta Neurologica Belgica, 106,* 19–26.

De Letter, M., Santens, P., De Bodt, M., Van Maele, G., Van Borsel, J., & Boon, P. (2007a). The effect of levodopa on respiration and word intelligibility in people with advanced Parkinson's disease. *Clinical Neurology and Neurosurgery, 109,* 495–500.

De Letter M., Santens, P., Estercam, I., Van Maele, G., De Bodt, M., Boon, P., & Van Borsel, J. (2007b). Levodopa-induced modifications of prosody and comprehensibility in advanced Parkinson's disease as perceived by professional listeners. *Clinical Linguistics and Phonetics, 21,* 783–791.

De Letter, M., Santens, P., & Van Borsel, J. (2003). The effects of levodopa on tongue strength and endurance in patients with Parkinson's disease. *Acta Neurologica Belgica, 103,* 35–38.

De Letter, M., Santens, P., & Van Borsel, J. (2005). The effects of levodopa on word intelligibility in Parkinson's disease. *Journal of Communication Disorders, 38,* 187–196.

De Letter, M., Van Borsel, J., Boon, P., De Bodt, M., Dhooge, I., & Santens, P. (2010). Sequential changes in motor speech across a levodopa cycle in advanced Parkinson's disease. *International Journal of Speech-Language Pathology, 12,* 405–413.

Djaldetti, R., & Melamed, E. (1998). Management of response fluctuations: Practical guidelines. *Neurology, 51*(Suppl. 2), S36–S40.

Dromey, C., Kumar, R., Lang, A. E., & Lozano, A. M. (2000). An investigation of the effects of subthalamic stimulation on acoustic measures of voice. *Movement Disorders, 15,* 1132–1138.

Fox, M. W., Ahlskog, J. E., & Kelly, P. J. (1991). Stereotactic ventrolateralis thalamotomy for medically refractory tremor in post-levodopa era Parkinson's disease patients. *Journal of Neurosurgery, 75,* 723–730.

Frost, E., Tripoliti, E., Hariz, M. I., Pring, T., & Limousin, P. (2010). Self-perception of speech changes in patients with Parkinson's disease following deep brain stimulation of the subthalamic nucleus. *International Journal of Speech-Language Pathology, 12,* 399–404.

Gardner, W. N., Langdon, N., & Parkes, J. D. (1987). Breathing in Parkinson's disease. *Advances in Neurology, 45,* 271–274.

Gentil, M., Chauvin, P., Pinto, S., Pollak, P., & Benabid, A. L. (2001). Effect of bilateral stimulation of the subthalamic nucleus on parkonsonian voice. *Brain and Language, 78,* 233–240.

Gentil, M., Garcia-Ruiz, P., Pollak, P., & Benabid, A. L. (1999). Effect of stimulation of the subthalamic nucleus on oral control of patients with parkinsonism. *Journal of Neurology, Neurosurgery and Psychiatry, 67,* 329–333.

Gentil, M., Pinto, S., Pollak, P., & Benabid, A. L. (2003). Effect of bilateral stimulation of the subthalamic nucleus on parkinsonian dysarthria. *Brain and Language, 85,* 190–196.

Gentil, M., Tournier, C-L., Pollak, P., & Benabid, A. L. (1999). Effect of bilateral subthalamic nucleus stimulation and dopatherapy on oral control in Parkinson's disease. *European Neurology, 42,* 136–140.

Ghika, J., Ghika-Schmid, F., Frankhauser, H., Assal, G., Vingerhoets, F., Albanese, A., . . . Favre, J. (1999). Bilateral contemporaneous posteroventral pallidotomy for the treatment of Parkinson's disease: Neuropsychological and neurological side effects. Report of four cases and review of the literature. *Journal of Neurosurgery, 91,* 313–321.

Goberman, A., & McMillan, J. (2005). Relative speech timing in Parkinson's disease. *Continuing Issues in Communication Science and Disorders, 2005,* 22–29.

Goetz, R. G., DeLong, M. R., Penn, R. D., & Bakay, R. A. (1993). Neurosurgical horizons in Parkinson's disease. *Neurology, 43,* 1–7.

Harel, B., Cannizzaro, M., & Snyder, P. J. (2004). Variability in fundamental frequency during speech in prodromal and incipient Parkinson's disease: A longitudinal case study. *Brain and Cognition, 56,* 24–29.

Ho, A. K., Bradshaw, J. L., & Iansek, R. (2008). For better or worse: The effect of levodopa on speech in Parkinson's disease. *Movement Disorders, 15,* 574–580.

Hoffman-Ruddy, B., Schulz, G., Vitek, J. L., & Evatt, M. (2001). A preliminary study of the effects of subthalamic nucleus (STN) deep brain stimulation (DBS) on voice and speech characteristics in Parkinson's disease. *Clinical Linguistics and Phonetics, 15,* 97–101.

Iacono, R. P., Shima, F., Lonser, R., Kuniyoshi, S., Maeda, G. S., & Yamada, S. (1995). The results, indications and physiology of posteroventral pallidotomy for patients with Parkinson's disease. *Neurosurgery, 36,* 1118–1125.

Jenkins, A. C. (1968). Speech defects following stereotaxic operations for the relief of tremor and rigidity in parkinsonism. *Medical Journal of Australia, 1,* 585–588.

Johansson, F., Malm, J., Nordh, E., & Hariz, M. (1997). Usefulness of pallidotomy in advanced Parkinson's disease. *Journal of Neurology, Neurosurgery and Psychiatry, 62,* 125–132.

Karlsson, F., Unger, E., Wahlgren, S., Blomstedt, P., Linder, J., Nordh, E., . . . van Doorn, J. (2011). Deep brain stimulation of caudal zona incerta and subthalamic nucleus in patients with Parkinson's disease: Effects on diadochokinetic rate. *Parkinsons Disease, Volume 2011,* Article ID60560.

Kelly, P. (1995). Pallidotomy in Parkinson's disease. *Neurology, 36,* 1154–1157.

Klostermann, F., Ehlen, F., Vesper, J., Nubel, K., Grosse, M., Marzinzik, F., . . . Sappok, T. (2008). Effects of subthalamic deep brain stimulation on dysarthrophonia in Parkinson's disease. *Journal of Neurology, Neurosurgery and Psychiatry, 79,* 522–529.

Kompoliti, K., Wang, Q. E., Goetz, C. G., Leurgans, S., & Raman, R. (2000). Effects of central dopaminergic stimulation by apomorphine on speech in Parkinson's disease. *Neurology, 25,* 458–462.

Krack, P., Fraix, V., Mendes, A., Benabid, A. L., & Pollak, P. (2002). Postoperative management of subthalamic nucleus stimulation for Parkinson's disease. *Movement Disorders, 17*(Suppl. 3), S188–S197.

Kumar, R., Lozano, A. M., Montgomery, E., & Lang, A. E. (1998). Pallidotomy and deep brain stimulation of the pallidum and subthalamic nucleus in advanced Parkinson's disease. *Movement Disorders, 13*(Suppl. 1), 73–82.

Laitinen, L. V., Bergenheim, A. T., & Hariz, M. I. (1992). Ventroposterolateral pallidotomy can abolish all parkinsonian symptoms. *Stereotactic Functional Neurosurgery, 58,* 14–21.

Lang, A. E., Lozano, A. M., Montgomery, E., Duff, J., Tasker, R., & Hutchinson, W. (1997). Posteroventral medial pallidotomy in advanced Parkinson's disease. *New England Journal of Medicine, 337,* 1036–1042.

Larson, K., Ramig, L., & Scherer, R. (1994). Acoustic and glottographic voice analysis during drug related fluctuations in Parkinson's disease. *Journal of Medical Speech-Language Pathology, 2,* 227–239.

Leanderson, R., Meyerson, B. A., & Persson, A. (1971). Effect of L-dopa on speech in parkinsonism: An EMG study of labial articulatory function. *Journal of Neurology, Neurosurgery and Psychiatry, 34,* 679–681.

Legg, C. F., & Sonnenberg, B. R. (1998). Changes in aspects of speech and language functioning following unilateral pallidotomy. *Aphasiology, 12,* 235–266.

Linhares, M. N., & Tasker, R. R. (2000). Micro-electrode guided thalamotomy for Parkinson's disease. *Neurosurgery, 46,* 390–395.

Louis, E. D., Winfield, L., Fahn, S., & Ford, B. (2001). Speech dysfluency exacerbated by levodopa in Parkinson's disease. *Movement Disorders, 16,* 562–565.

Lozano, A. M., Lang, A. E., Galvez-Jimenez, N., Miyasaki, J., Duff, J., Hutchinson, W. D., & Dostrovksy, J. O. (1995). Effect of GPi pallidotomy on motor function in Parkinson's disease. *Lancet, 346,* 1383–1387.

Lundgren, S., Saeys, T., Karlsson, F., Olofsson, K., Blomstedt, P., Linder, J., . . . Van Doorn, J. (2011). Deep brain stimulation of caudal zona incerta and subthalamic nucleus in patients with Parkinson's disease: Effects on voice intensity. *Parkinson's Disease, Volume 2011,* Article ID658956.

Matsumoto, K., Asano, T., Baba, T., Miyamoto, T., & Ohmoto, T. (1976). Long-term follow-up results of bilateral thalamotomy for parkinsonism. *Applied Neurophysiology, 39,* 257–260.

Mawdsley, C., & Gamsu, C. V. (1971). Periodicity of speech in Parkinson's. *Nature, 231,* 315–316.

Murdoch, B. E., Chenery, H. J., Bowler, S., & Ingram, J. C. (1989). Respiratory function in Parkinson's subjects exhibiting a perceptible speech deficit: A kinematic and spirometric analysis. *Journal of Speech and Hearing Disorders, 54,* 610–626.

Nakano, K. K., Zubick, H., & Tyler, H. R. (1973). Speech defects of parkinsonian patients: Effects of levodopa therapy on speech intelligibility. *Neurology, 23,* 865–870.

Narayana, S., Jacks, A., Robin, D. A., Poizner, H., Zhang, W., Franklin, C., . . . Fox, P. T. (2009). A noninvasive imaging approach to understanding speech changes following deep brain stimulation in Parkinson's disease. *American Journal of Speech-Language Pathology, 18,* 146–161.

Olanow, C. W., Gauger, L. L., & Cedarbaum, J. M. (1991). Temporal relationships between plasma and cerebrospinal fluid pharmacokinetics of levodopa and clinical effect in Parkinson's disease. *Annals of Neurology, 29,* 556–559.

O'Sullivan, J., Said, C., Dillon, L., Hoffman, M., & Hughes, A. (1998). Gait analysis in patients with Parkinson's disease and motor fluctuations: Influence of levodopa and comparison with other measures of motor function. *Movement Disorders, 13,* 900–906.

Petrovici, J. N. (1980). Speech disturbances following stereotaxic surgery in ventrolateral thalamus. *Neurosurgical Review, 3,* 189–195.

Plaha, P., Ben-Shlomo, Y., Patel, N. K., & Gill, S. S. (2006). Stimulation of the caudal zona incerta is superior to stimulation of the subthalamic nucleus in improving contralateral parkinsonism. *Brain, 129,* 1732–1747.

Poluha, P. C., Teulings, H. L., & Brookshire, R. H. (1998). Handwriting and speech changes across the levodopa cycle in Parkinson's disease. *Acta Psychologia, 100,* 71–84.

Rice, J. E., Antic, R., & Thompson, P. D. (2002). Disordered respiration as a levodopa-induced dyskinesia in Parkinson's disease. *Movement Disorders, 17,* 524–527.

Rigrodsky, S., & Morrison, E. B. (1970). Speech changes in parkinsonism during L-dopa therapy: Preliminary findings. *Journal of the American Geriatrics Society, 18,* 142–151.

Rousseaux, M., Krystkowiak, P., Kozlowski, O., Ozsancak, C., Blond, S., & Destée, A. (2004). Effects of subthalamic nucleus stimulation on parkinsonian dysarthria and speech intelligibility. *Journal of Neurology, 251,* 327–334.

Samara, K., Riklan, M., Levita, E., Zimmerman, J., Waltz, J., Bergmann, L., & Cooper, I. S. (1969). Language and speech correlates of anatomically verified lesions in thalamic surgery for parkinsonism. *Journal of Speech and Hearing Research, 12,* 510–540.

Samuel, M., Caputo, E., Brooks, D. J., Schrag, A., Scaravilli, T., Branston, N. M., . . . Quinn, N. P. (1998). A study of medial pallidotomy for Parkinson's disease: Clinical outcome, MRI location and complications. *Brain, 121,* 59–75.

Sanabria, J., Ruiz, P. G., Gutierrez, R., Marquez, F., Escobar, P., Gentil, M., & Cenjor, C. (2001). The effect of levodopa on vocal function in Parkinson's disease. *Clinical Neuropharmacology, 24,* 99–102.

Santens, P., De Letter, M., Van Borsel, J., De Reuck, J., & Caemaert, J. (2003). Lateralized effects of subthalamic nucleus stimulation on different aspects of speech in Parkinson's disease. *Brain and Language, 87,* 253–258.

Schneider, S. L., Duffy, J. R., & Uitti, R. J. (1999). *Motor speech changes following pallidotomy in patients with Parkinson's disease.* Paper presented at the American Speech-Language-Hearing Association Annual Convention, San Francisco, CA.

Schrag, A., Samuel, M., Caputo, E., Scaravilli, T., Troyer, N., Marsden, C. D., . . . Quinn, N. P. (1999). Unilateral pallidotomy for Parkinson's disease: Results after more than 1 year. *Journal of Neurology, Neurosurgery and Psychiatry, 67,* 511–517.

Schulz, G. M., & Grant, M. K. (2000). Effects of speech therapy and pharmacologic and surgical treatments on voice and speech in Parkinson's disease: A review of the literature. *Journal of Communication Disorders, 33,* 59–88.

Schulz, G. M., Greer, M., & Friedman, W. (2000). Changes in vocal intensity in Parkinson's disease following pallidotomy surgery. *Journal of Voice, 14,* 589–606.

Schulz, G. M., Peterson, T., Sapienza, C. M., Greer, M., & Friedman, W. (1999). Voice and speech characteristics of persons with Parkinson's disease pre- and post-pallidotomy surgery: Preliminary findings. *Journal of Speech, Language, and Hearing Research, 42,* 1176–1194.

Schuurman, P. R., Bosch, D. A., Bossuyt, P. M., Bonsel, G. J., van Someren, E. J., de Bie, R. M., . . . Speelman, J. D. (2000). A comparison of continuous thalamic stimulation and thalamotomy for suppression of severe tremor. *New England Journal of Medicine, 342,* 461–468.

Scott, R., Gregory, R., Hines, N., Carroll, C., Hyman, N., Papanasstasiou, V., . . . Aziz, T. (1998). Neuropsychological, neurological and functional outcome following pallidotomy for Parkinson's disease: A consecutive series of eight simultaneous bilateral and twelve unilateral procedures. *Brain, 121,* 659–675.

Selby, G. (1967). Stereotactic surgery for the relief of Parkinson's disease: A critical review. *Journal of the Neurological Sciences, 5,* 315–342.

Solomon, N. P., & Hixon, T. J. (1993). Speech breathing in Parkinson's disease. *Journal of Speech and Hearing Research, 36,* 294–310.

Solomon, N. P., McKee, A. S., Larson, K. J., Nawrocki, M. D., Tuite, P., Eriksen, S., & Low, W. C. (2000). Effects of pallidal stimulation on speech in three men with Parkinson's disease. *American Journal of Speech-Language Pathology, 9,* 241–256.

Solomon, N. P., Robin, D., & Luschei, E. S. (2000). Strength, endurance, and stability of the tongue and hand in Parkinson's disease. *Journal of Speech, Language, and Hearing Research, 43,* 256–267.

Steiger, M. J., Thompson, P. D., & Marsden, C. D. (1996). Disordered axial movement in Parkinson's disease. *Journal of Neurology, Neurosurgery and Psychiatry, 61,* 645–648.

Tasker, R. R., DeCarvalho, G. C., Li, C. S., & Kestle, J. R. (1996). Does thalamotomy alter the course of Parkinson's disease? *Advances in Neurology, 69,* 563–583.

Theodoros, D. G., Ward, E. C., Murdoch, B. E., Silburn, P., & Lethlean, J. (2000). The impact of pallidotomy motor speech function in Parkinson's disease. *Journal of Medical Speech-Language Pathology, 8,* 315–322.

Tornqvist, A. L., Schalen, L., & Rehncrona, S. (2005). Effects of different electrical parameter settings on the intelligibility of speech in patients with Parkinson's disease treated with subthalamic deep brain stimulation. *Movement Disorders, 20,* 416–423.

Tripoliti, E., Zrinzo, L., Martinez-Torres, I., Frost, E., Pinto, S., Foltynie, T., . . . Limousin, P. (2011). Effects of subthalamic stimulation on speech of consecutive patients with Parkinson's disease. *Neurology, 76,* 80–86.

Tripoliti, E., Zrinzo, L., Martinez-Torres, I., Tisch, S., Frost, E., Borrell, E., . . . Limousin, P. (2008). Effects of contact location and voltage amplitude on speech and movement in bilateral subthalamic nucleus deep brain stimulation. *Movement Disorders, 23,* 2377–2383.

Uitti, R. J., Wharen, R. E., Duffy, J. R., Lucas, J. A., Schneider, S. L., Rippeth, J. D., . . . Atkinson, E. J. (2000). Unilateral pallidotomy for Parkinson's disease: Speech, motor and neuropsychological outcome measurements. *Parkinsonism and Related Disorders, 6,* 133–143.

Wang, E., Verhagen Metman, L., Bakay, R., Arzbaecher, J., & Bernard, B. (2003). The effect of unilateral electrostimulation of the subthalamic nucleus on respiratory/ phonatory subsystems of speech production in Parkinson's disease: A preliminary report. *Clinical Linguistics and Phonetics, 17,* 283–289.

Wolfe, V. I., Garvin, J. S., Bacon, M., & Waldrop, W. (1975). Speech changes in Parkinson's disease during treatment with L-dopa. *Journal of Communication Disorders, 8,* 271–279.

Yorkston, K. M., & Beukelman, D. R. (1980). Assessment of intelligibility of dysarthric speech. *Journal of Communication Disorders, 13,* 15–31.

# 5

# Course of the Diseases

*BRUCE E. MURDOCH*

## Introduction

The clinical course of any disease has important implications for its management. Whether a patient is expected, as part of the disease course, to show gradual or rapid exacerbation of their clinical signs and symptoms, or a degree of recovery over time, has important ramifications for determining the type, quantity, and frequency of therapy and for the monitoring and interpretation of treatment outcomes. Although the majority of movement disorders presenting in the clinical caseload of speech-language pathologists represent progressive degenerative conditions, there are exceptions. While many movement disorders show a progressive increase in the patient's level of disability, in some movement disorders there is a tendency for initial signs and symptoms to decrease with age. For example, in Tourette syn-

drome (TS) a number of clinical signs and symptoms, such as tics, evident in childhood tend to resolve and decrease after adolescence. In other movement disorders, although initial signs and symptoms may somewhat resolve with time, they are replaced by an equally disabling set of other negative features. For example, in Huntington chorea (HC), the initial chorea may decline with time to be replaced by rigidity, dystonia, and parkinsonism.

Even within the same movement disorder syndrome, considerable individual variation in clinical course can be observed with a number of factors (e.g., age at diagnosis, initial presenting symptoms, etc.) apparently influencing the progress of the disease and prognosis. Furthermore, progress of the disease within any one individual may not be smooth and even with periods of slow progressive decline interrupted by exacerbations during which marked progression of symptoms occurs. Finally, in some diseases the clinical course of the disorder may be complicated by the addition of therapy-induced symptoms to their clinical profiles. For example, in Parkinson disease (PD) the clinical symptoms and progress of the disorder is regularly complicated by the appearance of levodopa-induced motor complications and neuropsychiatric disturbances. While it is not possible within the scope of the present chapter to examine the clinical course of all movement disorders, a description of the clinical course of the major movement disorders associated with the occurrence of motor speech and/or language disturbances is provided, including PD, HC, TS, and dystonia.

## Clinical Course of Parkinson Disease

Akinesia is the defining, obligatory, and principal disabling feature of PD. It is a symptom complex, comprising slowness of movement (bradykinesia), poverty of movement and small amplitude of movements (hypokinesia), difficulty initiating movement or with simultaneous motor acts, and, most specifically, fatiguing and decrementing amplitude of repetitive alternating movements. Almost all individuals with PD also display muscular rigidity to passive movement across a joint. Tremor is an optional extra for PD, although up to 80% of patients with PD display tremor at some stage. This is usually in the form of a 4- to 6-Hz rest tremor which lessens with movement to reappear after an interval when a new position of rest is achieved.

PD often begins insidiously, and most patients have difficulty deter-mining the date of the onset of their symptoms. Loss of dexterity for skilled movements or mild stiffness in one hand may precede the onset of noticeable tremor by many years. Patients often accept a decrease in their ability to carry out specific fine movements, a slowly progressive change in the gait, or a mild degree of fatigue in one or both arms or legs without seeking medical attention. Early, but often over-looked, manifestations of PD include: a slight loss in motor dexterity, unilateral fatigue or awkwardness, loss of usual vitality in facial expression, generalized slight slowness in otherwise rapidly executed tasks (e.g., shaving, dressing), and a slight reduction in overall motor activity.

PD is progressive in virtually all patients, although the degree and rate of progression varies from patient to patient. The better known classic symptoms of PD listed above appear as the disease progresses. Most patients are able to accurately date the appearance of tremor. As the disease progresses a fourth "cardinal" sign of PD usually appears, namely postural abnormality. Although it may or may not be evident early in the disease course, postural abnormality is typically a late feature in PD and involves the adoption of a flexed posture. In the erect position, the trunk is bent forward at both the lumbar and cervical spine. The arms are adducted, flexed at the elbows, and brought together in front so that the hands come closer to each other at about the level of the umbilicus. Dorsal kyphosis is common, and there is adduction of the legs with some flexion at the knees so that the patient develops a simian posture. Gait in the mid-stages of PD is frequently slow, being made up of small shuffling steps. When combined with a flexed posture the resulting "festinating" gait makes the patient appear as if he or she is trying to catch up with his or her center of gravity. As the disease progresses, there is often progressive difficulty with balance, so that some patients cannot stand by themselves. Patients with marked akinesia often walk with progressively smaller steps and may freeze after only a few steps. They are able to start moving only after a delay of several minutes only to freeze again after a few steps.

During the course of the disease a number of other manifestations are also evident. It has been estimated that around 90% of individuals with PD develop a speech disorder in the form of a hypokinetic dysarthria. (The clinical characteristics of hypokinetic dysarthria are described in Chapter 7.) Disordered speech may occur in the early stage of PD or as a late feature of the condition. There is even some evidence based on acoustic analysis to suggest that alterations in vocal function may precede the usual clinical manifestations and diagnosis of PD in some cases. As the disease progresses, the severity of the associated hypokinetic dysarthria also increases leading to increasing levels of phonatory and articulatory dysfunction with increasing compromise of associated prosodic aspects of the patient's speech. More specifically, speech becomes monotonous with decreased use of all vocal parameters for effecting stress and emphasis. Speech intensity decreases as does precision of articulation of consonants leading to a concomitant decrease in speech intelligibility. The patient's voice may stop in the middle of a sentence similar to the freezing phenomena seen in activities such as walking and there may be difficulty

in initiating speech production. In the late stages of PD the individual may no longer be able to use vocalization for communication.

In addition to speech, handwriting is often markedly affected. Early in the disease it is often shaky and tremulous and either small throughout or becomes progressively smaller as the patient continues to write. Letters at the beginning of a word may be normal size but decrease in size with each successive letter. Simultaneously, the speed of writing also slows and appears to require greater effort on the part of the patient. After many years, the end stage of PD is characterized by progressive tremor, rigidity, akinesia, and difficulty with postural reactions. These reactions result in the patient becoming chair- or bedridden and unable to care for themselves.

Hoehn and Yahr (1967) developed a nonlinear scale that is widely used clinically to describe the stages in the clinical course of PD. According to this scale, unilateral PD (stage 1), always progresses through stage 2 (bilateral PD), which typically lasts 5 to 10 years, until postural instability (stage 3) appears. Over time, fully developed disease (stage 4) evolves, and after many years the patient may eventually become chair—or even bedridden (stage 5); however, this progression is influenced by treatment, so that a patient on chronic levodopa treatment may fluctuate between stages 4 or even 5 when "OFF," to stage 2 or 3 when "ON." In addition, a range of other factors also appear to influence the clinical course of PD including age at diagnosis and initial symptoms, among others.

Analysis of a cohort of 800 patients with PD has identified two major subtypes: one characterized by tremor as the dominant parkinsonian feature and the second dominated by postural instability and gait disorder (PIGD). The tremor-dominant form of PD appears to be associated with a relatively preserved mental status, earlier age of onset, and a slower rate of progression and better prognosis than the PIGD subtype. The latter subtype, in contrast, is characterized by more severe bradykinesia, dementia, and a relatively rapid progressive course. The clinical course of PD appears to be influenced not only by the age of onset and the clinical presentation but also by a number of other factors including stress, pregnancy, intercurrent illness, and therapy. Furthermore, there is growing evidence that the rate of progression of PD is not linear over time, being more rapid initially and slowing in more advanced stages of the disease (Jankovic, 2005; Schapira & Obeso, 2006). Although therapeutic advances in the form of levodopa therapy and neurosurgical procedures (e.g., deep brain stimulation) have had a positive impact on quality of life in PD, epidemiologic studies have not been able to demonstrate that these procedures significantly prolong life. Several studies, however, have concluded that patients with PD have a nearly normal life expectancy (Parkinson Study Group, 1998).

### Clinical Course of Tourette Syndrome

Tourette syndrome (TS) is a distinctive disease of childhood and is the most common cause of tics. The cause of the condition is unknown, but the disorder appears to be inherited in the majority of cases. The diagnostic criteria for TS are complex and reflect the marked fluctuation in symptoms and severity observed in any one case over the clinical course of the disease. According to the diagnostic criteria for definite TS formulated by the Tourette Syndrome Classification Study Group (1993) the following features must be present: (1) both multiple motor and one or more vocal/phonic tics have to be present at some time during the illness, although not necessarily concurrently; (2) tics must occur many times a day, nearly every day, or intermittently throughout a period of more than 1 year; (3) the anatomic location, number, frequency, type, complexity, or severity of tics must change over time; (4) onset must be before age 21 years; (5) involuntary movements (motor tics) and noises (vocal/phonic tics) cannot be explained by other medical conditions; and (6) motor and/or phonic tics must be directly witnessed by a reliable examiner at some point during the illness or must be recorded by videotape or cinematography. These criteria are clearly reflective of the fact that the clinical course of TS changes regularly and considerably over time.

The onset of TS is usually heralded by simple tics involving the eyes. Indeed, in around 36 to 48% of patients, the initial symptom is eye blinking, followed by tics involving the face and head. Blink rate in TS is about double that of normal age-matched controls. During the course of the disease, nearly all cases exhibit tics involving the face or head, two-thirds have tics in the arms, and half have tics involving the trunk or legs. The average age at onset of tics is about 5.6 years. Tics usually become most severe at around age 10 to 12 years and by 18 years of age, half of the patients are tic free. It has been reported that even though tic disability and tic severity improves significantly after age 18 years, that in up to 90% of cases tics persist into adult life even though the patients themselves often consider themselves to be tic free.

Involuntary sounds (phonic tics) have been reported to be the initial symptom of TS in 12 to 37% of patients, throat clearing being the most common. Phonic tics (e.g., sniffing, snorting, etc.) and vocal tics (e.g., barking, making animal noises, etc.) can be quite troublesome and embarrassing for patients and those around them. Coprolalia, one of the most distressing and recognizable symptoms of TS, along with echolalia and palilalia, actually only occurs in less than half the cases. In addition to motor and vocal/phonic tics, patients with TS also exhibit a variety of behavioral symptoms, particularly obsessive-compulsive disorder (OCD) and attention deficit hyperactivity disorder (ADHD). The peak in OCD severity has been reported to occur 2 years after peak tic severity. Consequently, it is important to counsel parents about the possibility of OCD development in children who have recently been diagnosed with TS.

Although the long-term prognosis for TS is generally favorable for most patients, a minority of cases may exhibit persistent severe tic symptoms that may be resistant to medications. By far the majority of tics exhibited by adults represent recurrences of childhood-onset tics. Only in very rare cases do patients have their first tic occurrence during adulthood. In these latter cases it is important to rule out secondary causes such as infection, trauma, stroke, neuroleptic exposure, cocaine use, and peripheral nerve injury. In those cases where adult-onset tics do occur, evidence is available to suggest that compared with typical childhood-onset tics, the former type is associated with more severe symptoms, greater social morbidity, and less favorable response to medications. (See Chapter 10 for medical treatment of TS.)

## Clinical Course of Huntington Chorea

Huntington chorea (HC) is a slowly progressive autosomal-dominant neurodegenerative disorder that is manifest by progressive chorea, or at times other extrapyramidal symptoms, as well as progressive intellectual deterioration. Onset can occur at any time, but the disorder usually manifests in the fourth or fifth decade of life. The average age at onset is around 40 years. About 10% of HC cases have their onset before the age of 20 years. Whereas hyperkinesia, usually in the form of chorea, is typically present in adult-onset HC, parkinsonism (an akinetic-rigid syndrome) is characteristic of juvenile HC (onset less than 20 years of age). Juvenile HC typically presents with a combination of progressive parkinsonism, dementia, ataxia, and seizures. In contrast, adult HC usually presents with an insidious onset of clumsiness and choreic movements.

The clinical course of HC varies. As the disease progresses the signs and symptoms change, so disease duration can markedly modify the clinical presentation. Progress of the disease is inexorable, with death occurring 15 to 20 years from onset for the adult HC and about 4 to 5 years for the juvenile variant. The onset of HC is often difficult to discern clearly. Many patients report psychiatric problems or mild cognitive symptoms before developing any motor problems, although this is not always the case; however, definitive diagnosis of HC with the appearance of motor impairments. Subtle motor abnormalities seen early in the disease include general restlessness, abnormal eye movements, hyper-reflexia, impaired finger tapping, and fidgety movements of the fingers, hands, and toes during stress or when walking. Oculomotor abnormalities are a cardinal sign of the disorder and often the earliest motor sign. As the disease progresses obvious extrapyramidal signs develop and the chorea becomes more and more striking. Eventually all the patient's musculature is involved. The full-blown clinical picture includes not only facial grimacing (involving lips, tongue, and cheeks) but also jerks of the head, weaving movements of the arms and shoulders, twists and jerks of the body, as well as superimposed voluntary movements. An upward jerk of the arm may be fused into voluntary scratching of the head. The patient is virtually a stage on which numerous uncoordinated muscle movements take place. The patient's gait is often markedly involved and comprises jerky, lurching steps that are a combination of voluntary and involuntary movements. Muscular strength is unimpaired and the ability to initiate movements is intact, but the carrying out of a continuous movement is frequently impeded by superimposed jerks that result in a severe and distressing form of unco-ordination. Dysarthria in the form of a hyperkinetic dysarthria (see Chapter 7) and dysphagia are common features of more advanced HC. Indeed, aspiration pneumonia resulting from dysphagia is often the immediate cause of death of patients with HC. Although chorea dominates the clinical picture in the early and middle stages of adult HC with around 90% of cases showing choreic movements at these times, the late stage of adult HC is often dominated by dystonia, rigidity, and parkinsonism.

Progressive intellectual deterioration is another cardinal feature of HC. The patient often becomes irritable, more excitable, begins to lose his or her temper more easily, and develops other subtle personality changes. Progressive indifference resulting in severe apathy may occur. Inattention or decrease in the ability to concentrate is often noted by the patient or their associates. Judgment, comprehension, and memory become affected until the patient is ultimately demented. The psychiatric manifestations are at times quite prominent, with instances of manic-depressive or schizophrenic reaction having been reported. Although these manifestations are unusual, less marked alteration of personality, including paranoid ideation and impulsive behavior, are most frequent.

In addition to motor, cognitive, and behavioral abnormalities, most patients with HC lose weight during the course of their disease, despite increased appetite. The pathogenesis of weight loss in HC is unknown. The usual end state is one of progressive motor dysfunction, dementia, dysarthria, dysphagia, and incontinence eventually leading to institutionalization and death from aspiration, infection, and poor nutrition.

## Clinical Course of Dystonia

Dystonia is a heterogeneous movement disorder characterized by relatively slow and long-sustained involuntary muscle contractions frequently causing twisting and repetitive movements or abnormal postures. Both agonist and antagonist muscles contract simultaneously to cause the dystonic movements. The movements may be intermittent or sustained, rapid or slow, rhythmic or unpatterned, tremulous or jerky. Dystonic movements sometimes increase during attempted purposeful activities, nervousness, and emotional stress. They may also be task specific. Contorting, nonpatterned and powerful dystonic movements involve both axial and appendicular musculature and commonly are more proximal than distal. The disruption of the dystonic movements can be generalized (usually involving both legs and at least one other part), segmental (involving two or more contiguous body parts), multifocal (involving two or more noncontiguous body parts), or focal (involving a single body part). Focal dystonia is the most common form of dystonia.

Although dystonia can be classified in various different ways, clinically the most important and useful division is classifying patients into two categories: those with "primary dystonia" and those with "secondary/heredodegenerative dystonia."

## Primary Dystonia

Dystonia is the only clinical sign (with the exception of tremor) in primary dystonia, and there is no symptomatic cause or neurodegeneration. Primary dystonia almost always begins by affecting a single body part (i.e., focal dystonia). In most cases, dystonia remains as a focal dystonia without spreading to other parts of the body; however, within that single body part multiple muscles can be affected. For example, in patients with dystonia of the neck (cervical dystonia or torticollis), a combination of muscles is involved. In a sizable minority of patients, dystonia that starts in one part of the body can spread to other parts of the body. Most often, the spread is to contiguous body parts; hence, the spread is usually from focal to segmental dystonia. Age at onset appears to be very important in determining the clinical phenotype of patients with primary dystonia. As a general rule, the younger the age of onset, the more likely it is that the dystonia will spread. Young-onset dystonia (before the age of 28 years) most commonly manifests with limb-onset dystonia (usually involving one leg), followed by subsequent generalization, and was referred to in the older literature as dystonia musculorum deformans (DMD) or Oppenheim's dystonia. It is now known that about 70% of patients presenting in this way carry a single GAG deletion in the DYT1 gene on chromosome 9. It has an autosomal-dominant inheritance but a very low phenotypic penetrance such that only 30 to 40% of gene carriers ever develop dystonia, and in those who do this almost always happens before the age of 30 years. Greater than 90% of children who develop dystonia in the legs develop generalized dystonia within 10 years. As another general rule, primary dystonias are affected by age at onset with a caudal-to-rostral change in the site of onset as a function of age (O'Riordan et al., 2004).

Dystonia appearing in adult life is characterized by a focal or segmented distribution and the condition does not generalize. Examples of adult-onset dystonia in order of frequency of occurrence include cervical dystonia (spasmodic torticollis), cranial dystonia (e.g., blepharospasm, Meige syndrome), writer's cramp, laryngeal dystonia (spasmodic dysphonia), and other task-specific dystonias (e.g., musician's cramp). Adult-onset focal dystonias are sporadic in most cases and have a different etiology to early-onset DYT1 gene-related dystonia with this gene having been excluded in these disorders.

Primary dystonia commonly begins with a specific-action dystonia, that is, the abnormal movements appear in combination with a special action (i.e., a task-specific action) and are not presented at rest, in contrast to secondary dystonias, which are much more likely to begin with dystonia at rest. For example, a child who develops primary dystonia might have the initial symptom in one leg but only when walking forward. It could be absent when the child runs or walks backward. Other common examples are the task-specific dystonias that are seen with writing (writer's cramp), playing a musical instrument (musician's cramp), chewing, and speaking. Often, these task-specific dystonias produce occupational disability (e.g., musicians unable to play their instrument professionally). As the dystonic condition progresses, less specific voluntary motor actions of the involved limb can bring out the dystonic movements. For example, the affected leg of the child in the previous example might also activate the dystonia when it is tapping the floor. With further evolution, actions in other parts of the body can also induce dystonic movements of the involved leg, so-called overflow. Talking is the most common mechanism for causing overflow dystonia in other body parts. With still further worsening of the condition the affected limb can develop dystonic movements while it is at rest and eventually the leg may exhibit sustained postural abnormalities; thus, dystonia at rest is usually a more severe form of the condition than pure action dystonia. Much less common than action dystonia or overflow dystonia is the reverse phenomenon, that is, for dystonia at rest to be improved by talking or other voluntary active movements, so-called paradoxical dystonia. The focal dystonia that is most frequently decreased by voluntary motor activity is blepharospasm with about 60% of patients with blepharospasm obtaining some degree of relief when talking.

Patients with dystonia usually exhibit dystonic movements continually throughout the day whenever the affected body part is in use and, as a sign of greater severity, also when the body part is at rest. Dystonic movements tend to increase with fatigue, stress, and emotional states. They tend to be suppressed with relaxation, hypnosis, and sleep. Unless it is extremely severe, dystonia often disappears with deep sleep. An interesting and almost unique feature of dystonic movements is that they can often be diminished by tactile or proprioceptive "sensory tricks"; thus, touching the involved body part or an adjacent body part can often reduce the muscle contractions.

For example, patients with spasmodic torticollis often place a hand on the chin or side of the face to reduce nuchal contractions, and orolingual dystonia is often helped by touching the lips or placing an object in the mouth.

With the exception of spasmodic torticollis, pain is uncommon in dystonia. Approximately 75% of patients with spasmodic torticollis experience pain that appears to result from muscle contraction as it is relieved by botulinum toxin injection. Dystonia in most parts of the body, however, is rarely accompanied by pain.

## Secondary and Heredodegenerative Dystonias

The secondary dystonias are subdivided into several categories: those that are due to environmental causes and those associated with heredodegenerative diseases. Dystonias occurring secondary to environmental causes are usually due to structural brain damage that affects the basal ganglia, such as occurs in traumatic brain injury, stroke, or perinatal conditions. The leading cause of secondary dystonia occurring in the first year of life is cerebral palsy or a metabolic error such as glutaric aciduria. A number of cases of symptomatic dystonias, so-called delayed-onset dystonias, appear months to years after cerebral insult. Often, such a delayed onset is seen with perinatal or early childhood asphyxia but can also be seen following stroke, traumatic head injury, and a large variety of other static brain lesions.

Dystonia is also a feature of a wide range of heredodegenerative condi-tions. Of all the causes of heredodegenerative dystonia, Wilson disease is the most important. It is an autosomal-recessive disorder of copper metabolism that has onset of clinical signs mostly in the first two decades of life. Patients may present with acute liver failure, chronic hepatitis, or cirrhosis, most commonly in the first decade of life, and a few present with acute hemolytic anemia. Other features include joint and bone abnormalities, azure lunulae of the fingernails, aminoaciduria, cardiomyopathy, and ophthalmologic manifestations. The classic and best-known ophthalmologic finding is a dull, yellow-brown pigment at the limbus of the cornea called Kayser-Fleischer rings resulting from copper deposition. Neurologic symptoms are the initial presentation in approximately 60% of patients, the most common initial neurologic signs being dysarthria, dysphagia, bradykinesia, and behavioral disturbance. Speech involvement is a constant feature with neurological involvement, the speech disorder taking the form of a mixed ataxic–hypokinetic–spastic dysarthria. Parkinson disease symptoms may predominate with reduced facial expression, bradykinesia, and tremors. Dystonia is a frequent feature, the dystonia usually being generalized and involving the neck (torticollis) and face (grimacing), but it may be focal such as involving a hand. Ultimately, patients become severely rigid with a pseudobulbar palsy. Psychiatric disturbances also are present in 25 to 65% of patients, although no specific behavioral syndrome is characteristic. The condition ultimately ends in death unless treated by systematic chelation therapy with penicillamine.

## References

Hoehn, M. M., & Yahr, M. D. (1967). Parkinsonism: Onset, progression and mortality. *Neurology, 17,* 427–442.

Jankovic, J. (2005). Progression of Parkinson's disease: Are we making progress in charting the course? *Archives of Neurology, 62,* 351–352.

O'Riordan, S., Raymond, D., Lynch, T., Saunders-Pullman, R., Bressman, S. B., Daly, L., & Hutchinson, M. (2004). Age at onset as a factor in determining the phenotype of primary torsion dystonia. *Neurology, 63,* 1423–1426.

Parkinson Study Group: Mortality in DATATOP. (1998). A multicenter trial in early Parkinson's disease. *Annals of Neurology, 43,* 318–325.

Schapira, A.H., & Obeso, J. (2006). Timing of treatment initiation in Parkinson's disease: A need for a reappraisal. *Annals of Neurology, 59,* 559–562.

Tourette Syndrome Classification Study Group. (1993). Definitions and classification of tic disorders. *Archives of Neurology, 50,* 1013–1016.

# 6

# Principles of Management

*BRUCE E. MURDOCH*

## Introduction

It has long been recognized and accepted that movement disorders, in addition to affecting the normal operation of the limbs and trunk, may also disrupt the function of the speech production musculature leading to dysarthria. As in the case of motor impairments of the limbs, dysarthrias associated with movement disorder syndromes are commonly grouped into hyper- and hypokinetic as well as ataxic subtypes. (A detailed description of the clinical features of dysarthrias occurring in association with movement disorders is presented in Chapter 7.) More recently, it has also been recognized that in addition to speech impairments, movement disorder syndromes, such as Parkinson disease and Huntington chorea, among others, are also associated with subtle language and cognitive impairments. The clinical features of these language and cognitive deficits are discussed

in Chapter 9. The focus of the current chapter is to outline contemporary speech pathology management strategies applied to motor speech and language disorders seen in association with movement disorders. Such strategies must also take into account any concurrent medical treatments being administered to the client. Medical treatments applied to the major types of movement disorders are outlined in Chapter 10.

## Assessment and Treatment of Motor Speech Impairments Associated with Movement Disorders

### Assessment of Dysarthria

Formulation of a diagnosis and subsequent determination of specific treatment priorities for dysarthrias associated with movement disorders is dependent on careful and detailed assessment. A range of assessment techniques are available to assist the clinician in this process. Typically, comprehensive assessment of clients affected by neurologic speech impairments includes the following components: a detailed case history, an oromotor examination, and determination of the key features of the speech disorder and identification of their neurologic substrates based on a combination of perceptual, acoustic, and physiologic procedures. Dysarthrias associated with movement disorders are no exception to this rule.

### Case History

In general, case history taking involves the compilation of information pertaining to the onset and course of the particular motor speech deficit, the client's perception of the disorder, and the way in which the speech deficit impacts the client's functional abilities and quality of life. Essential background information collected as part of the case history, therefore, should include the following client details: age; education level; occupation; marital and family status; prior history of speech-language impairments (including developmental conditions experienced in childhood); onset and course of the movement disorder (length of time the client has had the condition, whether it is progressive or stable, etc.); associated deficits (e.g., drooling, swallowing impairments, involuntary movements, etc.); emotional disturbances; prior treatment and management regimens; medical treatments (including drug treatments, dosages, etc.); client's awareness and understanding of the disorder; and consequences of the disorder (e.g., disruption to work, school, social activities, etc.).

### Oromotor Examination

Visual and tactual observation of the speech production mechanism, by way of an oromotor examination, during performance of a range of nonspeech activities provides important information about the size, strength, symmetry, range, tone, steadiness, speed, and accuracy of movements of the face, jaw, tongue, and velum (soft palate). Each of these four components of the speech production system is observed in the following conditions: at rest; during sustained postures (e.g., retraction of the lips, protrusion of the tongue, etc.); and during movement (e.g., alternate pursing and retraction of the lips). While each structure is at rest the clinician should observe whether or not the structure is symmetric or deviated to one side (e.g., at rest does the face, tongue, jaw, and velum appear symmetric). Furthermore, while at rest the presence of any involuntary movements (e.g., twitching of the tongue muscle) and muscle wastage (atrophy) need to be noted as both of these features may be indicative of the presence of a neurologic impairment such as a lower motor neuron lesion. The strength of the tongue and jaw can be tested by having the client move these structures against a force applied by the clinician (e.g., the client can be asked to press their tongue against the cheek to oppose a force imposed externally on the cheek by the hand of the clinician). The presence and absence of both normal and pathologic reflexes can also be good indicators of the presence of disease in either the peripheral or central nervous systems. For example, the absence of a normal reflex, such as the gag reflex or jaw jerk, can indicate the presence of pathology. Likewise, the presence of primitive or pathologic reflexes (i.e., reflexes absent in non-neurologically impaired individuals), such as the sucking reflex, is also indicative of neurologic impairment.

### Determination of the Principal Features of the Speech Disorder

Techniques available for determining the principal features of the neurologic speech disorder exhibited by a client and their neuropathologic substrates can be broadly divided into three major categories:

1. Perceptual techniques. These assessments are based on the clinician's impression of the auditory-perceptual attributes of the client's speech.
2. Acoustic techniques. Assessments in this category are based on the study of the generation, transmission, and modification of sound waves emitted from the vocal tract.
3. Physiologic techniques. These methods are based on instrumental assessment of the functioning of the various subsystems of the speech production mechanism in terms of their movements, muscular contractions, and so forth.

**Perceptual Assessment.** Perceptual analysis of neurologic speech disorders has been the gold standard and preferred method by which clinicians have made differential diagnoses and defined treatment programs for their clients for many years. In fact, many

clinicians still rely almost exclusively on auditory-perceptual judgments of speech intelligibility, articulatory accuracy, or subjective ratings of various speech dimensions on which to base their diagnosis of dysarthria and apraxia of speech and plan their intervention. The use of auditory-perceptual assessments to characterize the different types of dysarthria and identify the spectrum of deviant speech characteristics associated with each was pioneered by Darley, Aronson, and Brown (1969a, 1969b; 1975). It was from the findings of their auditory-perceptual studies of dysarthria that the system of classification of dysarthria most frequently used in clinical settings was developed. Darley et al. (1969a,b) assessed speech samples taken from 212 dysarthric speakers with a variety of neurologic conditions on 38 speech dimensions which fell into seven categories: pitch, loudness, voice quality (including both laryngeal and resonatory dysfunction), respiration, prosody, articulation, and two summary dimensions related to intelligibility and bizarreness. A key component of their research was the application of the "equal-appearing intervals scale of severity" which utilized a seven-part scale of severity.

Tasks useful for eliciting speech for perceptual evaluation include: vowel prolongation (i.e., provides information relative to pitch, loudness, and vocal quality); alternating motion/diadochokinetic rates (i.e., provides information pertaining to speech and consistency of rapid and repetitive muscle movements (e.g., puh-puh-puh-puh) in relation to articulatory precision; efficiency of velopharyngeal closure; phonatory and respiratory support); sequential motion rates (i.e., involves rapid and sequential movements from one articulatory posture to another (e.g., puh-tuh-kuh); and contextual speech (i.e., provision of a conversational, narrative, or reading sample).

There is only one published diagnostic dysarthria test, the Frenchay Dysarthria Assessment (FDA) (Enderby, 1983). It consists of a rating scale which is applicable to: information provided by the patient pertaining to their speech disorder; clinician's perception of specific speech features; observations of non-speech structure and function; intelligibility; speaking rate; status of hearing; and vision, dentition, language, mood, posture, and sensation. It encompasses assessment tasks which required speech and non-speech activities relevant to each motor speech subsystem (i.e., respiration, lips, tongue, jaw, velopharynx, and larynx), as well as an evaluation of intelligibility. On the basis of assessment results, each patient's profile may be classified according to dysarthria subtype (e.g., flaccid, spastic, ataxic, hypokinetic, mixed, etc.).

In addition to rating scales, other perceptual assessments used to investigate neurologic speech disorders include the application of intelligibility measures, phonetic transcription studies, and articulation inventories. According to Duffy (2005a) "intelligibility is the degree to which a listener understands the acoustic signal produced by a speaker" (p. 96).

The assessment of speech intelligibility (i.e., ease with which acoustic signal may be understood) provides information regarding the impact of a motor speech disorder on a patient's general ability to communicate. The focus of this section is on methods of evaluating speech intelligibility, as published measures of speech intelligibility are widely available and clinically applied. It has been suggested, however, that less widely utilized measures of comprehensibility (i.e., how understandable the acoustic signal is in addition to other cues which may influence comprehension such as knowledge of topic, gestures, etc.) and efficiency (i.e., rate at which comprehensible or intelligible information is communicated) may also be helpful in establishing the functional limitations of a motor speech disorder (Duffy, 2005a, 2005b).

The most basic method of evaluating speech intelligibility may involve the clinician estimating a percentage of intelligibility on the basis of clinical observations. Published assessments, however, include the Assessment of Intelligibility of Dysarthric Speech (ASSIDS) (Yorkston & Beukelman, 1981a), which has been described as the most widely applied measure of speech intelligibility in dysarthric populations (Duffy, 2005); the Sentence Intelligibility Test (Yorkston & Beukelman, 1996); Word Intelligibility Test (Kent, 1989); as well as the intelligibility subtests of the FDA (Enderby, 1983).

The ASSIDS enables the quantification of single word and sentence intelligibility via the calculation of intelligibility scores (i.e., percentage of correctly identified words), as well as a communicative efficiency ratio in relation to normal speakers. The Sentence Intelligibility Test is a revised version of the sentence intelligibility component of the ASSIDS. Although it requires clinicians to transcribe sentences produced by patients, computerized software generates intelligibility scores. The Word Intelligibility Test involves single words that are composed of phonetic stimuli deemed to be potentially vulnerable in dysarthric populations. Patients are required to read phonetically contrasting words that are transcribed by the examiner, and an intelligibility score is then calculated on the basis of percentage of intelligible words generated.

Perceptual assessments have a number of advantages and disadvantages relative to acoustic and physiologic procedures. The major advantages of perceptual assessment are those that have led to its preferred use as the tool for characterizing and diagnosing dysarthric speech. Perceptual assessments are readily available and require only limited financial outlay. In addition, all students of speech-language pathology are taught how to test for and identify perceptual symptoms. Finally, perceptual assessments are useful for monitoring the effects of treatment on speech intelligibility and the adequacy of communication.

Clinicians need to be aware, however, that there are a number of inherent inadequacies with perceptual assessment that may limit their use in determining treatment priorities. First, accurate, reliable perceptual judgments are often difficult to achieve as they can be influenced by a number of factors including the skill and experience of the clinician and the sensitivity of the assessment. In particular, raters must have extensive structured experience in listening prior to performing perceptual ratings.

Second, perceptual assessments are difficult to standardize both in relation to the patient being rated and the environment in which the speech samples are recorded. Patient variability over time and across different settings prevents maintenance of adequate intra- and interrater reliability. Furthermore, the symptoms may be present in certain conditions and not others. This variability is also found in the patients themselves such that characteristics of the person being rated (e.g., their age, premorbid medical history, and social history) may influence speech as well as the neurologic problem itself.

A third factor that limits reliance on perceptual assessments is that certain speech symptoms may influence the perception of others. This confound has been well reported in relation to the perception of resonatory disorders, articulatory deficits, and prosodic disturbances.

Probably the major concern of perceptual assessments, particularly as they relate to treatment planning, is that they have restricted power for determining which subsystems of the speech motor system are affected. In other words, perceptual assessments are unable to accurately identify the pathophysiologic basis of the speech disorder manifest in various types of dysarthria. It is possible that a number of different physiologic deficits can form the basis of perceptually identified features, and that different patterns of interaction within a patient's overall symptom complex can result in a similar perceptual deviation (e.g., distorted consonants can result from reduced respiratory support for speech, inadequate velopharyngeal functioning, or weak tongue musculature). When crucial decisions are required in relation to optimum therapeutic planning, an over-reliance on only perceptual assessment may lead to a number of questionable therapy directions.

**Acoustic Assessment.** Acoustic analyses can be used in conjunction with perceptual assessments to provide a more complete understanding of the nature of the disturbance in dysarthric speech. In particular, acoustic assessment can highlight aspects of the speech signal that may be contributing to the perception of deviant speech production and can provide confirmatory support for perceptual judgments. For example, they may confirm the perception that speech is slow and demonstrate that the reduced rate of speech may be the result of increased interword durations and prolonged vowel and consonant production. As a further example, an acoustic analysis might be used to confirm the perception of imprecise consonant production and to show that such imprecision is the result of spirantization of consonants and reduction of consonant clusters. In addition to altered speech rate and consonant imprecision, other perceived deviant speech dimensions that can be confirmed by way of acoustic analysis include, among others, breathy voice, voice tremor, and reduced variability of pitch and loudness. Acoustic analysis is also useful for providing objective documentation of the effects of treatment and disease progression on speech production.

Acoustic measurements can be taken primarily from two different types of acoustic displays: oscillographic displays and spectrographic displays. An oscillographic display is a two-dimensional waveform display of amplitude (on the $y$-axis) as a function of time ($x$-axis). Oscillographic displays are easy to generate and can provide information on a variety of acoustic parameters such as segment duration (e.g., vowel duration, word duration, etc.), amplitude, fundamental frequency, and the presence of some acoustic cues of articulatory adequacy such as voice onset time, spirantization, and voiced/voiceless distinctions. Measurements from oscillographic displays can be made either manually or alternatively, by using computer-controlled acoustic analysis software. Some of the commonly used computerized systems and dedicated devices for acoustic speech analysis include: C Speech, CSL (Computerized Speech Lab), CSRE (Canadian Speech Research Environment), ILS-PC (Interactive Laboratory System), and MSL (Micro Speech Lab).

In contrast to the two-dimensional oscillographic display, a spectrographic display is actually a three-dimensional display, of both frequency and amplitude as a function of time, where time is displayed on the $x$-axis and frequency on the $y$-axis. There are two different types of spectrographic displays: wideband displays (also called broadband displays) and narrowband displays. Wideband spectrographic displays are used to determine accurate temporal measurements, whereas narrowband spectrograms are useful for making measurements of fundamental frequency and the prosodic aspects of speech.

While there is no "standard" set of parameters included in all acoustic analyses, there are, however, a number of different acoustic measures which can provide important information about the acoustic features of dysarthric speech. These parameters can be loosely arranged into groups of measures including: fundamental frequency measures, amplitude measures, perturbation measures, noise-related measures, formant measures, temporal measures, measures of articulatory capability, and evaluations of manner of voicing.

**Physiologic Assessment.** The use of instrumental procedures in the process of diagnosing speech disorders enables clinicians to extend their senses and objectify their perceptual observations. In particular, instrumentation has given the clinician the ability to determine the contributions of malfunctions in the various components of the speech production mechanism to the production of disordered speech. Indeed, modern instrumentation enables the clinician to assess and obtain information about the integrity and functional status of the muscle groups at each stage of the speech production process from respiration to articulation.

To be of value in determining treatment priorities, instrumental assessment should be comprehensive, covering as many components of the speech production mechanism as possible. A wide variety of different types of physiologic instrumentation have been described in the literature for use in the assessment of the functioning of the various components of the speech production apparatus. Each of these instruments has been designed to provide information on a specific aspect of speech production including muscular activity, structural movements, as well as airflows and air pressures generated in various parts of the speech mechanism. The features of the most commonly used physiologic instruments used to assess the functioning of the respiratory system, larynx, velopharynx (soft palate), and articulators (e.g., lips, tongue, etc.) are briefly outlined below.

**Instrumental Assessment of Speech Breathing.** Physiologic instruments used in the assessment of speech breathing can be divided into two major types: those that directly measure various lung volumes, capacities, and airflows (e.g., spirometers), and those that indirectly measure respiratory function by monitoring movements of the chest wall, the so-called kinematic assessments (e.g., mercury strain gauges, magnetometers, respiratory inductance plethysmographs, strain-gauge belt pneumographs).

Spirometers are specifically designed for the evaluation of respiratory volumes. The basic principle of a spirometer is to measure and record the volumes of air blown into either a tube or a fitted face mask, which is attached to the machine. By using this type of assessment, the investigator can obtain a number of valuable respiratory/airflow measures, including vital capacity, forced expiratory volume, functional residual capacity, inspiratory capacity, expiratory and inspiratory reserve volumes, as well as volume/flow relationships and tidal volume and respiration rate.

Kinematic devices allow the clinician to infer the airflow volume changes during respiration from rib cage and abdominal displacements. In that they do not require the need for restrictive mouth pieces and nose clips that can interrupt natural speech production and respiratory patterns, the kinematic method allows for more accurate measurements of the breath support during speech production.

Investigations of speech breathing using kinematic assessments have predominantly used four main types of kinematic instrumentation. These types include magnetometers (e.g., Solomon & Hixon, 1993); strain-gauge belt pneumograph systems (e.g., Manifold & Murdoch, 1993), mercury strain gauges (e.g., Cavallo & Baken, 1985), and respiratory inductance plethysmography (available commercially as the "Respitrace" system) (e.g., Sperry & Klich, 1992). Of these techniques, the Respitrace system is most commonly available in clinical settings.

One other important indicator of respiratory function for speech production is the ability of the subject to generate subglottal air pressure during speech. Subglottal air pressure is estimated using an Aerophone II (Kay Elemetrics, Montvale, N.J.) airflow measurement system (Figure 6–1). The Aerophone II consists of hand-held transducer module together with a powerful data acquisition and processing software program. The transducer module consists of miniaturized transducers capable of recording airflow, air pressure, and acoustic signals during speech. A face mask through which a thin flexible tube of silicon rubber is inserted to record intraoral pressure is attached to the hand-held transducer module.

**Instrumental Assessment of Laryngeal Function.** Physiologic evaluation of laryngeal function is carried out using both direct and indirect techniques. Endoscopy using a rigid endoscope or nasendoscopy using a flexible fiberscope both allow for direct observation of vocal fold movement. Both systems are telescopic-type devices that illuminate the laryngeal area and allow visual inspection of the laryngeal region. The rigid endoscope is inserted through the mouth into the region of the oropharynx, allowing direct obser-

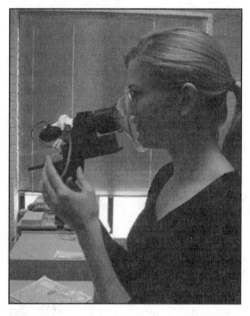

**FIGURE 6–1.** The Aerophone II airflow measurement system is shown.

vation of the vocal folds during phonation of sustained vowels. In comparison, the flexible fiberscope is inserted through the nasal cavity and then passed down through the pharyngeal area until the tip of the scope is positioned at approximately the level of the epiglottis to allow an unobstructed view of the vocal folds. As the oral cavity is not obstructed using the nasoendoscopic technique, visual record of laryngeal function can be obtained during normal speech production. Both the endoscope and nasoendoscope are connected to a video monitoring and recording system, which allows the visual image of the vocal folds to be recorded for later viewing and analysis. Videostroboscopy combines the use of a strobe light source in conjunction with the videoendoscopic procedures outlined above. Using the stroboscopic technique, the movements of the vocal folds during speech production can be "slowed" or "stopped" through the optical illusion of stroboscopy making identification of vocal fold dysfunction much easier.

The indirect methods of evaluating physiologic functioning of the larynx include electroglottography (electrolaryngography) and aerodynamic examination. Electroglottography is an electrical impedance method of estimating vocal fold contact during phonation that is designed to allow investigation of laryngeal microfunction (cycle-by-cycle periodicity and contact). The electroglottographic assessment is conducted using a Fourcin laryngograph interfaced with a Waveform Display System (Kay Elemetrics, model 6091). The system records the degree of vocal fold contact and the vocal fold vibratory patterns during phonation, these features being displayed in the form of an Lx waveform.

Aerodynamic measures allow examination of the macrofunctions of the larynx such as laryngeal airflow, glottal pressures, and glottal resistance. Esti-

mates of these parameters are obtained by way of an Aerophone II Airflow Measurement System (see Instrumental Assessment of Speech Breathing above).

**Instrumental Assessment of Velopharyngeal Function (Soft Palate).** The most commonly used instrument for assessment of nasality is the Nasometer (Kay Elemetrics) (Figure 6–2). The Nasometer is a computer-assisted instrument that provides a measure of nasality derived from the ratio of acoustic energy output from the nasal and oral cavities during speech. Acoustic energy is detected by two directional microphones (one placed in front of the nares and the other in front of the mouth) separated by a sound-separator plate. The instrument yields a "nasalance" score made up of a ratio of nasal-to-oral plus nasal acoustic energy calculated as a percentage.

**Instrumental Assessment of Articulatory Function.** The term "articulators" is used to represent collectively the muscle groups of the lips, tongue, and

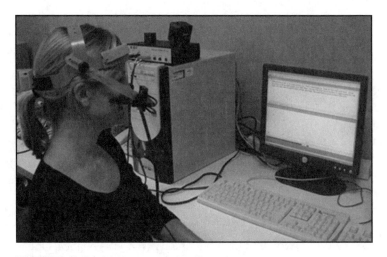

**FIGURE 6–2.** A nasometer is shown.

jaw. Although these structures are often grouped together due to their common influence over speech production at the articulatory stage, each one functions independently and contributes differently to speech production. Consequently, a variety of instrumental techniques have been developed in order to examine the degree of compression force exerted by each articulator during speech and nonspeech tasks, as well as to investigate force control properties, rate of individual articulatory movements, endurance capabilities of the individual articulators and the movement patterns during speech production of each separate aspect of the articulatory system

Of the various types of instrumentation used to assess the articulators, strain-gauge transducers, used to record articulator movement and force-generating capacities, have been the most frequently used. Because of their high levels of sensitivity, strain-gauge transducers are especially suited to detecting the subtle changes in movement that occur in speech production. In addition, they are relatively inexpensive, non-invasive, provide an immediate voltage analogue of movement, and can be adapted to assess lip, tongue, and jaw function during both speech and non-speech tasks. An example of a strain-gauge system for estimating lip strength is shown in Figure 6–3.

In addition to strain-gauge transducers, pressure or force transducers can also provide valuable information regarding the functioning of the articulatory system. For example, a miniaturized pressure transducer is frequently used to assess lip function. Because of its small size, the transducer is capable of being placed between the lips to generate interlabial pressure measurements during speech production without interfering with normal articulatory movements.

An equivalent commercially available instrument for estimating tongue strength and endurance is the Iowa Oral Performance Instrument (IOPI), which consists of an air-filled rubber bulb attached to a pressure transducer (Figure 6–4). For testing, the bulb is placed in the mouth and the subject is

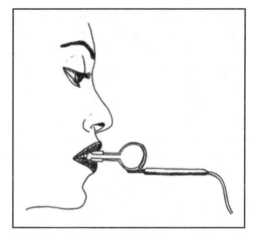

**FIGURE 6–3.** Example of a strain-gauge system for measuring lip strength.

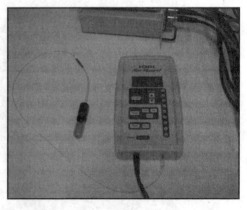

**FIGURE 6–4.** The Iowa Oral Performance Instrument is shown.

instructed to squeeze the bulb against the roof of the mouth with the tongue. When the bulb is squeezed by the tongue, the amount of pressure is displayed on a digital readout.

Electromyography (EMG) is another technique that has commonly been used (primarily by researchers rather than clinicians) to examine articulator function. Using this technique, the momentary changes in electrical activity that occur when a muscle is contracting are recorded by using various types of electrodes (e.g., surface, needle, or hook-wire) placed either overlying (surface electrodes) or within (e.g., hook-wire electrodes and needle electrodes) the muscle. The data obtained from EMG assessment have proven useful for investigating the neurophysiologic bases of various disorders, such as identifying the presence of increased muscle tone (hypertonicity) or abnormal variations in the activation or inhibition of muscle activity. In addition, EMG has been used to record muscle activity simultaneously with the speech move-ment patterns of these same muscles, in order to examine the motor control of the articulators.

Electropalatography is another technique for examining tongue function, which provides the clinician with information on the location and timing of tongue contacts with the palate during speech. With this technique, the client wears an acrylic palate with an array of contact sensors implanted on the surface (Figure 6–5). When contact occurs between the tongue and any of the electrodes, a signal is conducted via lead-out wires to an external processing unit, which then displays the patterns of contact on a computer screen.

In recent years the development and introduction of a technique called electromagnetic articulography (EMA) has provided a safe, non-invasive assessment tool with which the dynamic aspects of articulatory dysfunction in various neurologic speech disorders can be investigated. Importantly, the EMA technique does not require the use of ionizing radiation. Rather, the EMA

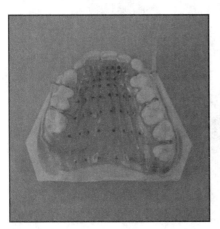
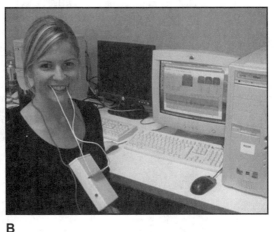

**A**                    **B**

**FIGURE 6–5. A.** Acrylic electropalatography palate with embedded touch sensors. **B.** Client fitted with an electropalatography palate.

system tracks articulatory movements during speech using weak alternating electromagnetic fields. Transmitter coils, housed in a plastic cube and positioned around the head, generate alternating magnetic fields at different frequencies, which in turn induce alternating signals in small receiver coils temporarily glued to the tongue, upper and lower lip, and jaw. The position of the receiver coils in relation to the transmitter coils is sampled over time and plotted on a computer, providing a visual representation of articulator movements in real time. From these data, quantitative kinematic parameters can be derived including the velocity, acceleration, distance, and duration of movements of the lips, tongue, and jaw during speech production. The most recently introduced EMA system, the AG500, is capable of tracking articulatory movements in three dimensions (Figure 6–6).

Evaluating the movements of the tongue is more difficult than assessing lip or jaw movement primarily because of the fact that the tongue functions within the confines of the mouth. In addition to the EMA technique described above, imaging techniques such cineradiography and ultrasound have proved useful for examining the complex patterns of tongue movement during speech.

## Treatment of Dysarthria

Subsequent to motor speech evaluation and differential diagnosis, appropriate treatment strategies may be implemented. As previously mentioned, dysarthrias associated with movement

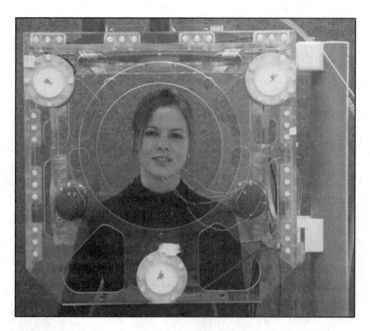

**FIGURE 6–6.** The AG500 Electromagnetic articulograph is shown.

disorders are typically classified as hypokinetic, hyperkinetic, or ataxic. The following section summarizes the relevant treatment approaches (i.e., behavioral, biofeedback, prosthetic) commonly used to remediate these motor speech disorders, typically within the context of affected motor speech subsystems. Surgical and pharmacologic management strategies are also briefly discussed, where relevant.

### Treatment of Hypokinetic Dysarthria

Hypokinetic dysarthria is typically characterized by phonatory, articulatory, and prosodic impairments; however, it can involve all motor speech subsystems (i.e., also encompass resonatory and respiratory disturbances as well) as a potential consequence of variability in disease state and progression. Treatment strategies have primarily focused on behavioral and instrumental techniques specially designed for this population, or have evolved from more traditional dysarthria therapy techniques; however, alternative techniques that may also have some bearing on speech function include surgical procedures and drug regimens.

**Treatment of Phonatory Dysfunction in Hypokinetic Dysarthria.** The treatment of phonatory dysfunction represents the mainstay of speech pathology intervention in Parkinson disease populations, and has typically incorporated behavioral, prosthetic, and biofeedback techniques. Behavioral strategies have largely focused on improving breathy vocal quality, reduced vocal intensity, monopitch, and monoloudness.

The Lee Silverman Voice Treatment (LSVT) program represents a contemporary and efficacious behavioral therapeutic approach aimed at recalibrating the amplitude of motor output in patients with parkinsonian dysarthria via the production of intensive, repetitive, and high-effort motor behavior. The program was developed around the central hypothesis that reduced phonatory and respiratory drive underlie the perceptual manifestations of reduced volume and prosodically flat speech perceived in the speech of Parkinson disease patients. The program focuses on increasing vocal effort via intensive (i.e., 16 sessions per month) and repeated maximum phonation drills which subsequently retrain respiratory and phonatory patterns, ranging from vowel to conversation-level production. Prolonged improvements in vocal loudness have been demonstrated for up to 24 months following treatment with this technique, and generalization of increased function across motor speech subsystems has also been reported including improvements in pitch, rate, facial expression, swallowing, and speech intelligibility.

**Treatment of Articulatory Dysfunction in Hypokinetic Dysarthria.** Articulatory dysfunction observed in Parkinson disease patients has been attributed to reductions in fine force control, rate, range, and strength of lip, tongue, and jaw musculature. Behavioral techniques aimed at remediating the articulatory deficits associated with hypokinetic dysarthria principally include articulation drills which focus on the production of frequently occurring articulation errors, as well as nonspeech tasks which concentrate on improving the strength, rate, and range of lip, tongue, and jaw movements.

Biofeedback tools have also been applied to the treatment of articulatory dysfunction in hypokinetic dysarthria. Electromyographic feedback from the lip muscles has been shown to be effective in normalizing labial muscle activity in patients with Parkinson disease. In addition, an electropalatography (i.e., device which provides information regarding the timing and location of tongue to palate contact during speech) may also be modified for articulatory biofeedback purposes in Parkinson disease patients.

**Treatment of Prosodic Dysfunction in Hypokinetic Dysarthria.** Increased speech rate is a common feature of hypokinetic dysarthric speech, and a range of behavioral and prosthetic approaches have been applied in treating this characteristic. Pacing techniques involving hand tapping, metronomes, pacing boards, and computerized pacing software have been successful in altering pause and articulation timing in patients with Parkinson disease. Other strategies, such as the utilization of short phrase lengths and breath group patterning, have also been effective in reducing the speech rate of these patients, as has the application of delayed auditory feedback techniques. Speech dysfluency in parkinsonian speech, such as phoneme repetition, initiation problems, and palilalia, may also be remediated via the rate control techniques mentioned above.

Impaired stress patterning and intonational contours are also commonly reported features of hypokinetic dysarthric speech. Therapeutic techniques aimed at improving stress patterning include contrastive stress drills, where sentence meanings are altered by producing alternative stress patterns. The manipulation of vocal intensity and pitch using conventional techniques, such as reading aloud items marked for pause time and intonation patterns, as well as biofeedback tools such as Visi-Pitch and Vocalite, have also been effective in altering intonational contours within hypokinetic dysarthric speech.

**Treatment of Resonatory Dysfunction in Hypokinetic Dysarthria.** Velopharyngeal dysfunction and associated nasality impairments in Parkinson disease patients are rare, with the majority of disturbances in this speech feature reported as mild. In cases of overt velopharyngeal dysfunction, however, a range of behavioral therapeutic techniques which aim to improve velopharyngeal valving can be applied, including: (1) oral opening and tongue movement exercises which improve the oral cavity's resonatory capacity; (2) speech rate reduction facilitating more effective velopharyngeal closure; and (3) contrastive nasal and non-nasal articulation drills. Biofeedback instruments that provide visual cues as to the effectiveness of velopharyngeal valving, such as the Nasometer (Kay Elemetrics) and accelerometry, may also be useful in remediating nasality disturbances in hypokinetic dysarthric speech.

**Treatment of Respiratory Dysfunction in Hypokinetic Dysarthria.** Respiratory dysfunction in Parkinson disease commonly involves the following: impaired breath support for speech, reduced vital capacity, short speech rushes, reduced overall volume and loudness decay, irregular breathing, shortened phonation time and phrase length, and incoordination of chest wall movements. Behavioral techniques utilized in the treatment of these impairments have typically included: exercises to improve breath control (e.g., progressive counting) and increase loudness, relaxing diaphragmatic breathing patterns, and establishing appropriate phrasing and breath grouping for speech. Most recently, the LSVT program has also been shown to be effective in increasing respiratory support for speech. The accent method and inspiratory checking techniques may be also be applied in cases where incoordinate speech breathing is a concern. The accent method trains patients to establish an abdominal pattern of speech breathing, whereas inspiratory checking involves establishing maximal respiratory volume and airflow for speech.

Biofeedback methods that provide information about subglottal air pressure/respiratory volume during speech may also be useful in remediating respiratory dysfunction in dysarthric Parkinson disease populations. Most recently, kinematic instrumentation, which provides feedback pertaining to chest wall movements during speech (i.e., rib cage versus abdomen), has been recommended for use in populations with speech breathing disorders, including those with hypokinetic dysarthria.

**Surgical and Pharmacologic Approaches to the Treatment of Hypokinetic Dysarthria.** Although the greatest effects of dopamine agonists, such as levodopa, selegiline (Deprenyl), and carbidopalevodopa (Sinemet), have been largely observed relative to nonspeech function in Parkinson disease patients, some limited benefits have also been reported in motor speech abilities (Duffy, 2005a, 2005b). Of particular note for the clinician are evident variations in motor performance following the administration of dopamine agonists which are thought to be drug-cycle dependent (see Chapter 7).

As discussed in Chapters 7 and 10, neurosurgical techniques, including thalamotomy, pallidotomy, and deep brain stimulation (DBS), are now commonly applied in the modern-day management of movement disorders such as Parkinson disease. Although not originally attempted with the aim of remediating speech deficits, some interesting effects from these procedures have been observed relative to the motor speech apparatus, including both improvements and decrements in function (see Chapter 7 for detailed discussion of effects). For example, unilateral pallidotomy has been reported to effect improvements in phonation and articulation in some Parkinson disease patients (Schulz, Peterson, Sapienza, Greer, & Friedman, 1999), while other studies have reported declines in speech intelligibility as a consequence of this procedure (Theodoros, Ward, Murdoch, Silburn & Lethlean, 2000; Uitti et al., 2000). Bilateral pallidotomy has been associated with improvements in force control of oral structures as well as enhanced postoperative lip movement, more relaxed facial musculature, and improved eating and drinking abilities (Barlow, 1998). Reports of significant worsening of dysarthria, saliva control difficulties, dysphagia, and hypophonia have also been documented (Scott et al., 1998). Thalamotomy has been consistently associated with post-operative development or worsening of dysarthria, particularly in the case of bilaterally placed lesions (Kelly, Ahlskog, Goerss, Daube, Duffy, & Kall, 1987; Shannon, 2000). Residual dysarthria is a commonly reported side effect of deep brain stimulation of the subthalamic nucleus (DBS-STN) (Limousin et al., 1998; Rousseaux, Krystkowiak, Kozlowski, Ozsancak, Blond, & Destée, 2004), despite reports of both improvements and decrements in speech intelligibility following this procedure (Rousseaux et al., 2004), as well as improvements in phonatory and articulatory speech subcomponents (Maruska, Smit, Koller, & Garcia, 2000; McFarlane, Hoh-Romeo, & Lavorato, 1991). General consensus, however, dictates that the above surgical procedures are more commonly harmful than beneficial to hypokinetic dysarthric symptoms, and that more significant improvements in limb function as opposed to motor speech function may be typically elicited by these techniques (Pinto, Ozsancak, Tripoliti, Thobois, Limousin Dowsey, & Auzou, 2004).

## Treatment of Hyperkinetic Dysarthria

Hyperkinetic dysarthria has been defined as a diverse group of speech disorders involving abnormal involuntary movements of the limbs, trunk, neck, or face which disturb the rate and rhythm of speech production. Given the considerable heterogeneity of hyperkinetic symptoms (i.e., relative to type and locality of abnormal movements produced), each of the motor speech subsystems may be affected in hyperkinetic dysarthria.

Pharmacologic intervention has provided the primary conventional treatment modality for the management of hyperkinetic dysarthria, with improvements in speech function associated with improvements in movement disorder (Beukelman, 1983). More recently, surgical procedures (e.g., thalamotomy, pallidotomy, and DBS) used to treat tremor, dystonia, and dyskinesia have also produced some benefit in the alleviation of hyperkinetic dysarthric symptoms (Duffy, 2005a,b).

At a subsystem level, phonatory and respiratory dysfunction have received significant attention in the treatment of hyperkinetic dysarthria; however, the mainstay of evaluated speech therapy techniques involve the application of behavioral, biofeedback, and prosthetic methods of increasing postural and/or articulatory stability, and hence speech intelligibility, as well as techniques which promote the monitoring/controlling of excessive movements. As such, the ensuing discussion on hyperkinetic dysarthria focuses upon individual treatment strategies versus levels of subsystem dysfunction.

**Pharmacologic Treatment of Hyperkinetic Dysarthria.** Botulinum toxin injections have produced perhaps the most dramatic effects in improving the functional speech abilities of patients with hyperkinetic dysarthria and associated oromandibular dystonia (Duffy & Yorkston, 2003), hemifacial spasm (Brin, 1998), spasmodic torticollis (Tsui, Eisen, & Mak, 1985), spasmodic dysphonia (Duffy, 2005), and palatal myoclonus (Varney, Demetroulakos, Fletcher, McQueen, & Hamilton, 1996). Other drug agents typically used to treat systemic hyperkinetic movement disorders have demonstrated indirect effects on motor speech mechanisms. For example, in treating limb tremor, the use of Inderal, primodone (Mysoline), carbamazepine (Tegretol), baclofen (Lioresal), methazolamide (Neptazane), trihexyphenidyl (Artane), and lithium have been reported to improve vocal and head tremor (Koller, Graner, & Mlcoch, 2001). Laryngeal and respiratory dystonias are reportedly receptive to Artane (Ludlow, Sedora, & Fujita, 1989). Oromandibular dystonias and spasmodic dysphonias have been reported to improve following administrations of Lioresal, Artane, lithium, and alprazolam (Xanax) (Rosenfeld, 1991). Palatal myoclonus is reportedly responsive to clonazepam, carbamazapine, or trihexyphenidyl (Frucht, 2003) and choreic dysarthria responsive to Lioresal, resperine, and haloperidol (Haldol) (Rosenfeld, 1991).

**Behavioral Treatment of Hyperkinetic Dysarthria.** The most useful behavioral strategies for this population include the introduction of postural strategies that reduce involuntary movements and subsequently facilitate functional speech production (Duffy, 2005a, 2005b). In addition, rate reduction therapy has also been reported to improve speech intelligibility in patients with action myoclonus where increased speech rate results in increased myoclonic activity (Duffy, 2005a, 2005b). Augmentative and alternative communication techniques have also been suggested for those patients in whom functional speech intelligibility is difficult to achieve (Beukelman, 1983).

In reference to patients with adductor spasmodic dysphonia (ADSD), behavioral techniques that encourage the production of a breathy phonation onset or increased vocal pitch have been effective (Duffy, 2005a, 2005b). In contrast, patients with abductor spasmodic dysphonia have benefited from exercises which encourage the production of hard glottal attack at the commencement of phonation, or the voicing of voiceless consonants (Duffy, 2005a, 2005b). There is also some evidence to suggest (i.e., at least in the case of ADSD), that behavioral strategies may be most effective following Botox injections (Murray & Woodson, 1995).

**Instrumental Biofeedback Techniques Used in the Treatment of Hyperkinetic Dysarthria.** The majority of studies that have applied biofeedback techniques to the treatment of hyperkinetic dysarthria have utilized instrumentation which aims to alleviate involuntary muscle movements by providing EMG information pertaining to muscle activity. For example, hemifacial spasms have been able to be reduced in patients with hyperkinetic dysarthria (Rubow, Rosenbek, Collins, & Celesia, 1984), as have excessive oral and facial movements in cases of tardive dyskinesia with EMG feedback techniques (Fudge, Thailer, & Alpert, 1991; Sherman, 1979). Attempts to normalize breathing patterns have also been successful in a case of generalized dystonia, with the aid of visual feedback via inductance plethysmography (LaBlance & Rutherford, 1991). Although worthy of further investigation, the limited amount of outcome data pertaining to the effects of biofeedback approaches in the treatment of hyperkinetic dysarthria prohibits the general application of such techniques to the management of this disorder (Duffy, 2005a, 2005b).

**Prosthetic Devices Used in the Treatment of Hyperkinetic Dysarthria.** Bite blocks have been reportedly successful in improving the speech of patients with oromandibular dystonia and other hyperkinetic movements that disrupt jaw stability. Preventing excessive jaw movements and enhancing orofacial postural control as a consequence of applying a bite block has resulted in improved speech proficiency in a small number of patients with hyperkinetic dysarthria.

## Treatment of Ataxic Dysarthria

In comparison with the treatment of other types of dysarthria, the management of ataxic dysarthria has a primary focus on improving overall control of the motor speech apparatus as well as integration of speech movements, in contrast to the remediation of specific deficits in muscle strength and tone. Surgical and prosthetic treatment approaches have also been labeled as largely irrelevant to the population with ataxic dysarthria (Duffy, 2005a, 2005b). Some benefits of pharmacologic therapy have been documented, however, including the reduction of vocal tremor with clonazepam (Cannito & Marquardt, 1997).

**Treatment of Articulatory Dysfunction in Ataxic Dysarthria.** Articulatory deficits typically seen in cases of ataxic dysarthria include: imprecise consonant production, vowel distortion, and irregular breakdowns in articulation, resulting from impaired coordination of the range, speed, force, and timing of lip, tongue, and jaw musculature. Recommended articulatory treatment strategies include: phoneme drills focusing on improving articulatory coordination, integral stimulation, intelligibility drills, exaggeration of articulatory movements, phonetic placement and derivation, as well as minimal contrasts (Duffy, 1995). Biofeedback techniques, such as electropalatography and articulography which provide information pertaining to the range, force, and timing of lip, tongue, palate, and/or jaw movements, have also been suggested.

**Treatment of Phonatory Dysfunction in Ataxic Dysarthria.** Phonatory instability and incoordination producing abnormal alterations in pitch and loudness, as well as harsh vocal quality, represent the phonatory characteristics of a speaker with ataxic dysarthria. Treatment approaches which focus on the coordination of breathing and phonation have been recommended on the premise that phonation and respiration are integrally connected (Murdoch & Theodoros, 1998). Vocal drills involving the manipulation of pitch and loudness have also been suggested, including hand-drawn or simulated electronic feedback on instrumentation such as the VisiPitch (Murray, 1983).

The issue of vocal quality is addressed with strategies that aim to reduce vocal fold tension and increase coordination of breathing and voicing to facilitate regular vibration of the vocal folds (Murdoch & Theodoros, 1998). An additional technique used to equilibrate vocal fold muscle power and expiration is the accent method, which aims to produce rhythmic phonation (Kotby, 1995).

**Treatment of Respiratory Dysfunction in Ataxic Dysarthria.** Respiratory disturbances that manifest as a consequence of ataxic dysarthria are reportedly the result of incoordinate movement of chest wall components during speech (Murdoch, Chenery, Stokes, & Hardcastle, 1991). As a result, treatment strategies that aim to remediate respiratory dysfunction within this population typically focus on the stabilization and coordination of chest wall movements during expiration (Murdoch & Theodoros, 1998). Chest wall activity (i.e., rib cage and abdominal wall movements) may be demonstrated with biofeedback techniques such as the Respitrace (i.e., oscillographic display). Other more traditional behavioral approaches include: inspiratory checking, controlled exhalation tasks, vowel prolongations, timing speech at the onset of expiration, appropriate termination of speech during expiration, and optimal breath grouping (Duffy, 1995).

**Treatment of Prosodic Dysfunction in Ataxic Dysarthria.** In contrast to the treatment regimens of other dysarthric subtypes which tackle prosodic disturbances near the termination of therapy, prosodic impairments represent a starting point for patients with ataxic dysarthria (Duffy, 1995). Treatment generally aims to reduce speech rate and to consequently improve speech intelligibility as well as to produce more naturally sounding speech via the development of appropriate stress and intonation patterns (Duffy, 2005a, 2005b).

Given that ataxic dysarthria is characterized by abnormal timing of the components of the motor speech apparatus, it has been postulated that reducing speech rate permits better coordination of speech subsystems (Murdoch & Theodoros, 1998). Numerous behavioral rate reduction techniques have

been successfully applied to the treatment of ataxic dysarthria, including: alphabet (Beukelman & Yorkston, 1977) and pacing boards (Helm, 1979); timed and cued production of single words (Yorkston, Hammen, Beukelman, & Traynor, 1990); hand tapping, metronomic and word-by-word reading strategies (Rosenbek & LaPointe, 1978); as well as additive rhythmic and rhythmic cuing of utterances (Yorkston & Beukelman, 1981b; Beukelman, Yorkston, & Tice, 1988; Yorkston et al., 1990).

Biofeedback techniques have also been reportedly successful in reducing speech rate within ataxic dysarthric speakers. For example, oscillographic feedback provides a means of controlling articulatory and pause durations (Berry & Goshorn, 1983; Yorkston & Beukelman, 1981b) as well as vocal intensity (Caligiuri & Murry, 1983), subsequently improving speech intelligibility. In addition, the IBM Speech Viewer has also been demonstrated as effective in improving the modulation of fundamental frequency in patients with ataxic dysarthria (Bougle, Ryalls, & Le Dorze, 1995). Furthermore, clinician-driven rate reduction techniques (i.e., clinician instructs patient to reduce speaking rate during reading of unfamiliar passage until optimal rate at which maximal intelligibility is determined) (Yorkston & Beukelman, 1981b) and self-monitoring techniques (Yorkston & Beukelman, 1981b) may also represent efficacious rate reduction methods.

Prosodic impairments may also be improved via the application of contrastive stress and intonation drills (Rosenbek & LaPointe, 1978), and durational contrasts (Yorkston, 1999; Yorkston & Beukelman, 1981b). These drills alter the meaning of utterances on the basis of pitch and loudness levels used, as well as syllable and pause length, respectively.

**Treatment of Resonatory Dysfunction in Ataxic Dysarthria.** Incoordinate movements of the soft palate provide the pathophysiologic basis for disorders of nasality (i.e., hypernasality, hyponasality, or mixed nasality), which may be seen in patients with ataxic dysarthria, as opposed to weakness of the palatal muscles (Murdoch & Theodoros, 1998). Resonatory treatment techniques may include such approaches as articulation drills that encourage the contrastive as well as overemphasized production of nasal and nonnasal consonants as a means of improving the force, timing, and range of palatal movement as well as increasing speech intelligibility (Rosenbek & LaPointe, 1978). In addition, exaggerated movements of the lips, tongue, and jaw may also be promoted in an effort to enhance oral resonance (Rosenbek & LaPointe, 1978).

---

**Assessment and Treatment of Language Impairments Associated with Movement Disorders**

---

The language profiles of clients with movement disorders characteristically involve deficits of higher level function which are intrinsically related to frontal lobe or cognitive function. Typically these individuals present with relatively normal profiles on tests of primary language function, yet demonstrate difficulty on tasks that assess metacognitive and metalinguistic processes. When intact, these processes permit the conscious and effective manipulation of the semantic system via the interaction of primary language as well as cognitive and executive processes. Failure to adequately evaluate these skills within this population, by way of the exclusive application of traditional aphasia assessments which appraise primary comprehension and production abilities, may serve to mask more complex language deficits that exist as a result of the subcortical lesions that underlie their movement disorder.

## Assessment of Language Impairments

As in the case of neurologic speech disorders outlined above, prior to initiation of any treatment for acquired language disorders the clinician must complete a detailed case history and comprehensive assessment of the communication disorder. In the early stages post-onset, a bedside evaluation is most often based largely on observation by the clinician rather than the administration of formal language tests. As part of the bedside assessment the speech-language pathologist should consider factors such as: the patient's ability to comprehend spoken language (e.g., do they follow the conversation, can they follow one, two- and three-stage commands such as "point to the floor then to the ceiling"); naming abilities; and the patient's ability to repeat words of increasing complexity and sentences.

Once the client is medically stable, observation can then be supplemented with a range of formal tests. In general, these tests fall into one of two major categories: tests that evaluate basic language skills, and tests of functional and pragmatic language abilities.

### Tests of Basic Language Function

These tests identify the presence of language deficits but do not ascertain the impact of these deficits on functional communication abilities. In this way tests included in this category sample neurologic language disorders such as aphasia at what the World Health Organization (WHO) refers to as the "impairment level." Tests of basic language function can be divided into two groups: tests of general language that assess primary comprehension and production abilities, and high-level language tests that assess more complex language function.

**Tests of General Language Abilities.** Examples of tests of general language abilities commonly used by speech-language pathologists include: Neurosensory Center Comprehensive Examination for Aphasia (NCCEA) (Spreen & Benton, 1977); Boston Naming Test (BNT) (Kaplan, Goodglass, & Weintraub, 1983); Boston Diagnostic Aphasia Examination (BDAE) (Goodglass, Kaplan, & Barresi, 2001); Western Aphasia Battery (WAB) (Kertesz, 1982); Porch Index of Communicative Abilities (PICA) (Porch, 1967); Examining for Aphasia-4 (EFA-4) (LaPointe & Eisenson, 2008); Reading Comprehension for Aphasia (RCBA-2) (LaPointe & Horner, 1998); and Aphasia Diagnostic Profile (ADP) (Helm-Estabrooks, 1992). A detailed description of each of these assessments is beyond the scope of this chapter; however, in order to demon-strate the range of language tasks covered by this type of assessment, further description of the components of the NCCEA, BNT, EFA-4, and RCBA-2 is provided below.

**Neurosensory Center Comprehensive Examination for Aphasia.** The NCCEA constitutes a detailed assessment of language functions, incorporating subtests that evaluate primary as well as high-level linguistic abilities. Principally designed for the assessment of aphasic individuals, the NCCEA is composed of 20 language tasks which specifically evaluate the status of immediate verbal memory, verbal production and fluency, receptive language, reading, writing, and basic articulatory proficiency. Overall, the assessment provides a descriptive versus taxonomic classification of linguistic abilities (Table 6–1 provides a description of individual NCCEA subtests).

**Boston Naming Test.** The BNT is a reliable measure of confrontation naming abilities and provides information about the effectiveness of semantic and phonemic cues in facilitating word retrieval. Subjects are instructed to name 60 constituent black-and-white line drawings of various objects ranging in frequency from *bed* to *abacus* and are permitted up to 20 seconds to respond to each item. A semantic cue is given if the subject provides a response that represents a misinterpretation of the target or a lack of recognition. A phonemic cue is provided subsequent to any failure to respond or incorrect response to a semantic cue, or in the event of recognition of the item but an inability to produce its name.

**Table 6–1.** Description of Individual Neurosensory Center Comprehensive Examination for Aphasia Subtests

1. Visual object naming (VN): requires subjects to verbally label objects presented on a tray.

2. Description of object use (DOU): requires subjects to provide a description of use pertaining to a range of presented objects following the probe, "What do you use this for?"

3. Tactile naming right hand (TNR): a range of objects are individually placed into the subject's right hand under a covering screen, and the subject is instructed to name the objects accordingly.

4. Tactile naming left hand (TNL): as per TNR; however, objects are placed in left hand.

5. Sentence repetition (SR): requires subjects to repeat spoken sentences of increasing length but of minimal grammatical complexity.

6. Repetition of digits (REPD): requires subjects to repeat a series of spoken digit strings ranging from three to seven numbers.

7. Reversal of digits (REVD): subjects are instructed to reverse a series of spoken digit strings ranging from three to seven numbers.

8. Phonemic fluency (WF): requires subjects to generate as many words as possible beginning with the letters F, A, and S, each within 60-s intervals.

9. Sentence construction (SC): subjects are instructed to produce grammatically correct sentences incorporating two or three stimulus words provided by the examiner.

10. Object identification by name (IDNAME): subjects are instructed to point to a range of objects on command.

11. Token (TT): subjects are required to point to or move a number of colored tokens relative to a series of spoken instructions of increasing length and grammatical complexity.

12. Oral reading of names (ORNAME): subjects are instructed to read object names from a series of flash cards.

13. Oral reading of sentences (ORSENT): subjects are instructed to read sentences of increasing difficulty extracted from the token test, from a series of flash cards.

14. Reading names for meaning (RNM): typically administered after subtest 12 (ORNAME), subjects are required to point to range of objects corresponding to written names on a series of flash cards.

15. Reading sentences for meaning (RSM): typically administered after subtest 13 (ORSENT), subjects are required to follow simple commands written on a series of flash cards.

16. Visual graphic naming (VGN: subjects are instructed to write the names of a range of presented objects.

17. Written naming (WN): relates to performance on the VGN task. Items are scored according to accuracy of writing and spelling.

**Table 6–1.** *continued*

18. Writing to dictation (WD): subjects are required to write their name and two dictated sentences.

19. Writing to copy (WC): subjects are instructed to copy two sentences presented on flash cards.

20 Articulation (ART): subjects are required to repeat a series of real words and non-words containing a variety of consonant–vowel blends.

*Source:* From Spreen and Benton (1977).

**Examining for Aphasia-4.** Use the EFA-4 to identify the presence of acquired aphasia, determine the severity of symptoms and their impact on quality of life, target goals for treatment, and document progress during treatment.

The subtests include Visual Recognition, Auditory Recognition, Tactile Recognition, Auditory Verbal Comprehension, Silent Reading Comprehension, Nonverbal Tasks, Verbal Tasks, Meaningful Speech, and Meaningful Writing. Components of the test include: examiner's manual, picture book, 25 diagnostic-form examiner record booklets, 25 short-form examiner record booklets, 25 diagnostic-form response forms, 25 short-form response forms, 25 diagnostic summary forms, 25 personal history forms, and an object kit.

**Reading Comprehension for Aphasia.** The RCBA-2 provides a systematic evaluation of the nature and degree of reading impairment in adults with aphasia, including oral-reading comprehension, measures reading comprehension, and guides the direction and focus of the therapy. Presented in large, bold print materials, the RCBA-2 is individually administered in 30 minutes with 20 subtests covering single-word comprehension for visual confusions, auditory confusions, and semantic confusions; functional reading; synonyms; sentence comprehension; short paragraph comprehension; paragraphs; and morpho-syntactic reading with lexical controls. The test kit includes examiner's manual, stimulus picture book, supplementary picture books, 25 profile/summary forms, and storage box.

**Tests of High-Level Language Function.** Tests included in this category assess those aspects of language function most highly dependent on frontal lobe function and in so doing evaluate those processes that permit conscious and effective manipulation of the semantic system via the interaction of primary language, cognitive, and executive processes in the brain. Examples of tests of high-level language function commonly used by speech-language pathologists include: Test of Language Competence-Expanded Edition (TLC-E) (Wiig & Secord, 1989); the Word Test-Revised (TWT-R) (Huisingh, Barrett, Zachman, Blagden, & Orman, 1990); Wiig-Semel Test of Linguistic Concepts (WSTLC) (Wiig & Semel, 1974); and semantic fluency tasks. As these tests assess a different aspect of high-level language function, the major features of each are briefly summarized below.

**Test of Language Competence—Expanded Edition.** The TLC-E is an assessment of language proficiency and metalinguistic ability, consisting of a range of subtests which probe the semantic system, semantic-syntactic interfaces, and pragmatics. Designed and standardized on two levels (i.e., Level 1: children 5 to 9 years; Level 2: pre-adolescents and adolescents aged 9 to 18+ years), the TLC-E assesses language competence by way of complex tasks that demand divergent language production, cognitive-linguistic flexibility, and planning for production. Subtests included in the TLC-E Level 2 include: Ambiguous Sentences (AS); Listening Comprehension: Making Inferences (MI); Oral Expression: Recreating Sentences (RS); Figurative Language (FL); and Remembering Word Pairs (RWP) subtests.

The AS subtest assesses the ability to identify and interpret the alternative meanings of lexical and structural ambiguities. Lexically, ambiguous sentences contain lexical elements with more than one possible meaning (e.g., *He bought the glasses*, where *glasses* may refer to *eyeglasses* or *drinking glasses*). Structural ambiguities may be classified as either surface or deep subtypes. Surface structure level ambiguities contain adjacent words that may be grouped in two or more distinct ways (e.g., *Mary likes small dogs and cats*, where *small dogs and cats* may refer to *all small dogs* and *small cats* or rather *small dogs* and *cats in general* [regardless of size]). Deep structure level ambiguities contain more than one logical relationship between words and phrases (e.g., *The turkey is ready to eat*, where the *turkey* may *be ready to eat something* or *ready to be eaten*). Subjects are presented with a series of ambiguous sentences in both spoken and written form and instructed to provide two distinct interpretations for each item. Responses are scored quantitatively according to essential meaning criteria.

The MI subtest assesses a client's ability to utilize causal relationships or chains in short paragraphs to make logical inferences. Clients are provided with a series of paired propositions including a lead-in (e.g., *Jack went to a Mexican restaurant*) and concluding sentence (e.g., *He left without giving a tip*). On the basis of this information they are then instructed to make logical inferences pertaining to the event chain, by selecting two plausible intervening clauses from four possible choices (e.g., (a) *The restaurant closed when he arrived*, (b) *He only had enough money to pay for the meal*, (c) *The food and service were excellent*, or (d) *He was dissatisfied with the service*). All test stimuli are provided in spoken as well as written form. The correct responses for the above example would be (b) and (d).

The RS subtest evaluates the ability to formulate grammatically complete sentences utilizing key semantic elements within defined contexts. Clients are provided with a situational context (e.g., *At the ice cream store*) and three words (e.g., *some, and, get*) in spoken and written/pictorial form, and are instructed to generate a complete sentence that reflects the relevant situational context, utilizing all three words. Responses are scored according to holistic scoring rules pertaining to semantic, syntactic, and pragmatic accuracy, as well as the number of target words successfully used.

The FL subtest evaluates the ability to interpret metaphorical expressions and to correlate structurally related metaphors according to shared meanings. Clients are provided with a series of metaphorical expressions (e.g., *She sure casts a spell over me*) accompanied by defined situational contexts (e.g., *A boy talking about a girl at a school dance*), and are instructed to provide a novel verbal interpretation of the metaphor. Once clients have explained the metaphor in their own words, they are instructed to identify a match for the sample metaphor from four possible choices. Response choices include: a metaphoric match (e.g., *She is totally bewitching to me*), an oppositional foil (e.g., *I am out from under her spell*), a literal foil (e.g., *She spells much better than I*) and a nonrelated foil (e.g., *In her life, every day is Halloween*). All test stimuli are presented in spoken as well as written form. Metaphorical explanations are recorded verbatim and scored according to specified interpretation rules. The final score represents a composite of the verbal interpretation score and the matched selection score.

The RWP supplemental subtest assesses the ability to recall paired word associates. Associations are classified as one of four possible categories, including: paradigmatic (e.g., *coat–sock*), spatial (e.g., *plane–cloud*), temporal (e.g., *moon–bed*), and unrelated (e.g., *antler–egg*). Clients are provided with two presentations (i.e., elicitation lists A and B) of 16 spoken word pairs considered to be representative of common and familiar vocabulary. Subsequent to the oral presentation of each elicitation list, the examiner provides one of the words from each pair. Clients are then instructed to recall its associate. The sum of correctly recalled pairs relative to elicitations list A and B represents the total score.

**The Word Test-Revised.** The Word Test-Revised (TWT-R) represents an assessment of expressive vocabulary and semantics, originally designed for use with the school-age child. TWT-R specifically probes the ability to identify and express critical semantic features of the lexicon by way of tasks that involve categorization, definition, verbal reasoning, and lexical selection. Subtests of TWT-R include: Associations (ASS), Synonyms (SYN), Semantic Absurdities (SEMAB), Antonyms (ANT), Definitions (DEF), and Multiple Definitions (MULDEF).

The ASS subtest requires clients to identify a semantically unrelated word within a group of four spoken words and to provide an explanation for the selected word in relation to the category of semantically related words. For example, from the group of words *knee, shoulder, bracelet*, and *ankle* the word *bracelet* is considered semantically unrelated because it is not a body part. Responses are scored according to word choices as well as criteria pertaining to acceptable and unacceptable explanations.

The SYN subtest requires clients to generate synonyms for verbally presented stimuli. Answers are again scored in reference to acceptable and unacceptable response criteria. For example, in response to the stimulus *donate*, acceptable responses include words with similar sets of semantic features such as *give/contribute*, whereas unacceptable responses include *offer/fund*.

The SEMAB subtest evaluates a client's ability to identify and repair semantic incongruities. Clients are presented orally with a series of semantically absurd sentences (e.g., *My grandfather is the youngest person in my family*) and instructed to repair the evident incongruity by generating a semantically appropriate sentence. Scoring is again based upon acceptable response criteria. Acceptable responses demand the simultaneous identification of the resident semantic incongruity, the replacement of inappropriate with appropriate vocabulary and the maintenance of the integrity of essential elements within the generated sentence (e.g., *My grandfather is the oldest person in my family*). Incorrect repairs (e.g., *My grandfather is the biggest person in my family*), explanation of the semantic absurdity despite prompting (e.g., *My grandfather can't possibly be the youngest person in my family*), or semantic negation (e.g., *My grandfather is not the youngest person in my family*) are all classified as unacceptable responses.

The ANT subtest requires clients to generate antonyms for verbally presented stimuli. Answers are scored in reference to acceptable and unacceptable response criteria. In response to stimulus *first*, *last* would be classified as an acceptable response as it encapsulates reversible critical semantic dimensions of the stimulus word, whereas *second* would be classified as an unacceptable response.

The DEF subtest evaluates a client's ability to identify and describe the critical semantic features of a word. Subjects are provided with a series of stimulus words and instructed to explain their meaning. Answers are again scored according to acceptable and unacceptable response criteria, in relation to specific critical semantic elements. For example, in providing a definition of the word *house*, the attributes *person + lives* are defined as critical semantic elements. *Where my family lives* therefore, would be classified as a complete/acceptable definition; however,

*Where you play* would be classified as an incomplete/unacceptable response.

The MULDEF subtest requires clients to provide two distinct meanings for a series of spoken homophonic words in relation to specific referents, probing flexibility in vocabulary use. Scoring is again based on acceptable and unacceptable response criteria. For example, germane definition references pertaining to the word *rock* include a *stone, music,* or an *action*. Acceptable task responses would include *It's a hard piece of earth, Music you play,* or *Moving back and forth. A hard thing* or *A thing you throw*, however, would be classified as unacceptable responses, as they fail to incorporate specified semantic referents.

**Wiig-Semel Test of Linguistic Concepts.** The WSTLC assesses the auditory comprehension of complex linguistic structures. Consisting of 50 yes/no questions, correct responses are contingent upon the undertaking of logical semantic operations in the manipulation of a range of complex linguistic relationships, including passive, comparative, temporal, spatial, and familial structures.

**Semantic Fluency Tasks.** Semantic fluency tasks involve having the client generate as many items as possible within specified semantic categories, in 60-second intervals. The semantic categories can include items such as exotic animals (e.g., lion, giraffe, etc.), tools (hammer, screwdriver, etc.), vegetables, etc. In some cases a semantic category may be restricted by specifying that named items must start with a particular letter (e.g., Name all the vegetables that start with the letter "c"—cabbage, carrots, cauliflower, etc.).

### Tests of Functional and Pragmatic Language Abilities

As indicated above, a primary limitation of tests of basic language function is that they primarily focus on the evaluation of language abilities from an impairment perspective (i.e., identify the presence of language deficits but fail to ascertain the impact of these deficits on the functional communication skills). Alternatives or adjuncts to the assessments outlined above include measures of communication activity limitation and participation restriction. Assessments of communication activity limitation encompass measures of functional and pragmatic communication abilities, which enable the evaluation of a client's ability to plan, deliver, and understand communication content within a range of interactive contexts. Pragmatic assessments typically appraise the ability to use language within natural contexts, including knowledge of language structure, knowledge of the environment and social rules, as well as the ability to adapt to changing environmental demands (Penn, 1999). In contrast, functional communication assessments largely aim to evaluate the quality of communication attempts (Manochiopining, Sheard, & Reed, 1992), or the impact of communication disorders on social and vocational roles, otherwise referred to as participation restrictions. Although a more in-depth discussion of these assessment tools is beyond the scope of this chapter, the incorporation of such measures is considered critical to any thorough clinical evaluation of language dysfunction, as opposed to an exclusive impairment-driven approach. The reader is referred to Table 6–2 for some suggested functional and prag-

matic assessments that may be applied in the management of aphasia and related neurologic language disorders. In recent years several scales that aim to evaluate quality of life and burden for aphasic individuals and close relatives (e.g., spouses) have been developed including the Burden of Stroke Scale (Doyle, 2002) and the Quality of Communicative Life Scale (Paul, Frattali, Holland, Thompson, Caperton, & Slater, 2004).

## Treatment of Language Impairments

Communication has been described as essential to all activities of daily living and critical to maintaining psychosocial well-being and positive quality of life. Akin to any communication deficit, the efficacious treatment of language disorders associated with movement disorders relies on comprehensive assessment at impairment, activity, and participation levels. On the basis of these findings, appropriate therapeutic goals and treatment programs can then be developed.

A range of treatment approaches, largely adopted from the school of cognitive neuropsychology, can be applied to the rehabilitation of language disorders associated with movement disorders, including restorative, compensatory, and behavioral treatment approaches.

### Restorative Treatment Approaches

Restorative approaches operate on the premise that the repetitive undertaking of specific exercises which train particular neuronal circuits will improve functional abilities as a consequence of

**Table 6–2.** Suggested Functional and Pragmatic Communication Assessments That Can Be Applied to the Management of Subcortical Language Disorders

| *Functional Assessments* | |
| --- | --- |
| Functional Communication Profile | (Sarno, 1975) |
| Everyday Communication Needs Assessment (ECNA) | (Worrall, 1999) |
| Functional Assessment of Communication Skills for Adults (ASHA FACS) | (Frattali, Thompson, Holland. Wohl, & Ferketic, 1995) |
| Communicative Effectiveness Index (CETI) | (Lomas, Pickard, Betser, Elbard, Finlayson, & Zoghaib, 1989) |
| Communicative Adequacy in Daily Situations | (Clark & White, 1995) |
| The Communication Profile | (Payne, 1994) |
| *Pragmatic Assessments* | |
| The Profile of Communicative Appropriateness | (Penn, 1985) |
| The Edinburgh Functional Communication Profile (revised) | (Wirz, Skinner, & Dean, 1990) |
| Communicative Abilities in Daily Living (CADL) – Revised | (Holland, Frattali, & Fromm, 1999) |

neuronal growth. In this manner, cognitive skills are re-established within the context of their premorbid status.

In applying this approach, specific linguistic deficits are determined by psychometric/impairment-based assessment and rehabilitation programs implemented involving the repeated execution of structured tasks which target areas of deficit. In relation to language rehabilitation, such tasks may involve: lexical-semantic processing exercises (e.g., identifying synonyms and antonyms, defining words according to semantic criteria, categorization tasks); complex comprehension exercises (e.g., following instructions of increasing complexity, story retelling, defining multiple meaning words); or word retrieval exercises (e.g., word association tasks, synonym and antonym generation).

Limitations of this approach, however, exist and include a potential difficulty for some patients to generalize skills taught during structured clinical tasks to real-world situations, and may be related to an incomplete understanding of the relationship between the targeted deficit and the training task utilized. It has been suggested that the modification of such tasks to include functionally relevant stimuli on an individual basis may alleviate this downfall to some extent, as would combining this approach with the development of compensatory strategies.

### Compensatory and Behavioral Treatment Approaches

Compensatory approaches operate on the premise that function cannot be restored once lost. Alternatively, skills and strategies are developed in order to establish functional competence. Behavioral treatment approaches adopt behavior modification techniques which aim to reinforce desired behaviors and to extinguish undesirable behaviors, or to positively reinforce the learning of new skills. In applying compensatory approaches, patients are taught self-initiated methods by which to overcome language deficits such as the use of aids (e.g., notebooks containing word cues in the case of word-finding difficulties) and external cues (e.g., requests for repetition of information in the case of comprehension deficits), with a view to automatization over time. Functional skills training may entail activity-based tasks within relevant communicative environments (e.g., telephone answering routines, role playing, direct instructions and scripting, fading of cues). Functional skills training may also extend to environmental manipulation techniques, whereby the patient's communicative environment is modified in order to maximize communicative success (e.g., providing communication strategies for potential communication partners, such as allowing increased

time for a response or reducing environmental distractions to enhance comprehension).

## References

Barlow, S. M. (1998). The effects of postero-ventral pallidotomy on force and speech aerodynamic in Parkinson's disease. In M. P. Cannito, K. M. Yorkston, & D. R. Beukelman (Eds.), *Neuromotor speech disorders: Nature, assessment and management*. Baltimore, MD: Brookes.

Berry, W. R., & Goshorn, E. L. (1983). Immediate visual feedback in the treatment of ataxic dysarthria: A case study. In W. R. Berry (Ed.), *Clinical dysarthria* (pp. 253–265). San Diego, CA: College-Hill Press.

Beukelman, D. R. (1983). Treatment of hyperkinetic dysarthria. In W. H. Perkins (Ed.), *Current therapy of communication disorders: Dysarthria and apraxia* (pp. 101–103). New York, NY: Thieme-Stratton.

Beukelman, D. R., & Yorkston, K. M. (1977). A communication system for the severely dysarthric speaker with an intact language system. *Journal of Speech and Hearing Disorders, 42*, 265–270.

Beukelman, D. R., Yorkston, K. M., & Tice, B. (1988). *Pacer/Tally.* Tucson, AZ: Communication Skill Builders.

Bougle, R., Ryalls, J., & Le Dorze, G. (1995). Improving fundamental frequency modulation in head trauma patients: A preliminary comparison of speech-language therapy conducted with and without IBM's Speech Viewer. *Folia Phoniatrica et Logopaedica, 47*, 24–32.

Brin, M. F. (1998). Pharmacological treatment of movement disorders. In I. Germano (Ed.), *Neurosurgical treatment of movement disorders* (pp. 83–104). Park Ridge, IL: Thieme.

Caligiuri, M. P., & Murry, T. (1983). The use of visual feedback to enhance prosodic control in dysarthria. In W. R. Berry

(Ed.), *Clinical dysarthrias* (pp. 267–282). San Diego, CA: College-Hill Press.

Cannito, M. P., & Marquardt, T. P. (1997). Ataxic dysarthria. In M. R. McNeil (Ed.), *Clinical management of sensorimotor speech disorders.* New York, NY: Thieme.

Cavallo, S. A., & Baken, R. J. (1985). Prephonatory laryngeal and chest wall dynamics. *Journal of Speech and Hearing Research, 28,* 79–87.

Clark, L. W., & White, K. (1995). Nature and efficiency of communication management in Alzheimer's disease. In R. Lubinski (Ed.), *Dementia and communication* (pp. 238–256). San Diego, CA: Singular.

Darley, F. L., Aronson, A. E., & Brown, J. R. (1969a). Differential diagnostic patterns of dysarthria. *Journal of Speech and Hearing Research, 12,* 246–269.

Darley, F. L., Aronson, A. E., & Brown, J. R. (1969b). Clusters of deviant speech dimensions in the dysarthrias. *Journal of Speech and Hearing Research, 12,* 462–496.

Darley, F. L., Aronson, A. E., & Brown, J. R. (1975). *Motor speech disorders.* Philadelphia, PA: W. B. Saunders.

Doyle, P. J. (2002). Measuring health outcomes in stroke survivors. *Archives of Physical Medicine and Rehabilitation, 83*(12 Suppl. 2), S39–S43.

Duffy, J. R. (1995). *Motor speech disorders: Substrates, differential diagnosis and management.* Baltimore, MD: Mosby-Year Book.

Duffy, J. R. (2005a). *Motor speech disorders: Substrates, differential diagnosis and management.* St. Louis, MO: Elsevier Mosby.

Duffy, J. R. (2005b). *Motor speech disorders: Substrates, differential diagnosis, and management* (2nd ed.). St. Louis, MO: Elsevier Mosby.

Duffy, J. R., & Yorkston, K. M. (2003). Medical interventions for spasmodic dysphonia and some related conditions: A systematic review. *Journal of Medical Speech Language Pathology, 11,* ix.

Enderby, P. (1983). *Frenchay dysarthria assessment.* San Diego, CA: College-Hill Press.

Frattali, C., Thompson, D., Holland, A., Wohl, C., & Ferketic, M. (1995). *American Speech-Language and Hearing Association Functional Assessment of Communication Skills for Adults.* Rockville, MD: American Speech-Language Hearing Association.

Frucht, S. J. (2003). Myoclonus. In J. H. Noseworthy (Ed.), *Neurological therapeutics: Principles and practice* (Vol. 1, pp. 2913–2920). New York, NY: Martin Dunitz.

Fudge, R. C., Thailer, S. A., & Alpert, M. (1991). The effects of electromyographic feedback training on suppression of the oral-lingual movements associated with tardive dyskinesia. *Biofeedback and Self-Regulation, 16,* 117–129.

Goodglass, H., Kaplan, E., & Barresi, B. (2001). *The Boston Diagnostic Aphasia Examination* (3rd ed.). Philadelphia, PA: Lippincott Williams & Wilkins.

Helm, N. A. (1979). Management of palilalia with a pacing board. *Journal of Speech and Hearing Disorders, 44,* 350–353.

Helm-Estabrooks, N. (1992). *Aphasia Diagnostic Profile.* Chicago, IL: Riverside Press.

Holland, A., Frattali, C., & Fromm, D. (1999). *Communicative Activities of Daily Living.* Austin, TX: Pro-Ed.

Huisingh, R., Barrett, M., Zachman, L., Blagden, C., & Orman, J. (1990). *The Word Test-Revised: A test of expressive vocabulary and semantics.* Illinois, IL: Linguisystems.

Kaplan, E., Goodglass, H., & Weintraub, S. (1983). *Boston Naming Test.* Philadelphia, PA: Lippincott Williams & Wilkins.

Kelly, P. J., Ahlskog, J. E., Goerss, S. J., Daube, J. R., Duffy, J. R., & Kall, B. A. (1987). Computer-assisted stereotactic ventralis lateralis thalamotomy with microelectrode recording control in patients with Parkinson's disease. *Mayo Clinic Proceedings, 62,* 655–664.

Kent, R. (1989). Toward phonetic intelligibility testing in dysarthria. *Journal of Speech and Hearing Disorders, 54,* 482.

Kertesz, A. (1982). *The Western Aphasia Battery.* New York, NY: Grune & Stratton.

Koller, W., Graner, D., & Mlcoch, A. (2001). Essential voice tremor: Treatment with propranolol. *Neurology, 35,* 106–108.

Kotby, M. N. (1995). *The accent method of voice therapy*. San Diego, CA: Singular.

LaBlance, G. R., & Rutherford, D. R. (1991). Respiratory dynamics and speech intelligibility in dysarthric speakers with generalised dystonia. *Journal of Communication Disorders, 24,* 141–156.

LaPointe, L. L., & Eisenson, J. (2008). *Examining for Aphasia-4*. Austin, TX: Pro-Ed.

LaPointe, L. L., & Horner, J. (1998). *Reading Comprehension for Aphasia-2*. Austin, TX: Pro-Ed.

Limousin, P., Krack, P., Pollak, P., Benazzouz, A., Ardouin, C. M., Hoffman, D., & Benabid, A. L. (1998). Electrical stimulation of the subthalamic nucleus in advanced Parkinson's disease. *New England Journal of Medicine, 339*(16), 1105–1111.

Lomas, J., Pickard, L., Betser, S., Elbard, H., Finlayson, A., & Zoghaib, C. (1989). The Communicative Effectiveness Index: Development and psychometric evaluation of a functional communication measure for adult aphasia. *Journal of Speech and Hearing Disorders, 54,* 113–224.

Ludlow, C. L., Sedora, S. E., & Fujita, M. (1989). Inspiratory speech with respiratory dystonia. In N. Helm-Estabrooks, & J. L. Aten (Eds.), *Difficult diagnoses in communication disorders*. Boston, MA: College-Hill.

Manochiopining, S., Sheard, C., & Reed, V. A. (1992). Pragmatic assessment in adult aphasia: A clinical review. *Aphasiology, 6,* 519–534.

Manifold, J., & Murdoch, B. E. (1993). Speech breathing in young adults: Effect of body type. *Journal of Speech and Hearing Research, 36,* 657–671.

Maruska, K. G., Smit, A. B., Koller, W. C., & Garcia, J. M. (2000). Sentence production in Parkinson's disease treated with deep brain stimulation and medication. *Journal of Medical Speech Language Pathology, 8,* 265–270.

McFarlane, S. C., Hoh-Romeo, T. L., & Lavorato, A. S. (1991). Unilateral vocal fold paralysis: Perceived vocal quality following three methods of treatment.

*American Journal of Speech Language Pathology, 1,* 45–48.

Murdoch, B. E., Chenery, H. J., Stokes, P., & Hardcastle, W. J. (1991). Respiratory kinematics in speakers with cerebellar disease. *Journal of Speech and Hearing Research, 34,* 768–780.

Murdoch, B. E., & Theodoros, D. G. (1998). Ataxic dysarthria. In B. E. Murdoch (Ed.), *Dysarthria: A physiological approach to assessment and treatment* (pp. 242–265). Cheltenham, UK: Stanley Thornes.

Murray, T. (1983). Treatment of ataxic dysarthria. In W. H. Perkins (Ed.), *Current therapy of communication disorders: Dysarthria and apraxia* (pp. 79–89). New York, NY: Thieme-Stratton.

Murray, T., & Woodson, G. (1995). Combined-modality treatment of adductor spasmodic dysphonia with botulinum toxin and voice therapy. *Journal of Voice, 9,* 460–465.

Paul, D., Frattali, C., Holland, A., Thompson, C., Caperton, C., & Slater, S. (2004). *Quality of communication life scale*. Rockville, MD: American Speech-Language Hearing Association.

Payne, J. C. (1994). *Communication Profile: A functional skills survey*. Tucson, AZ: Communication Skill Builders.

Penn, C. (1985). The Profile of Communicative Appropriateness: A clinical tool for the assessment of pragmatics. *South African Journal of Communication Disorders, 32,* 18–23.

Penn, C. (1999). Pragmatic assessment and therapy for persons with brain damage: What have clinicians gleaned in two decades. *Brain and Language, 68,* 535–552.

Pinto, S., Ozsancak, C., Tripoliti, E., Thobois, S., Limousin Dowsey, P., & Auzou, P. (2004). Treatments for dysarthria in Parkinson's disease. *Lancet Neurology, 3,* 547–556.

Porch, B. E. (1967). *Porch Index of Communicative Ability*. Palo Alto, CA: Consulting Psychologists Press.

Rosenbek, J. C., & LaPointe, L. L. (1978). The dysarthrias: Description, diagnosis, and treatment. In D. Johns (Ed.), *Clinical management of neurogenic communication disorders* (pp. 97–152). Boston, MA: Little Brown & Co.

Rosenfeld, D. B. (1991). Pharmacologic approaches to speech motor disorders. In D. Vogel, & M. P. Cannito (Eds.), *Treating disordered speech motor control: For clinicians by clinicians* (pp. 111–152). Austin, TX: Pro-Ed.

Rousseaux, M., Krystkowiak, P., Kozlowski, O., Ozsancak, C., Blond, S., & Destée, A. (2004). Effects of subthalamic nucleus stimulation on parkinsonian dysarthria and speech intelligibility. *Journal of Neurology, 251,* 327–334.

Rubow, R. T., Rosenbek, J. C., Collins, M. J., & Celesia, G. C. (1984). Reduction of hemifacial spasm and dysarthria following EMG biofeedback. *Journal of Speech and Hearing Disorders, 49,* 26–33.

Sarno, M. T. (1975). *The Functional Communication Profile.* New York, NY: NYU Medical Center, Institute of Rehabilitation Medicine.

Schulz, G., Peterson, C. M., Sapienza, M., Greer, M., & Friedman, W. (1999). Voice and speech characteristics of persons with Parkinson's disease pre- and post-pallidotomy surgery: Preliminary findings. *Journal of Speech Language and Hearing Research, 42,* 1176–1194.

Scott, R. B., Gregory, R., Hines, N., Carroll, C., Hyman, N., Papanasstasiou, V., . . . Aziz, T. (1998). Neuropsychological, neurological and functional outcome following pallidotomy for Parkinson's disease: a consecutive series of eight simultaneous bilateral and twelve unilateral procedures. *Brain, 121,* 659–675.

Shannon, K. M. (2000). Surgical treatment of Parkinson's disease. In C. H. Adler, & J. E. Ahlskog (Eds.), *Parkinson's disease and movement disorders: Diagnosis and treatment guidelines for the practicing physician* (pp. 185–196). New York, NY: Humana Press.

Sherman, R. A. (1979). Successful treatment of one case of tardive dyskinesia with electromyographic feedback from the masseter muscle. *Biofeedback and Self-Regulation, 4,* 367–370.

Solomon, N., & Hixon, T. (1993). Speech breathing in Parkinson's disease. *Journal of Speech and Hearing Research, 36,* 294–310.

Sperry, E. E., & Klich, R. J. (1992). Speech breathing in senescent and younger women during oral reading. *Journal of Speech and Hearing Research, 35,* 1246–1255.

Spreen, O., & Benton, A. L. (1977). *Neurosensory Center Comprehensive Examination for Aphasia.* Victoria, Australia: University of Victoria.

Theodoros, D. G., Ward, E. C., Murdoch, B. E., Silburn, P., & Lethlean, J. B. (2000). The impact of pallidotomy on motor speech function in Parkinson's disease. *Journal of Medical Speech Language Pathology, 8,* 315–322.

Tsui, J. K., Eisen, E., & Mak, J. (1985). A pilot study in the use of botulinum toxin in spasmodic torticollis. *Canadian Journal of Neurological Sciences, 12,* 31–316.

Uitti, R., Wharen, R., Duffy, J. A., Lucas, J. A., Schneider, S. L., Rippeth, J. D., . . . Atkinson, E. J. (2000). Unilateral pallidotomy for Parkinson's disease: Speech, motor, and neuropsychological outcome measurements. *Parkinsonism and Related Disorders, 6,* 133–143.

Varney, S. M., Demetroulakos, J., Fletcher, M., McQueen, W., & Hamilton, M. (1996). Palatal myoclonus: Treatment with *Clostridium botulinum* toxin injection. *Otolaryngology-Head and Neck Surgery, 114,* 317–320.

Wiig, E. H., & Secord, W. (1989). *Test of Language Competence-expanded edition.* New York, NY: Psychological Corporation.

Wiig, E. H., & Semel, E. (1974). Development of comprehension of logical grammatical sentences by grade school children. *Perceptual and Motor Skills, 38,* 171–176.

Wirz, S. L., Skinner, C., & Dean, E. (1990). *Revised Edinburgh Functional Communication Profile.* Tucson, AZ: Communication Skill Builders.

Worrall, L. (1999). *The Everyday Communication Needs Assessment*. London, UK: Winslow Press.

Yorkston, K. M. (1999). *Management of motor speech disorders in children and adults* (2nd ed.). Austin, TX: Pro-Ed.

Yorkston, K. M., & Beukelman, D. R. (1981a). *Assessment of Intelligibility of Dysarthric Speech*. Tigard, OR: CC Publications.

Yorkston, K. M., & Beukelman, D. R. (1981b). Ataxic dysarthria: Treatment sequences based on intelligibility and prosidic considerations. *Journal of Speech and Hearing Disorders, 46*, 398–404.

Yorkston, K. M., & Beukelman, D. R. (1996). *Sentence Intelligibility Test*. Lincoln, NE: Tice Technology Services.

Yorkston, K. M., Hammen, V. L., Beukelman, D. R., & Traynor, C. D. (1990). The effect of rate control on the intelligibility of naturalness of dysarthric speech. *Journal of Speech and Hearing Disorders, 55*, 550–560.

# 7

# Speech Impairments Associated with Movement Disorders: Neuromotor Control Systems

*BRUCE E. MURDOCH*

## Introduction

Movement disorders can be defined as neurologic syndromes in which there is either an excess of movement or a paucity of voluntary and automatic movements, unrelated to weakness or spasticity. The former are commonly referred to as hyperkinesias (excessive movements), dyskinesias (unnatural movements), or abnormal involuntary movements. Although the term "dyskinesias" is most frequently used, all three terms are interchangeable. The five major categories of dyskinesias include chorea, dystonia, myoclonus, tics, and tremor. The group of move-

ment disorders characterized by a paucity of movement are referred to as hypokinesias (decreased amplitude of movement) or alternatively as bradykinesia (slowness of movements) or akinesia (loss of movement). Parkinson disease is the most common cause of such paucity of movement with other hypokinetic disorders representing only a small portion of patients. Overall movement disorders can be conveniently divided into parkinsonism and all other types, with each of these two groups having approximately the same number of individuals.

By far the majority of movement disorders are associated with pathologic changes in the basal ganglia or their connections. There are some general exceptions to this general rule. Pathology of the cerebellum or its pathways typically results in impairment of coordination (asynergia, ataxia), misjudgment of distance (dysmetria), and intention tremor. Myoclonus and many forms of tremors do not appear to be related primarily to basal ganglia pathology and often arise elsewhere in the central nervous system, including the cerebral cortex (cortical reflex myoclonus), brainstem (cerebellar outflow tremor, reticular reflex myoclonus, rhythmic brainstem myoclonus such as palatal myoclonus), spinal cord (rhythmic segmental myoclonus), and cerebellum (progressive myoclonic ataxia). It is not known for certain which part of the brain is associated with tics, although the basal ganglia and the limbic structures have been implicated.

It is thought that many of the movement disorders that arise from disruption to the basal ganglia or cerebellum are the outcome of disrupted basal ganglia or cerebellar outputs to areas of the cerebral cortex involved in the control of movement. Models of basal ganglia—thalamocortical and cerebellocortical circuits therefore have become central to research and theoretical approaches aimed at understanding the role of the basal ganglia and cerebellum in speech motor functions. Consequently, central to any attempt to understand the role of these subcortical structures in speech motor control is a knowledge of their basic neuroanatomy. The following section aims to provide an update of the functional neuroanatomy of the basal ganglia and cerebellum necessary for understanding models of subcortical mechanisms in speech motor control and the neu-ropathologic basis of speech disorders seen in association with movement disorders.

## Functional Neuroanatomy of the Basal Ganglia and Cerebellum

### Basal Ganglia

Anatomically, the term "basal ganglia" refers to the deep gray matter nuclei within the cerebral hemispheres (telencephalon) which include the caudate nucleus, putamen, globus pallidus, and amygdala. Basic anatomy and discussion of functions of the basal ganglia have been introduced earlier in this book, but details of the impact of these structures on movement disorders will be described here. Physiologically and clinically, however, the basal ganglia represent a functional system of interconnected gray matter components which include the caudate nucleus, putamen, globus pallidus (GP) (which is divided into a lateral [external] part and a medial [internal] component, abbreviated GPe and GPi, respectively) in the cerebral hemispheres; the subthalamic nucleus (STN) (located in the diencephalon, the substantia nigra (composed of the substantia nigra pars compacta [SNc] and substantia nigra pars reticulata [SNr]) located in the mesencephalon; and the red nucleus also located in the mesencephalon. The caudate nucleus and putamen are collectively called the corpus striatum (striatocapsular region) or often abbreviated as the striatum. Collectively, the putamen and globus pallidus are often referred to as the lenticular (or lentiform) nucleus. The relative position of the basal ganglia to other structures within the cerebral hemispheres is shown in Figures 7–1 and 7–2.

The caudate nucleus is the most medial part of the basal ganglia. It is an elongated mass of gray matter that is bent over on itself and throughout its length follows the lateral ventricle. The nucleus is divided into a head, body, and tail (see Figure 7–1). The head of the caudate nucleus bulges into the anterior horn of the lateral ventricle and lies rostral to the thalamus. The body extends along the dorsolateral surface of the thalamus. The remainder of the caudate nucleus is drawn out into a highly arched tail that, conforming to the shape of the lateral ventricle, turns

into the temporal lobe and terminates in relation to the amygdaloid nucleus (see Figure 7–1). Throughout much of its extent, the caudate nucleus is separated from the lenticular nucleus by the internal capsule.

The lenticular nucleus is located in the midst of the cerebral white matter. Its shape is somewhat similar to that of a biconvex lens, hence the name lenticular or lentiform (see Figure 7–1). The largest portion of the lenticular nucleus is the putamen, which is a rather thick, convex mass located just lateral to the globus pallidus and internal capsule. Its lateral surface is separated from the cerebral cortex by the claustrum, the external capsule, and the extreme capsule (see Figure 7–2). The globus pallidus is the smaller and most medial part

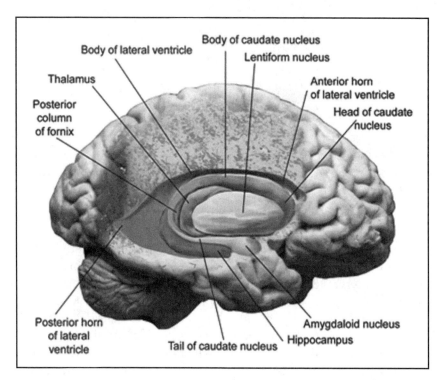

**FIGURE 7–1.** Lateral view of the right cerebral hemisphere dissected to show the position of the different basal ganglia. (From Murdoch, 2010)

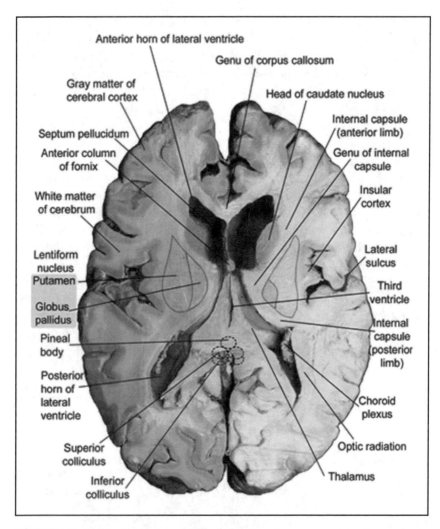

**FIGURE 7–2.** Horizontal section of the cerebrum as seen from above showing the relationship of the different basal ganglia. (From Murdoch, 2010)

of the lenticular nucleus and is subdivided into medial and lateral parts of a small band of white fibers called the medial medullary lamina.

Although midbrain structures, the STN and substantia nigra are functionally related to the basal ganglia. The STN is a small gray mass located inferiorly to the thalamus. It receives afferent fibers from the GPe, motor, premotor, and prefrontal cortex and thalamus and projects efferent fibers to both the internal and external segments of the globus pallidus as well as the substantia nigra. The substantia nigra is a gray matter mass located within the midbrain which contains dopaminergic neurons. It receives inputs from the cerebral cortex, globus pallidus, caudate nucleus, subthalamic nucleus, and other midbrain nuclei, and projects to the cerebral cortex, globus pallidus, red nucleus, subthalamic nucleus, thalamus, amygdaloid nucleus, reticular formation, and superior colliculus.

### Circuitry and Associated Neurotransmission Mechanisms

Although the connections of the basal ganglia are not yet fully understood, with new findings continuing to be made, the basic anatomy of the circuitry connecting these structures was clearly described by Alexander, DeLong, and Strick (1986). Essentially, according to their description, information originating in the cerebral cortex passes through the basal ganglia and returns via the thalamus to specific areas of the frontal lobe, this feedback circuit often being referred to as the cortico-striato-pallido-thalamo-cortical loop.

In general, the basal ganglia can be considered to be composed of a group of "input" structures (the caudate nucleus, putamen, and ventral striatum) that receive direct input essentially from areas of the cerebral cortex, and "output" structures (the internal segment of the GP [GPi], the SNr and the ventral pallidum) that project back to the cerebral cortex via the thalamus. Over the past two decades, notions of the organization of the basal ganglia, the thalamus, and connections with various cortical regions have been revised. Originally, the striatum was considered to serve primarily to integrate diverse inputs from the entire cerebral cortex and to "funnel" these influences via the ventrolateral thalamus to the primary motor cortex alone. Consistent with the view held at the time that they functioned primarily in the domain of motor control, the basal ganglia were thus seen as a mechanism for "funneling" information into the motor system. Based on recent research, it is now clear that output from the basal ganglia terminates in thalamic regions that gain access to a wider region of the frontal lobe than just the primary motor cortex. Rather, these subcortical nuclei appear to project to many or most of the same cortical areas that send efferents to them. Consequently, the original notion of the basal ganglia acting as a mechanism to "funnel" information to the motor cortex has been superseded by the view of the striatum as a "multi-lane throughway" which forms part of a series of multisegregated circuits connecting the cortex, the basal ganglia, and the thalamus (Alexander et al., 1986; Graybiel & Kimura, 1995; Middleton & Strick, 2000); thus, basal ganglia anatomy is characterized by their participation in multiple "loops" with the cerebral cortex each of which follows the basic route of cortex→striatum→globus pallidus/substantia nigra→thalamus→cortex in a unidirectional fashion.

Alexander et al. (1986) identified at least five separate, parallel cortico-basal ganglia circuits according to the specific region of the frontal lobe that serves as a target for their thalamocortical projections. One of these cortico-basal ganglia circuits projected to the skeletomotor areas of the frontal cortex while another projected to the oculomotor areas. The three remaining circuits projected to nonmotor areas of the frontal cortex, including the dorsolateral prefrontal area (area 46), the lateral orbitofrontal cortex (area 12), and the anterior cingulate/medial orbitofrontal cortices (areas 24 and 13) (Mink, 2007).

Importantly, these circuits appear to be, to a large extent, functionally segregated (Alexander et al., 1986; DeLong & Wichmann, 2007) suggesting that structural convergence and functional integration occur within rather than between each of the identified circuits. Given the segregated nature of the corticobasal ganglia circuits, collectively they may be viewed as having a unified role in modulating the operations of the entire frontal lobe, thereby influencing such diverse frontal lobe processes as motor activities, behavioral, cognitive, language, and even limbic processes. This anatomical arrangement, whereby the output from the basal ganglia gains access to multiple areas of the frontal lobe, including nonmotor areas, has profound consequences for the possible functional roles of the basal ganglia system and provides a basic neuroanatomic mechanism whereby these subcortical structures can influence aspects of behavior, cognition, and language, as well as motor function.

The corticobasal ganglia circuit that has received the greatest attention in the literature, and which is of greatest relevance to movement disorders associated with motor speech impairments, is the "skeletomotor circuit" (Alexander, Crutcher, & DeLong (1990) (Figure 7–3). At the cortical level this circuit comprises the pre- and postcentral sensorimotor areas, while at the subcortical level it comprises sensorimotor areas in the basal ganglia and the ventral anterior and ventrolateral thalamus. Cortical projections of the motor circuit terminate largely in the putamen. According to current models of the organization of the basal ganglia, putaminal output is directed over two separate projection systems, the so-called direct and indirect pathways. The direct pathway originates from striatal neurons that contain gamma-aminobutyric acid (GABA) plus the peptide substance P and/or dynorphin and conveys activity from the NS monosynaptically to the GPi and SNr. In contrast, the indirect pathway arises from striatal neurons that contain GABA and enkephalin and conveys activity to the GPi and SNr polysynaptically via a sequence of connections involving the external segment of the globus pallidus (GPe) and the STN. In both cases the returning thalamocortical connections seem to reach precisely the regions of the frontal cortex that contribute as inputs to the NS (Strick, Dunn, & Picard, 1995). A diagrammatic representation of the basic circuitry of the basal ganglia is presented in Figure 7–3.

Imbalance between the activity in the direct and indirect pathways and the resulting alterations in the activity of the GPi and SNr are thought to account for the hypo- and hyperkinetic features of basal ganglia disorders, including hypo- and hyperkinetic dysarthria. The possible roles of the direct and indirect pathways to the development of hypo- and hyperkinetic movement disorders are discussed later. It is noteworthy, however, that based on the findings of single-axon training studies in primates, the simple dual (direct/indirect) division of basal ganglia circuitry has recently been challenged (Parent, Lévesque, & Parent, 2001). Using a single-cell-labeling procedure, Parent et al. (2001) showed that striatal axons are highly collateralized, suggesting that the basal ganglia should not be regarded as a simple dual (direct/indirect) neuronal system, but rather should be viewed as a widely distributed network.

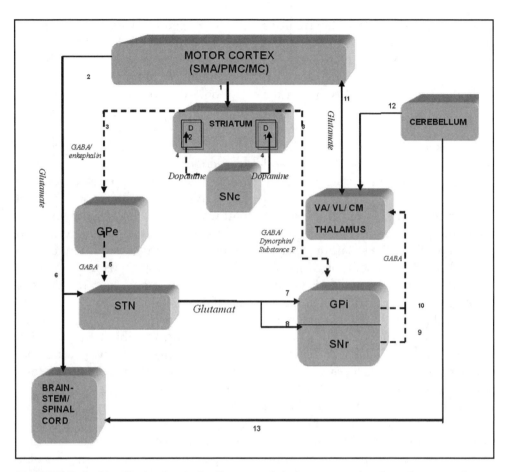

**FIGURE 7–3.** Modified schematic diagram of skeletomotor circuit under normal conditions based on DeLong (1990) and Mink (2007). **SMA**, supplementary motor area; **PMC**, premotor cortex; **MC**, motor cortex; **D1**, striatal output neuron receptor type D1; **D2**, striatal output receptor type D2; **SNc**, substantia nigra compacta; **GPe**, globus pallidus externus; **STN**, subthalamic nucleus; **GPi**, globus pallidus internus; **SNr**, substantia nigra reticulata; **VA**, ventral anterior nucleus of thalamus; **VL**, ventral lateral nucleus of thalamus; **CM**, centrum medianum. *Solid arrow* indicates excitatory pathway; *dashed arrow* indicates inhibitory pathway. *1* corticostriatal pathway; *2* corticobulbar and corticospinal pathways; *3* striatopallidal pathways; *4* nigrostriatal pathways; *5* pallidosubthalamic pathway, *6* corticosubthalamic pathway; *7* subthalamopallidal pathway; *8* subthalamonigral pathway; *9* nigrothalamic pathway; *10* pallidothalamic pathway; *11* thalamocortical and corticothalamic pathways; *12* cerebellothalamic pathway; *13* cerebellorubral pathway. Glutamate, GABA (gamma-amino butyric acid), enkephalin, dynorphin, and substance P are all active neurotransmitters. (From Murdoch, 2010)

The nature of the neurotransmitters utilized by the neurons that comprise the corticobasal ganglia circuits provides further insight as to the possible functional roles of these circuits. The cerebral cortex is connected to the striatum by way of excitatory neurons that use glutamate as a transmitter. In contrast, as noted above, the neurons connecting the striatum to the global pallidus use GABA, which exerts an inhibitory effect on targets in the medial and lateral globus pallidus and in the SNr, though these neurons also contain neuropeptides such as substance P and enkephalin. The globus pallidus neurons are themselves inhibitory and consequently there are two inhibitory synapses in series between the striatum and the thalamus. In effect these two inhibitory synapses in series act as an excitation. When the striatum is active the globus pallidus neurons disinhibit the thalamocortical projection via the direct pathway and thus presumably facilitate the initiation of movement (or some other frontal lobe activity). Briefly, the suggested mechanism for this initiation of movement is as follows: Corticostriatal activation of the direct pathway produces a GABA-mediated inhibition of GPi/SNr neurons, leading in turn to disinhibition of their thalamic target, thereby facilitating the thalamic projection to the precentral motor fields. The overall effect of this sequence is positive feedback for cortically initiated movements. Suppression of unwanted movements (activities) probably ensues through inhibition of the thalamocortical projections via the indirect pathway (Wichmann, Bergman, & DeLong, 1994) because projections from the STN to the GPi are excitatory. Put simply, corticostriatal stimulation of the GABA-enkephalin neurons in the indirect pathway inhibits the GPi and secondarily facilitates the STN. The latter results in increased excitatory drive onto the GPi/SNr which respond by increasing their output, thereby further inhibiting their thalamic and brainstem targets. The overall effect of this sequence is to provide negative feedback for movement, thereby acting to inhibit undesired movements or to signal a halt to movements in progress.

Both excitatory and inhibitory influences converge on the globus pallidus and their balance probably determines the activity in the thalamocortical projections. The most important neuromodulator of the balance between the activity of the direct and indirect pathways at the level of the striatum is dopamine. The dopaminergic input to the striatum is provided by the nigrostriatal projections from the SNc. Release of dopamine from terminals of the nigrostriatal projections appears to facilitate transmission over the direct pathway and to inhibit transmission over the indirect pathway via dopamine subtype $D_1$ and $D_2$ receptors, respectively (see Figure 7–3) (Gerfen, 1995). Consequently, reduced basal ganglia output from the GPi/SNr leading to increased activity of thalamocortical projection neurons is the outcome of striatal dopamine release. The role of abnormal striatal dopamine release in the occurrence of hypo- and hyperkinetic speech disorders is discussed in the section dealing with subcortical models of hypo- and hyperkinetic dysarthria.

## Cerebellum

The cerebellum is located in a dorsal position to the pons and medulla oblongata and is composed of two large cerebellar hemispheres which are connected by a mid-portion called the vermis. As in the case of the cerebral hemispheres, the cerebellar hemispheres are covered by a layer of gray matter of cortex. Unlike the cerebral cortex, however, the cerebellar cortex tends to be uniform in structure throughout its extent. The cerebellar cortex is highly folded into thin transverse folds or folia. A series of deep and definite fissures divides the cerebellum into a number of lobes. Although the lobe system of the cerebellum is classified differently by different authors, three lobes are commonly recognized: anterior, posterior, and flocculonodular (Figure 7–4). The posterior lobe, also referred to as the neocerebellum, lies between the other two lobes and is the largest portion of the cerebellum. Phylogenetically it is the newest portion of the cerebellum and is most concerned with the regulation of voluntary move-ments. In particular it plays an essential role in the coordination of phasic movements and is the most important part of the cerebellum for the coordination of speech movements.

The central core of the cerebellum, like that of the cerebral hemispheres, is made up of white matter. Located within the white matter, on either side of the midline, are four gray masses called the cerebellar or deep nuclei. These are the dentate nucleus, the globose and emboliform nuclei (collectively referred to as the interpositus), and the fastigial nucleus. The majority of the Purkinje cell axons, which carry impulses away from the cerebellar cortex, terminate in these nuclei. These structures can be appreciated in Figure 7–5.

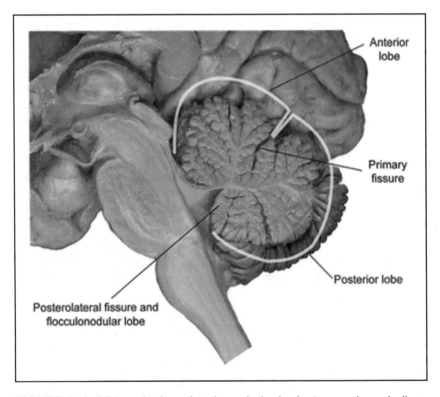

**FIGURE 7–4.** Mid-sagittal section through the brainstem and cerebellum. (From Murdoch, 2010)

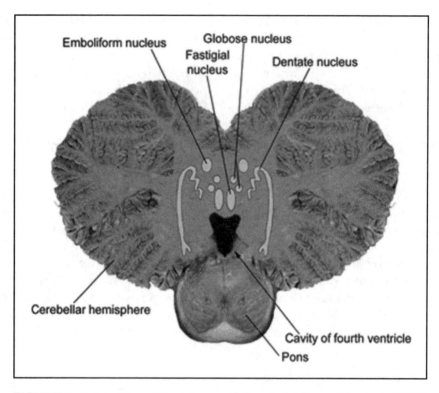

**FIGURE 7–5.** Location of the intracerebellar nuclei. (From Murdoch, 2010)

In order to be able to perform its primary function of synergistic coordination of muscular activity, the cerebellum requires extensive connections with other parts of the nervous system. Axonal inputs and outputs enter and exit the cerebellum via three fiber bundles or peduncles: superior, middle, and inferior (Figure 7–6). Damage to the pathways making up these connections can cause cerebellar dysfunction and possible ataxic dysarthria in the same way as damage to the cerebellum itself. Briefly, the cerebellum functions in part by comparing input from the motor cortex with information concerning the momentary status of muscle contraction, degree of tension of the muscle tendons, positions of parts of the body, and forces acting on the surfaces of the body originating from muscle spindles, Golgi tendon organs, and so forth, and then sending appropriate messages back to the motor cortex to ensure smooth, coordinated muscle function. Consequently, the cerebellum requires input from the motor cortex, muscle and joint receptors, and receptors in the internal ear detecting changes in the position and rate of rotation in the head, skin receptors, and so forth. Conversely, pathways carrying signals from the cerebellum back to the cortex are also required to complete the cerebrocerebellar loop.

The traditional view of cerebrocerebellar loops is that they receive information from widespread cortical areas in the frontal, parietal, and temporal lobes with the major afferent pathway connecting the cerebral cortex and the cerebellum being the corticopontine–

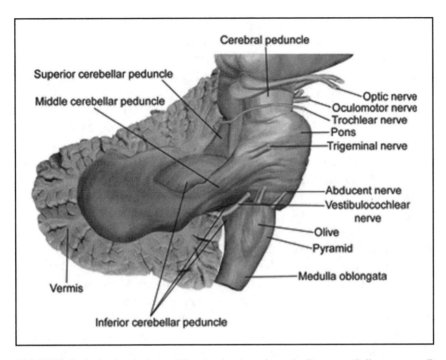

Cerebral peduncle

Superior cerebellar peduncle

Middle cerebellar peduncle

Optic nerve
Oculomotor nerve
Trochlear nerve
Pons
Trigeminal nerve

Abducent nerve
Vestibulocochlear nerve

Olive
Pyramid

Medulla oblongata

Vermis

Inferior cerebellar peduncle

**FIGURE 7–6.** Lateral view of the brainstem (cerebellum partially removed) showing the three cerebellar peduncles connecting the cerebellum to the brainstem. (From Murdoch, 2010)

cerebellar pathway. This pathway originates primarily from the motor cortex and projects to the ipsilateral pontine nuclei, from where secondary fibers project mainly to the cortex of the neocerebellum. Other afferent pathways project to the cerebellum from structures in the brainstem such as the olive (olivocerebellar tracts), the red nucleus (rubrocerebellar tracts), the reticular formation (reticulocerebellar tract), the midbrain (tectocerebellar tract) and the cuneate nucleus (cuneocerebellar tract), as well as from the spinal cord (spinocerebellar tracts).

Efferent pathways from the cerebellum originate almost entirely from the deep nuclei and project to many parts of the central nervous system, including the cerebral cortex (via the thalamus), basal ganglia, red nucleus,

brainstem reticular formation, and vestibular nuclei. Traditionally the output of cerebellar processing is thought to be directed at only a single cortical area, namely the primary motor cortex, consistent with the belief the corticocerebellar circuits function primarily in the domain of motor control. In recent years, however, this point of view has been challenged. For instance, anatomical evidence is now available that demonstrates that the site of termination of cerebellar efferents is not restricted to only the subdivisions of the ventrolateral thalamus that innervate the primary motor cortex. Rather, the regions of the thalamus that receive cerebellar input are now recognized as including those regions that project to many motor as well as nonmotor areas of the cerebral cortex (Middleton

& Strick, 1997, 2001). In support of the anatomical evidence, functional neuroimaging studies have demonstrated that, in addition to motor activities, the cerebellum is involved in functions that include higher cognitive functions such as language and attention (Schmahmann, 2001). As yet clinical data on the cerebellar representations of speech motor control do not provide a coherent picture. Although some studies have emphasized the importance of medial cerebellar structures to speech, others suggest a predominant contribution from the lateral parts of the cerebellum (Ackermann & Hertrich, 2000). Several investigations have linked ataxic dysarthria to bilateral damage to the cerebellum, whereas others have reported dysarthria in association with unilateral lesions (Ackermann & Ziegler, 1992). Although Lechtenberg and Gilman (1978) observed a significantly higher prevalence of dysarthria in patients with a left cerebellar lesions, Ackermann, Vogel, Petersen, and Poremba (1992) in a study of speech deficits associated with ischemic cerebellar lesions reported that three of their four dysarthric subjects had unilateral right-sided ischemia. The findings of these latter authors demonstrated that lesions of the cerebellar cortex without involvement of the dentate nucleus can cause dysarthria.

## Speech Impairments Associated with Movement Disorders

The occurrence of dysarthria in association with neurologic conditions caused by pathologic changes in the basal ganglia (e.g., Parkinson disease, Huntington disease) or cerebellum is well documented and is widely regarded as indicative of a role for subcortical structures in the motor control of the speech production mechanism. Pathologic changes involving the basal ganglia and cerebellum produce well-described alterations in motor function such as tremor, rigidity of the muscles, akinesia, or dysmetria which in turn may affect the normal functioning of the speech production mechanism leading to dysarthria. It is thought that many of these symptoms may be due to disruption of the basal ganglia or cerebellar outputs to areas of the cerebral cortex involved in the control of movement. In recent years, several models have been proposed in an attempt to further elucidate the possible contribution of subcortical structures to motor control and to explain the occurrence of movement disorders subsequent to basal ganglia and cerebellar lesions. These models are fully described and discussed later.

As in the case of movement disorders of basal ganglia origin affecting limb and trunk muscles, dysarthrias associated with lesions in the basal ganglia take the form of hypo- and hyperkinetic movement disorders. In general, hypokinetic disorders (e.g., Parkinson disease) are associated with increased basal ganglia output, whereas hyperkinetic movement disorders (e.g., Huntington disease) are associated with decreased output. Hypokinetic disorders are characterized by significant impairments in movement initiation (akinesia) and reduction in the velocity of voluntary movements (bradykinesia) and are usually accompanied by muscular rigidity and tremor at rest. By contrast, hyperkinetic disorders are characterized by excessive motor activity in the form of involuntary movements (dyskinesia) with varying degrees of hypotonia. With regard to their effect on the speech production mechanism, these disorders manifest as hypokinetic dysarthria (classically associated with Parkinson disease) and hyperkinetic dysarthria (seen in association with a range of hyperkinetic conditions such as Huntington disease, dystonia, etc.).

Ataxic dysarthria is the motor speech disorder classically associated with brain lesions involving the cerebellum or its connections. As in the case of the basal ganglia dysarthrias mentioned above, the clinical features of ataxic dysarthria follow from the neuromotor abnormalities associated with damage to the cerebellum, in particular ataxia. In contemporary neurologic literature, the term "ataxia" is used to define motor disturbances of cerebellar origin associated with a variety of clinical symptoms including dysmetria-hypermetria, asynergia, postural and gait instability, intention tremor, and space-time motor incoordination.

## Hypokinetic Dysarthria

Hypokinetic dysarthria is most commonly associated with Parkinson disease. In fact, the term "hypokinetic dysarthria" was first used by Darley, Aronson, and Brown (1969a, 1969b) to describe the resultant complex pattern of perceptual speech characteristics associated with parkinsonism. More recently an acoustically similar form of dysarthria has also been observed in persons with progressive supranuclear palsy (Steele-Richardson-Olszewski

syndrome) (Hanson & Metter, 1980; Metter & Hanson, 1986).

### Clinical Characteristics

In contrast to other forms of dysarthria, the clinical characteristics of hypokinetic dysarthria were identified by a systematic analysis of patients with a specific disease, namely, idiopathic Parkinson disease. Overall, the speech characteristics associated with hypokinetic dysarthria follow largely from the generalized pattern of hypokinetic motor disorders which includes marked reductions in the amplitude of voluntary movement (akinesia), initiation difficulties, slowness of movement (bradykinesia), muscular rigidity, tremor at rest, and postural reflex impairments. According to Darley, Aronson, and Brown (1975), marked limitation of the range of movement of the muscles of the speech mechanism is the outstanding characteristic of hypokinesia as it affects speech. These authors stated that the reduced mobility, restricted range of movement, and supranormal rate of the repetitive movements of the muscles involved in speech production lead to the various manifestations of hypokinetic dysarthria.

Although impairments in all aspects of speech production (i.e., respiration, phonation, resonance, articulation, and prosody) involving the various subsystems of the speech production mechanism have been identified in individuals with Parkinson disease, these individuals are most likely to exhibit disturbances of prosody, phonation, and articulation (Darley et al., 1975; Chenery, Murdoch, & Ingram, 1988; Zwirner & Barnes, 1992). The reported features of the speech disturbance in Parkinson disease commonly include monotony of pitch and loudness, decreased use of all vocal parameters for effecting stress and emphasis, breathy and harsh voice quality, reduced vocal intensity, variable rate including short rushes of speech or accelerated speech, consonant imprecision, impaired breath support for speech, reduction in phonation time, difficulty in the initiation of speech activities, and inappropriate silences (Darley et al., 1969a, 1969b; Ludlow & Bassich, 1983, 1984; Scott, Caird, & Williams, 1985; Chenery et al., 1988). Reduced pitch and loudness variation were among the most prominent speech deficits observed in patients with Parkinson disease in the perceptual-based studies of Darley et al. (1969a, 1969b; 1975). Based on their average perceptual rating scores, the following hierarchy of deviant speech dimensions was observed in 32 patients with Parkinson disease: (1) monopitch, (2) reduced stress, (3) monoloudness, and (4) imprecise consonants.

The reported findings, however, have not always been consistent with respect to the type of disturbances, the frequency of occurrence, and the degree of severity of the abnormal perceptual, acoustic, and physiologic features present in the speech of persons with hypokinetic dysarthria. For example, Darley et al. (1975) reported that in 15 of their 32 patients with Parkinson disease, the average perceived speech loudness levels were lower than those of other dysarthric groups, suggesting that reduced speech loudness is a distinctive feature of speech in Parkinson disease and as such may have a useful role in the differential diagnosis of hypokinetic dysarthria. Nevertheless, reduced speech loudness does not

appear to be present in all dysarthric patients with Parkinson disease. Ludlow and Bassich (1984) reported that only 42% (5 of 12) of their dysarthric patients with Parkinson disease were perceived to have reduced speech loudness. Similarly, in a more recent study Gamboa et al. (1997) reported that only 49% of dysarthric patients with Parkinson disease (20 of 41) self-reported that they had developed hypophonia. It has been suggested that these values may underestimate the actual proportion of dysarthric patients with Parkinson disease who are hypophonic, given that many of these people appear to be able to compensate for their hypophonia during formal speech testing. Other patients with Parkinson disease may have perceptual deficits that make it difficult for them to accurately identify hypophonia in their own speech (Ho, Bradshaw, & Iansek, 2000).

### Respiratory Function

A number of the perceptual features identified in hypokinetic dysarthria, such as reduction in overall loudness, decay of loudness, reduced phrase length, short rushes of speech, and reduced phonation time, have been attributed to the impairment of respiration (Darley et al., 1975). In support of these assumptions, Chenery et al. (1988) identified a mild impairment of respiratory support for speech in the majority (89%) of their subjects with Parkinson disease. In addition, more than half of their subjects demonstrated reductions in phrase lengths, short rushes of speech, reduced loudness, and decay of loudness during speech. Similarly, Ludlow and Bassich (1984) identified a reduction in overall loudness in 42%

of their subjects, and the majority of the cases with Parkinson disease demonstrated a variable rate of speech which could be partially attributed to respiratory insufficiency.

Patients with Parkinson disease have been identified by several investigators to exhibit significant reductions in their vital capacity (Cramer, 1940; de la Torre, Mier, & Boshes, 1960). In particular, de la Torre, Mier and Boshes (1960) found that two-thirds of their subjects with Parkinson disease recorded vital capacities 40% below the expected values. Laszewski (1956) reported that the majority of his subjects exhibited a marked reduction in vital capacity, with little measurable thoracic excursion during inhalation or exhalation. During a sustained phonation task, Mueller (1971) found that subjects with Parkinson disease expended significantly smaller volumes of air than control subjects. Using spirographic analysis, Hovestadt, Bogaard, Meerwaldt, van der Meche and Stigt (1989) revealed that, on nonspeech tasks, peak inspiratory and expiratory flow and maximum expiratory flow at a 50% level were significantly below normal for patients with relatively severe Parkinson disease. In contrast, neither Murdoch, Chenery, Bowler, and Ingram (1989) nor Solomon and Hixon (1993) identified significant overall reductions in vital capacity and lung volumes in their groups of subjects with Parkinson disease.

Recent studies involving kinematic investigations of respiratory function in Parkinson disease have also identified incoordinaton of the components of the chest wall during speech breathing. Murdoch et al. (1989) identified irregularities in chest wall movement during the production of sustained vowels and syllable repetitions. These abnormal chest wall movements took the form of abrupt changes in the relative contribution of the chest wall components and featured both ribcage and abdominal paradoxical movements. In addition, Murdoch et al. (1989) found that the subjects with Parkinson disease demonstrated a wide range of relative volume contributions of the ribcage and abdomen during speech breathing, with a predominance of ribcage involvement. Solomon and Hixon (1993), using different instrumentation, however, recorded smaller ribcage than abdominal contribution to lung volume change in speech breathing of patients with Parkinson disease and found that ribcage and abdominal paradoxing were not specific to subjects with Parkinson disease alone. Both studies, however, identified a significantly greater breathing rate and minute ventilation in subjects with Parkinson disease compared with control subjects.

## Laryngeal Function

Phonatory disturbance is often the initial symptom of the ensuing speech disorder associated with Parkinson disease. In fact, Logemann, Fisher, Boshes, and Blonsky (1978) identified laryngeal problems as being the most prominent deviant features in their group of 200 subjects with Parkinson disease, occurring in 89% of cases. Similarly, about half of the deviant speech dimensions identified by Darley et al. (1975) and Ludlow and Bassich (1983) as being the most distinguishing features of hypokinetic dysarthria can be associated with phonatory disturbance. The deviant perceptual features associated with laryngeal dysfunction in Parkinson disease include disorders of vocal quality and impairment of the overall levels and variability of pitch and loudness.

Descriptions of the vocal quality of the hypokinetic speaker have included a number of deviant vocal parameters including hoarseness, harshness, breathiness, vocal tremor, and glottal fry. Inconsistencies in the frequency of occurrence of these deviant phonatory features are apparent across many of the reported perceptual studies. In relation to hoarseness and harshness, the perceptual findings would appear to be equivocal with respect to the prominence of either feature in the vocal output of persons with hypokinetic dysarthria. Hoarseness was perceived to be present in 45% of patients in Logemann and Fisher's (1981) study, one-third of subjects examined by Ludlow and Bassich (1984), in each subject in the Chenery et al. (1988) study, and in 84% of the subjects with Parkinson disease assessed by Murdoch, Manning, Theodoros, and Thompson (1995). Hoarseness, however, was not found to be a prominent deviant dimension in the study reported by Darley et al. (1975). Instead harshness was listed among the ten most deviant speech features identified by these latter authors. A harsh vocal quality has been perceived to be present in 77 to 84% of patients with hypokinetic dysarthria (Ludlow & Bassich, 1984; Chenery et al., 1988; Zwirner & Barnes, 1992). Although there is some degree of inconsistency in the reported frequency of occurrence of breathiness in hypokinetic dysarthria, it would appear that a breathy vocal quality is also a relatively common characteristic of this type of dysarthria (Darley et al., 1975). Breathiness has been reported to occur in approximately 50 to 95% of patients with hypokinetic dysarthria (Chenery et al., 1988; Murdoch et al., 1995; Zwirner & Barnes, 1992). Glottal fry has been identified in 60 to 85% of cases with hypokinetic dysarthria, whereas pitch unsteadiness or vocal tremor has been reported to be present in approximately 65% of subjects with Parkinson disease (Chenery et al., 1988; Murdoch et al., 1995). The findings of acoustic studies suggest that the disorders of vocal quality perceived to be present in patients with Parkinson disease result from phonatory inefficiency due to abnormal positioning of the vocal folds, irregular vocal-fold activity, and problems with the synchronization of phonation and articulation.

In addition to deviations in vocal quality, the hypokinetic dysarthria associated with Parkinson disease is characterized perceptually by the presence of monotony of pitch and loudness as well as a reduction in overall pitch and loudness levels. Both monotony of pitch and loudness have been identified as prominent features of verbal output of subjects with Parkinson disease, being the first and third most deviant perceptual speech features of hypokinetic dysarthria, respectively, as documented by Darley et al. (1975). Later perceptual studies have confirmed the presence of monotony of pitch and loudness in the majority of subjects with Parkinson disease (Ludlow & Bassich, 1984; Chenery et al., 1988; Zwirner & Barnes, 1992). Similarly, acoustic findings have provided consistent evidence of a reduction in the variability of pitch and loudness in the speech output of these subjects (Flint, Black, & Campbell-Taylor, 1992; King, Ramig, Lemke, & Harii, 1994; Metter & Hanson, 1986).

Unfortunately, few studies reported in the literature have been based on physiologic investigation of laryngeal function in persons with Parkinson disease. Collectively, those studies that have been reported have shown that individuals with Parkinson disease demonstrate abnormal vocal-fold posturing and vibratory patterns and laryngeal aerodynamics (Gerratt, Hanson & Berke, 1987; Hanson, Gerratt, & Ward, 1983; Hirose, Sawashima & Niimi, 1985; Murdoch et al., 1995). Physiologic studies utilizing photoglottography (PGG) and electroglottography (EGG) have identified abnormal vocal-fold vibratory patterns in patients with Parkinson disease (Gerratt et al., 1987; Hanson et al., 1983). Essentially these studies have demonstrated a proportionately greater amount of time spent in opening relative to closing duration with no well-defined closed period (Gerratt et al., 1987; Hanson et al., 1983). Hanson et al. (1983) noted that only 15% of the glottal cycle was spent in the "closed period." In addition, these latter authors found that the waveform shape varied widely from cycle to cycle, suggesting variability in the control of vocal-fold posture. Abnormalities in the laryngeal aerodynamics of persons with Parkinson disease as identified by instrumental studies are also generally consistent with impaired laryngeal function in this group. Murdoch et al. (1995) identified a hyperfunctional pattern of laryngeal activity in subjects with Parkinson disease characterized by increased glottal resistance and reduced subglottal pressure, average phonatory sound pressure level, and phonatory flow rate compared with matched control subjects. It was suggested by Murdoch et al. (1995) that the aerodynamic findings in their study reflected the presence of rigidity in the laryngeal musculature. In addition, their study indicated that dysarthric speakers with Parkinson disease were not homogeneous, but rather exhibited differential impairment within the laryngeal subsystem. Overall, the laryngeal subsystem of the speech production mechanism in subjects with Parkinson disease would appear to demonstrate a greater degree of variability in perceptual, acoustic, and physiologic features than other subsystems of the speech production apparatus.

## Velopharyngeal Function

Controversy surrounds the existence of a resonatory disturbance in persons with Parkinson disease. Several authors have reported low incidences of perceived hypernasality in groups of subjects with Parkinson disease (Darley et al., 1975; Logemann et al., 1978; Theodoros, Murdoch, & Thompson, 1995). At the same time, hypernasality has been identified as one of the most useful perceptual features for differentiating between hypokinetic dysarthria and normal speech (Ludlow & Bassich, 1983). For some individuals with Parkinson disease hypernasality has been found to be the most prominent deviant speech feature (Hoodin & Gilbert, 1989a, 1989b).

Physiologic evaluation of velopharyngeal functioning using a variety of direct and indirect instrumental techniques has provided objective evidence of dysfunction of the velopharyngeal valve in subjects with Parkinson disease. Hirose, Kiritani, Ushijima, Yoshioka, and Sawashima (1981) conducted a study in which velar movements were directly observed by means of an x-ray microbeam system that tracked a lead pellet attached to the nasal side of the velum. During the rapid repetition of the monosyllable /ten/, Hirose and colleagues (1981) identified a gradual decrease in the degree of displacement of the velum. In effect, the lowering and elevation of the velum for the nasal and nonnasal consonants, respectively, were found to be incomplete towards the end of the speech task. At a rapid rate of repetition, the interval between each utterance was noted to be inconsistent and the displacement and rate of velar movements were found to be markedly reduced (Hirose et al., 1981).

In a study involving the use of videofluoroscopy to examine velar movements during speech in patients with Parkinson disease, Robbins, Logemann, and Kirshner (1986) identified a significant reduction in velar elevation, which was considered to reflect a reduced range of velar movement. Nasal accelerometry has also revealed a significantly greater degree and increased frequency of hypernasality in the speech output of a group of hypokinetic speakers with Parkinson disease (Theodoros et al., 1995). Specifically, the individuals with Parkinson disease, as a group, recorded significantly higher Horii Oral Nasal Coupling (HONC) indexes compared with the controls. Of the 23 individuals with Parkinson disease, 17 (74%) were identified by Theodoros et al. (1995) as exhibiting increased nasality.

Clinicians, therefore, should be alert to the existence of resonatory disturbance in Parkinson disease and be aware that this abnormality may manifest, to varying degrees, in some individuals and not others. Further research, involving the simultaneous use of both direct and indirect instrumental measures together with perceptual evaluation, is required to determine the exact nature of velopharyngeal function in hypokinetic dysarthria.

### Articulatory Function

By far the majority of speakers with hypokinetic dysarthria exhibit disorders of articulation. Articulatory impairments, such as consonant and vowel imprecision and prolongation of phonemes, have been observed, with consonant imprecision identified as the most common articulatory disturbance (Chenery et al., 1988; Darley et al., 1975; Logemann et al., 1978; Zwirner & Barnes, 1992). Consonant articulation has been found to be characterized by errors in the manner of production involving incomplete closure for stops and partial construction of the vocal tract for fricatives, resulting in the abnormal production of stop-plosives, affricates, and fricatives (Canter, 1965; Logemann & Fisher, 1981).

In addition to abnormalities of articulation, disordered speech rate is also frequently observed in patients with Parkinson disease. Perceptually, individuals with Parkinson disease have been noted to demonstrate both a faster (Chenery et al., 1988; Darley et al., 1975; Enderby, 1986; Zwirner & Barnes, 1992) and a slower overall rate of speech than normal (Chenery et al., 1988; Zwirner & Barnes, 1992), with most studies suggesting that the speech rate of these patients is generally variable (Hoodin & Gilbert, 1989a; Ludlow & Bassich, 1983; Scott et al., 1985). In addition, subjects with Parkinson disease have been noted to demonstrate short rushes of speech, or what is perceived as an "accelerated" speech pattern (Chenery et al., 1988; Darley et al., 1975; Zwirner & Barnes, 1992). The production of short rushes of speech in the verbal output of speakers with Parkinson disease was found by Darley et al. (1975) to be one of the most prominent features of hypokinetic dysarthria. Furthermore, this deviant speech dimension was identified in 84% of the subjects with Parkinson disease assessed by Chenery et al. (1988). In some cases, a progressive acceleration of speech within a speech segment has also been perceived to be present (Chenery et al., 1988; Scott et al., 1985).

Acoustic analysis of the speech rate disturbance in Parkinson disease has generally confirmed the perceptual impression of a variety of rate disturbances being evident in these subjects. Studies have demonstrated a normal rate of speech production (Ackermann & Ziegler, 1991; Flint et al., 1992), a normal to increased rate (Kent & Rosenbek, 1982; Weismer, 1984), and an increased rate (Hammen, Yorkston, & Beukelman, 1989; Lethlean, Chenery, & Murdoch, 1990), whereas some groups of subjects with Parkinson disease have been found to exhibit rate disturbance on a continuum from slower to faster than normal (Metter & Hanson, 1986). Interestingly, however, although many individuals with Parkinson disease demonstrate a faster than normal rate of speech, Ludlow and Bassich (1984) found that when specifically required to increase their speech rate, the subjects were often unable to do so.

Physiologic investigations of the articulatory function of patients with Parkinson disease have identified the presence of abnormal patterns of muscle activity, reductions in the range and velocity of articulatory movement, as well as impaired strength, endurance, and fine force control of the articulators and tremor in the orofacial structure. These investigations have included a wide variety of instrumental techniques including direct recordings of muscle activity such as electromyography (Hirose, 1986; Hunker, Abbs, & Barlow, 1982; Moore & Scudder, 1989) and a range of kinematic procedures including strain-gauge transduction systems (Abbs, Hunker, & Barlow, 1983; Connor, Ludlow, & Schulz, 1989), lead-pellet tracking (Hirose, Kiritani, & Sawashima, 1982), electromagnetic articulography (Ackermann, Grone, Hoch, & Schonle, 1993), and optoelectrics (Svensson, Hennington, & Karlsson, 1993). Overall, the most common physiologic findings relating to the articulatory subsystem of subjects with Parkinson disease include a reduction in the amplitude of displacement of the articulators and a decrease in velocity of movement (Forrest & Weismer, 1995). The physiologic findings of reduced amplitude and velocity of the articulatory movements provide support for the "articulatory undershoot" hypothesis proposed to explain the articulatory imprecision evident in persons with Parkinson disease (Hunker et al., 1982).

In summary, the findings of the perceptual, acoustic, and physiologic studies related to articulatory function in Parkinson disease have generally been consistent in identifying articulatory deficits in this group. Further research, however, is needed to determine the specific relationships among the deviant perceptual, acoustic, and physiologic speech features to define the precise nature of articulatory dysfunction. Such an approach requires a comprehensive perceptual, acoustic, and physiologic assessment of the articulatory subsystem of individual speakers with hypokinetic dysarthria.

### Prosodic Function

According to Darley et al. (1975), prosodic disturbances constitute the most prominent features of hypokinetic dysarthria. Descriptions of the speech of persons with Parkinson disease frequently refer to the dysprosodic aspects of speech production in relation to stress and intonation, fluency, and rate. Impairment of stress patterning, variable rate, short rushes of speech or "accelerated" speech, difficulty in the initiation of speech, phoneme repetition, palilalia, inappropriate silences, and monotony of pitch and loudness have been identified in these individuals (Chenery et al., 1988; Darley et al., 1975; Ludlow & Bassich, 1983, 1984; Zwirner & Barnes, 1992).

## Hyperkinetic Dysarthria

Hyperkinetic dysarthria is a collective name for a diverse group of speech disorders in which the deviant speech characteristics are the product of abnormal involuntary movements that disturb the rhythm and rate of motor activities, including those involved in speech production. These involuntary movements, which may involve the limbs, trunk, neck, face, and so forth, may be rhythmic or irregular and unpredictable, rapid, or slow. The abnormal involuntary movements involved vary considerably in their form and locus across the different diseases of the basal ganglia. Consequently, there is considerable heteroge-

neity in the deviant speech dimensions that manifest as the speech disorders termed "hyperkinetic dysarthria." Any or all of the major subcomponents of the speech production apparatus may be involved, including the respiratory system, phonatory valve, resonatory valve, and articulatory valve. Disturbances in prosody are also present.

In that the various different types of hyperkinetic dysarthria are each associated with one of the hyperkinetic movement disorders (Freed, 2000), clinically the hyperkinetic dysarthrias are usually described in the context of the underlying movement disorders causing the speech disturbance. With this construct in mind, Darley et al. (1975) distinguished between two categories of hyperkinetic disorders: quick hyperkinesias and slow hyperkinesias. Quick hyperkinesias include myoclonic jerks (e.g., palatopharyngolaryngeal myoclonus), tics, chorea, and ballism, and are characterized by rapid, abnormal, involuntary movements that are either unsustained or sustained only very briefly, and are random in occurrence with respect to the particular body part affected. In contrast, the abnormal involuntary movements seen in slow hyperkinesias build up to a peak slowly and are sustained for at least 1 s or longer. In some instances the abnormal muscle contractions seen in association with slow hyperkinesias are sustained for many seconds or even minutes, with muscle tone waxing and waning to produce a variety of distorted postures. The three major conditions included in the category of slow hyperkinesias are athetosis, dyskinesia (lingual–facial–buccal dyskinesia), and dystonia. The major types of hyperkinetic disorders are outlined in Table 7–1.

**Table 7–1.** Major Types of Hyperkinetic Disorder

| Disorder | Symptoms | Effect on Speech |
|----------|----------|------------------|
| Myoclonic jerks | Characterized by abrupt, sudden, unsustained muscle contractions which occur irregularly. Involuntary contractions may occur as single jerks of the body or may be repetitive. Two forms may affect speech: palatal myoclonus and action myoclonus. | Speech disorder in palatal myoclonus usually characterized by phonatory, resonatory, and prosodic abnormalities, for example, vocal tremor, rhythmic phonatory arrests, intermittent hypernasality, prolonged intervals, and inappropriate silences. |
| Tics | Tourette syndrome characterized by development of motor and vocal tics plus behavioral disorders. Vocal tics include simple vocal tics (for example, grunting, coughing, barking, hissing, etc.) and complex vocal tics (for example, stuttering-like repetitions, palilalia, echolalia, and copralalia). Brief, unsustained, recurrent, compulsive movements. Usually involves a small part of the body, for example, facial grimace. | Action myoclonus: speech disrupted as a result of fine, arrhythmic, erratic muscle jerks, triggered by activity of the speech musculature. |
| Chorea | A choreic movement consists of a single, involuntary, unsustained, isolated muscle action producing a short, rapid, uncoordinated jerk of the trunk, limb, face, tongue, diaphragm, etc. Contractions are random in distribution and timing is irregular. Two major forms: Sydenham chorea and Huntington disease. | A perceptual study of 30 patients with chorea demonstrated deficits in all aspects of speech production (Darley et al., 1969a). |
| Ballism | Rare hyperkinetic disorder characterized by involuntary, wide-amplitude, vigorous, flailing movements of the limbs. Facial muscles may also be affected. | Least important hyperkinetic disorders with regard to occurrence of hyperkinetic dysarthria. |

*continues*

**Table 7–1.** *continued*

| Disorder | Symptoms | Effect on Speech |
|---|---|---|
| Athetosis | Slow hyperkinetic disorder characterized by continuous, arrhythmic, purposeless, slow, writhing-type movements that tend to flow one into another. Muscles of the face, neck, and tongue are involved, leading to facial grimacing, protrusion, and writhing of the tongue and problems with speaking and swallowing. | Descriptions of the speech disturbance in athetosis largely related to athetoid cerebral palsy rather than hyperkinetic dysarthria in adults. |
| Dyskinesia | Two dyskinetic disorders are included under this heading: tardive dyskinesia and levodopa-induced dyskinesia. Basic pattern of abnormal involuntary movement in both of these conditions is one of slow, repetitive, writhing, twisting, flexing and extending movements often with a mixture of tremor. Muscles of the tongue, face, and oral cavity are most often affected. | Accurate placement of the articulators of speech may be severely hampered by the presence of choreoathetoid movements of the tongue, lip pursing and smacking, tongue protrusion, as well as sucking and chewing behaviors. |
| Dystonia | Characterized by abnormal involuntary movements that are slow and sustained for prolonged periods of time. Involuntary movements tend to have an undulant, sinuous character that may produce grotesque posturing and bizarre writhing, twisting movements. | Dystonias affecting the speech mechanisms may result in respiratory irregularities and/ or abnormal movement and bizarre posturing of the jaw, lips, tongue, face, and neck. In particular, focal cranial/ orolingual–mandibular dystonia and spasmodic torticollis have the most direct effect on speech function. |

## Quick Hyperkinesias: Myoclonic Jerks

Myoclonic jerks are abrupt, sudden, unsustained muscle contractions that occur irregularly. These involuntary muscle contractions may occur as single jerks of a body part or may be repetitive, with the muscles of the limbs, face, oral cavity, soft palate, larynx, and diaphragm being affected, among others. In those instances where the involuntary movements are repetitive, they can be either rhythmic or nonrhythmic in nature. According to Simon, Arminoff, and Greenberg (1999), myoclonic jerks are classified according to their distribution, relationship to precipitating stimuli, or etiology. Although myoclonic jerks are sometimes focal, involving only isolated muscles (focal myoclonus), they may also be multifocal, occurring simultaneously in larger groups of muscles (generalized myoclonus).

Myoclonic jerks may occur as a normal phenomenon in healthy persons as an isolated abnormality, or in association with lesions located in a variety of different sites in the central nervous system, ranging from the cerebral cortex (e.g., cortical reflex myoclonus) to the spinal cord (e.g., spinal myoclonus). Myoclonus may also occur as part of a convulsive disorder (epilepsy) or in association with diffuse metabolic, infectious, or toxic disturbances of the nervous system such as diffuse encephalitis and toxic encephalopathies. Although often occurring spontaneously, myoclonic jerks may also be induced by various sensory stimuli (e.g., visual, auditory, or tactile stimuli) or in some instances by voluntary muscle activity (action myoclonus).

The muscles of the speech mechanism may be affected by myoclonic jerks in the same way as the muscles of the limbs. Myoclonic jerks may involve the muscles of the soft palate, larynx, and diaphragm either individually or in combination. In those rare cases where it occurs in isolation, palatal myoclonus usually involves the rhythmic contraction of the soft palate which may result in temporary hypernasality and articulatory imprecision. Laryngeal myoclonus most frequently occurs in combination with palatal myoclonus (Drysdale, Ansell, & Adeley, 1993) where it can have the additional effect of temporarily interrupting phonation. Diaphragmatic myoclonus can cause slight interruptions to airflow and is usually most easily detected in sustained phonation tasks.

In particular two forms of myoclonus have a marked effect on speech: palatopharyngolaryngeal myoclonus (sometimes simply referred to as palatal myoclonus) and action myoclonus. Palatopharyngolaryngeal myoclonus is characterized by continuous synchronous jerks of the soft palate at the rate of 1 to 4 Hz with other brainstem-innervated muscles, particularly the larynx and pharynx. The condition can be either symptomatic or idiopathic (essential rhythmic palatal myoclonus), with the symptomatic condition most often the result of cerebrovascular lesions involving the brainstem or cerebellum (Deuschl, Mischke, & Schenck, 1990); however, a variety of other conditions, including tumors, multiple sclerosis, encephalitis, and degenerative diseases, can also lead to palatal myoclonus. Hyperkinetic dysarthria due to palatopharyngolaryngeal myoclonus rarely exists as an isolated speech disturbance, but more frequently occurs in conjunction with another type of dysarthria. Although palatopharyngolaryngeal myoclonus has direct effects on the speech musculature, speech deficits may not be readily perceived during conversational speech because of the low amplitude and brevity of the myoclonic movements (Duffy, 2013). Where a speech disturbance is apparent, it is usually characterized by phonatory, resonatory, and prosodic abnormalities such as vocal tremor, momentary rhythmic phonatory arrests, intermittent hypernasality, prolonged intervals of phonation, and inappropriate silences (Aronson, 1990; Darley et al., 1975).

Action myoclonus is differentiated from other myoclonic conditions such as palatopharyngolaryngeal myoclonus by the fact that it is triggered by muscle activity. In this condition speech function is disrupted as a result of fine, arrhythmic, erratic muscle jerks that are triggered by muscle activity associated with a conscious attempt at a task requiring precision of movement (e.g., speech production) (Lance & Adams, 1963). The muscle jerks may present one at a time or in a series and are usually less than 200 ms in duration (Lance & Adams, 1963). Documentation of the speech impairment associated with action myoclonus is restricted to one unpublished report. Aronson, O'Neill, and Kelly (1984; cited in Duffy, 1995) identified articulatory and phonatory impairments in a study of four cases. Despite demonstrating normal orofacial features at rest, myoclonic spasms of the lips were evident when speech was attempted, resulting in a reduced speech rate. Phonatory disturbances observed in these four cases included repetitive fluctuations in phonation and adductor vocal arrests that were synchronized with the myoclonic jerks of the lip muscles.

### Quick Hyperkinesias: Tics

Tics are brief, unsustained, recurrent, compulsive movements that involve a relatively small part of the body and occur out of a background of normal motor activity. They usually occur spontaneously without provocation by any particular stimulus and generally are considered as involuntary movements. Although tics may be briefly controlled voluntarily, such periods of suppression are often followed by a period of more intensive involuntary contraction.

Tics can be classified into four groups depending on whether they are simple or multiple and transient or chronic. Transient simple tics are very common in children, usually terminating spontaneously within 1 year, and generally require no treatment. Chronic simple tics can develop at any age but often begin in childhood, and treatment is not necessary in most cases. The syndrome of multiple motor and vocal tics is generally referred to as Tourette syndrome. First described by Frenchman Gilles de la Tourette in 1885, the first signs of Tourette syndrome consist of motor tics in 80% of cases and vocal tics in 20% (Alsobrook & Pauls, 2002; Simon et al., 1999). The condition primarily affects boys (4:1 ratio) and development of motor and vocal tics is accompanied by a variety of behavioral disorders, including obsessive-compulsive disorder, attention-deficit hyperactivity disorder, and other forms of general behavioral disturbances such as conduct disorder, panic attacks, multiple phobias, mania, etc. In those cases where the initial sign is a motor tic, it most commonly involves the face, taking the form of sniffing, barking, blinking, or forced eye closure. The motor tics progressively involve the face, neck, upper limbs, and eventually the entire body. Vocal tics include both simple and complex vocal tics. Simple vocal tics include grunting, coughing, barking, throat clearing, hissing, and snorting (Serra-Mestres, Robertson, & Shetty, 1998). This may occur as isolated events or be embedded with involuntary verbal utterances. In addition, complex vocal tics, such as stuttering-like repetitions, unintelligible sounds, palilalia (repetition of self-generated words or phrases), and echolalia, have also been reported. Copralalia (involuntary, compulsive swearing), although not universal, is another characteristic complex vocal tic observed in Tourette syndrome. Soft neurologic signs, such as mild incoordination in motor skills and slight asymmetry of motor function, including deep tendon reflexes, are also occasionally evident on examination of the child. The incidence of Tourette syndrome is less than 1 in 100,000 (Friedhoff, 1982), and drug therapy utilizing antidopaminergic agents has been shown to be effective in some cases.

### Quick Hyperkinesias: Chorea

The term "chorea" is derived from the Greek word for dance and was originally applied to the dance-like gait and continual limb movements seen in acute infectious chorea. A chronic (or choreiform) movement consists of a single, unsustained, isolated muscle action producing a short, rapid, uncoordinated jerk of the trunk, limb, face, tongue, diaphragm, and so forth. They are random in their distribution and their timing is irregular and unpredictable. Choreiform movements range in severity from gross displacements of body parts to subtle abnormal involuntary movements. Choreiform contractions are slower than myoclonic jerks, each lasting from 0.1 to 1 second, and can occur at rest, during sustained postures, or may be superimposed on voluntary movements. When superimposed on normal movements, the abnormal involuntary movements can cause characteristic symptoms such as dance-like gait. When superimposed on the normal movements of the speech

mechanism during speech production, choreic movements can cause momentary disturbances in the course of contextual speech.

A variety of different conditions may be associated with the occurrence of chorea, including metabolic and toxic conditions (e.g., hepatic encephalopathy, Wilson disease, hyperthyroidism, and dopaminergic medications), inflammatory/infectious disorders (e.g., Sydenham chorea, encephalitis), vascular lesions involving the basal ganglia or thalamus, and degenerative conditions (e.g., Huntington disease). Pregnant women can also on occasion manifest choreiform movements. Chorea can also occur as an idiopathic disorder. Two of the most common choreiform disorders are Sydenham chorea and Huntington disease. Sydenham chorea occurs principally in children and adolescents, and Huntington disease occurs principally in adults. Both disorders are characterized by hyperkinesia, as well as speech, language, cognitive, and psychiatric disorders.

**Sydenham Chorea.** First described by Thomas Sydenham in 1686 as St Vitus dance, Sydenham chorea is a movement disorder occurring primarily in association with β-hemolytic streptococcal throat infections or with rheumatic heart disease (Goldenberg, Ferraz, Fonseca, Hilário, Bastos, & Sachetti, 1992; Simon et al., 1999). The symptom complex of the condition includes involuntary, purposeless, rapid movements which are often associated with incoordination, muscle weakness, and/or behavioral abnormalities. These spontaneous movements may involve any portion of the body and occur at rest but disappear during sleep. The condition usually occurs in childhood or adolescence, with onset usually being noted between the ages of 5 and 10 years. Females are affected more than males and the onset of choreic involuntary movements may be either acute or insidious. The prognosis for Sydenham chorea is good and recovery is the general rule with symptoms usually subsiding within 4 to 6 months (Simon et al., 1999). The course of the condition, however, is extremely variable with some cases recovering within a few weeks while others have persistence of the abnormal involuntary movements over a period of years. Frequent relapses occur in some patients with Sydenham chorea. Pathologic changes in Sydenham chorea have been variously reported in the cerebral cortex, cerebellum, thalamus, caudate nucleus, putamen, and midbrain. These changes consist of widespread neuronal degeneration, vascular changes, and, rarely, focal brain lesions from embolization resulting from endocarditis. Neuropathologic and radiologic findings in the acute stage are rare, and no consistent neuropathologic lesions have been identified in Sydenham chorea.

Hyperkinetic dysarthria associated with Sydenham chorea has received little attention in the research literature. Furthermore, the few studies reported have largely only documented the presence of dysarthria in persons with Sydenham chorea rather than providing specific details as to the clinical features of the condition. Nausieda, Grossman, Koller, Weiner, and Klawans (1980) reported the findings of a retrospective study of 240 individuals with Sydenham chorea noting that 39% had dysarthria. Swedo et al. (1993) examined 11 moderately affected children reporting that all exhibited a dysarthria that manifested as "slurred or incoherent

speech . . . with two children rendered mute" (p. 707). In all but two of the children, the dysarthria subsided within months of initiation of medical treatment and was noted not to be present at an 18-month follow-up assessment. Further studies reporting the presence of dysarthria in Sydenham chorea were conducted by Goldenberg et al. (1992) who examined 187 children in Brazil, and Kulkarni and Anees (1996) who examined 60 children in India.

**Huntington Disease.** Huntington disease is a chronic degenerative neurologic disorder that is manifested by progressive chorea or, at times, other extrapyramidal symptoms as well as progressive intellectual deterioration. The condition is inherited as an autosomal-dominant trait, with onset of symptoms typically occurring in the fifth decade of life. As the condition is a progressive disorder, the degree of choreiform movements gradually becomes greater and greater as the condition advances and is usually fatal within 10 to 15 years post-onset. Pathologically, Huntington disease is marked by a loss of neurons in the caudate nucleus and putamen, and these structures are grossly shrunken and atrophic. The globus pallidus is usually well preserved as is the substantia nigra. Although major pathologic changes are seen in the striatum and cerebral cortex, some changes have also been noted in the cerebral white matter, thalamus, and hypothalamus. (A description of the changes in the basal ganglia circuitry in Huntington disease is given later.)

The clinical picture in the advanced stages of Huntington disease includes facial grimacing (involving the lips, tongue, and cheeks), jerks of the head, weaving movements of the arms and shoulders, twists and jerks of the body, as well as superimposed voluntary movements (e.g., an involuntary upward jerk of the arm may be fused into a scratching of the head). The patient's gait at this stage is often markedly involved, consisting of jerky lurching steps that represent a combination of voluntary and involuntary movements. Muscular strength, however, is unimpaired. Unlike Parkinson disease, the ability to initiate voluntary movements is intact; however, the conduct of a continuous movement (e.g., walking or speech production) is frequently impeded by superimposed muscle jerks.

The pervasive choreiform movements evident in patients with Huntington disease and other forms of chorea have a profound effect on the individual's attempts at speech production because of the sudden, rapid, and unpredictable nature of the involuntary movements which interfere with respiratory, laryngeal, velopharyngeal, and articulatory speech activity. The labored and effortful speech is presumed to be a manifestation of inaccuracy in the direction of movement, irregularity in rhythm, range, force and muscle tone, and a reduced rate of individual and repetitive movements of the muscles of the speech mechanism (Darley et al., 1969b). Hyperkinetic dysarthria associated with chorea is distinguished from other types of dysarthria by the sporadic and transient nature of the abnormal speech features. Individuals with chorea may, in fact, demonstrate normal speech intelligibility, punctuated by distorted speech production during periods of hyperkinesias.

To date, relatively few studies based on perceptual, acoustic, and/or physiologic assessments have documented the clinical features of hyperkinetic dysarthria associated with Huntington disease. The most comprehensive perceptual study to have been reported was performed by Darley et al. (1969a). They reported that all basic motor speech processes were disturbed. The ten most deviant speech dimensions observed in patients with chorea by Darley et al. (1969a) were, in rank order: (1) imprecise consonants, (2) prolonged intervals, (3) variable speaking rate, (4) monopitch, (5) harsh voice quality, (6) inappropriate silences, (7) distorted vowels, (8) excess loudness variation, (9) prolonged phonemes, and (10) monoloudness. In particular, they reported that choreic patients were most distinctive from other patients with dysarthria in the area of prosodic alterations, being more deviant than any other neurologic group on the speech dimensions of excess loudness variation, variable rate, and prolonged intervals. According to Darley et al. (1975), the prosodic changes appear to represent an attempt by the choreic speaker to avoid articulatory and phonatory interruptions by variably altering their rate of speech, prolonging their phonemes, and prolonging the intervals between words, equalizing the stress on syllables and introducing inappropriate silences.

Hartelius, Carlstedt, Ytterberg, Lillvik, and Laakso (2003) also examined the speech of speakers with mild and moderate Huntington disease and, consistent with Darley et al. (1969a,b), observed significant speech deviations in all areas of speech production tested. The most severe speech deviations observed by this group were in phonation, oral motor performance including oral diadochokinesis, and prosody. Although no correlation was found between age or gender and severity of dysarthria, a significant difference in the severity of dysarthria was found between the group with mild Huntington disease and the group with moderate Huntington disease. The most frequently occurring perceptual deviations found in continuous speech were mainly related to speech timing and phonation and were hypothesized to reflect the underlying excessive and involuntary movement pattern.

Imprecise consonant and distorted vowel production and irregular articulatory breakdowns have been reported to characterize the articulation of patients with chorea (Darley et al., 1975) and are consistent with the expected adverse effects of choreiform movements on lip, tongue, and jaw function. Support for this conclusion has been provided by several acoustic studies of the speech output of patients with Huntington disease. Zwirner and Barnes (1992) identified greater than normal variability in the first and second formants of a sustained vowel, reflecting abnormal jaw movements (first formant) and aberrations of tongue position and shape (second formant). In addition, Ackermann, Hertrich, and Hehr (1995) found that, on an oral diadochokinetic task, their patients with Huntington disease exhibited increased syllable durational variability and, in some cases, incomplete articulatory gestures that could be attributed to the effects of choreic activity.

The excessive loudness variation exhibited by patients with Huntington disease was considered to be a characteristic of this form of hyperkinetic dysarthria by Darley et al. (1969a, 1969b). In some cases, voice stoppages or arrests were observed in these patients. Objective acoustic assessments of voice in patients with Huntington disease have identified high phonatory instability (increased variability in fundamental frequency and sudden reductions in frequency of approximately one octave) consistent with involuntary laryngeal movements (Ramig, 1986; Ramig, Scherer, Titze, & Ringel, 1988; Zwirner & Barnes, 1992; Zwirner, Murry, & Woodson, 1991).

Hypernasality when present in patients with Huntington disease is usually only mild and intermittent, reflecting the variable nature of the choreiform movements affecting soft palate function. Darley et al. (1969a) reported that only approximately 40% of their patients with Huntington disease exhibited hypernasality. Likewise, these researchers only observed abnormal respiratory patterns in 6 of their 30 patients with chorea, the abnormal respiratory pattern taking the form of sudden, forced, and involuntary inspiration and/or expiration; however, Darley et al. (1969a) found this abnormal respiratory pattern to be unique to this form of hyperkinetic dysarthria.

### Quick Hyperkinesias: Ballism (Hemiballismus)

Hemiballismus is a rare hyperkinetic movement disorder characterized by involuntary, wide-amplitude, vigorous, flailing movement of the limbs, particularly the arm, on one side of the body. Facial muscles may also be affected. The most consistent neuropathologic finding associated with hemiballismus is vascular damage to the subthalamic nucleus or its immediate connections on the side contralateral to the involuntary movement disorder. Ballism can also be caused by other conditions including infections, drugs, autoimmune disorders, primary brain tumors, and acquired immunodeficiency syndrome. Ballism is the least important of all the quick hyperkinesias in relation to the occurrence of hyperkinetic dysarthria.

### Slow Hyperkinesias: Athetosis

Athetosis is a slow hyperkinesia characterized by continuous, arrhythmic, purposeless, slow, writhing-type movements that tend to flow one into the other. The abnormal movements cease only during sleep and the affected muscles are always hypertonic and may show transient stages of spasms. Athetoid movements particularly involve the distal musculature of the limbs. The muscles of the face, neck, and tongue, however, may also be affected leading to facial grimacing, protrusion, and writhing of the tongue, and problems with speaking and swallowing.

Athetosis occurs most often as part of a congenital complex of neurologic signs that results from disordered development of the brain, birth injury, or other etiologic factors, and represents a subcategory of cerebral palsy (Morris, Grattan-Smith, Jankelowitz, Fung, Clouston, & Hayes, 2002). The term, therefore, is rarely used to describe movement disorders acquired in adulthood with many neurologists regarding athetosis as synonymous with dystonia when referring to the acquired condition. Consequently, the majority of reports in the literature relating to the occurrence and nature of speech disorders associated with athetosis are largely based on studies of children or adults with cerebral palsy. Intelligibility of connected speech has been reported to be markedly decreased though phonemic competence is intact, suggesting that athetoid individuals lack the neuromuscular control for articulatory pre-

cision (Platt, Andrews, & Howie, 1980). The articulatory abnormalities noted in individuals with athetosis include wide-ranging jaw movements, inappropriate tongue placement, intermittent velopharyngeal closure, retrusion of lower lip, and prolonged transition time for articulatory movements (Kent & Netsell, 1978).

### Slow Hyperkinesias: Dyskinesia (Lingual–Facial–Buccal Dyskinesia)

The term "dyskinesia" is often used in a general way to refer to abnormal, involuntary, hyperkinetic movements without regard to etiology (Miller & Jankovic, 1990). Although when used in this way all involuntary movements could be described as dyskinetic, only two dyskinetic disorders are usually considered under this heading: tardive dyskinesia and levodopa-induced dyskinesia. As both of these conditions may be limited to the bulbar musculature, they are sometimes referred to as "focal dyskinesias." Furthermore, because the muscles of the tongue, face, and oral cavity are most often affected, these two disorders are also termed "lingual–facial–buccal" dyskinesias. The basic pattern of abnormal involuntary movement in both of these conditions is one of slow, repetitive, writhing, twisting, flexing, and extending movements, often with a mixture of tremor.

**Tardive Dyskinesia.** Tardive dyskinesia is a late-onset, acquired movement disorder resulting from long-term neuroleptic treatment (treatment with a pharmacologic agent having antipsychotic action) (Jeste & Wyatt, 1982). Although neuroleptic drugs have been prescribed for psychiatric disorders since the 1930s, the condition was first described by Schonecker (1957) when the term "tardive dyskinesia" was coined. Also sometimes referred to as Meige syndrome, tardive dyskinesia is regarded by some neurologists as a form of focal dystonia involving the cranial–cervical region (Ferguson, 1992). The syndrome occurs relatively late in the course of neuroleptic therapy.

The abnormal involuntary movements seen in tardive dyskinesia are usually of the choreoathetoid type, and are sometimes stereotyped and principally affect the tongue, lips, and jaw, and, to a lesser degree, the larynx and respiratory musculature (Feve, Angelard, & Lacau St Guily, 1995). The limbs and trunk are also occasionally involved. A combination of tongue twisting and protrusion as well as lip smacking and puckering and chewing movement in a repetitive and stereotypic fashion is often observed (Jankovic, 1995). In addition, the soft palate may also elevate and lower involuntarily. When asked to do so, patients with tardive dyskinesia may be able to suppress the involuntary mouth movements. These movements may also be suppressed by voluntary actions such as putting food in the mouth or talking.

Speech production is often markedly affected in tardive dyskinesia due to the abnormal involuntary, rhythmic movements of the orofacial, lingual, and mandibular structures. The accurate placement of the articulators of speech may be severely hampered by the presence of choreoathetoid movements of the tongue, lip pursing and smacking, tongue protrusion, and sucking and chewing behaviors (Matthews & Glaser, 1984; Vernon, 1991). According to Darley et al. (1969a, 1969b) articulatory deviations were the

most prominent features of the hyperkinetic dysarthria exhibited by their patients with tardive dyskinesia. Other perceptually based studies have also identified prosodic, phonatory, and respiratory impairments, in addition to articulatory disorders, in small groups of subjects with tardive dyskinesia (Gerratt, 1983; Gerratt, Goetz, & Fisher, 1984). In a perceptual study of 12 patients with tardive dyskinesia, Gerratt et al. (1984) reported that these patients exhibited marked disturbances in the temporal organization of speech (prosodic impairment) and phonation, while articulatory deficits (irregular articulatory breakdowns and imprecise consonants) were perceived to be less severely impaired. Respiratory dysfunction, involving respiratory dysrhythmia, involuntary grunts, and gasping sounds, have also been reported in patients with tardive dyskinesia (Faheem, Brightwell, Burton, & Struss, 1982; Weiner, Goetz, Nausieda, & Klewans, 1978).

The most comprehensive perceptual study of the hyperkinetic dysarthria associated with tardive dyskinesia was conducted by Khan, Jampala, Dong, and Vedak (1994). They reported that the 17 male psychiatric patients with tardive dyskinesia examined in their study demonstrated significantly reduced phonation times, levels of speech intelligibility, and speech rate compared with ten neuroleptically treated patients without tardive dyskinesia. La Porta, Archambault, Ross-Chouinard, and Chouinard (1990) phonetically analyzed the speech of two subjects with tardive dyskinesia during reading, sentence repetition, and spontaneous conversation tasks. Both cases were found to produce high frequencies of abnormal consonants, compared with a single control subject who had received long-term neuroleptic treatment but did not exhibit tardive dyskinesia. Specifically, the two patients with tardive dyskinesia made the most errors on alveolar, alveodental, and palatal phonemes, consistent with abnormal movements of the tongue in tardive dyskinesia. Interestingly, La Porta, Archambault, Ross-Chouinard, and Chouinard (1990) found that vowel production was unimpaired in these two subjects.

Support for the above perceptual findings in relation to articulation and phonation has come from acoustic investigations of the dysarthria associated with tardive dyskinesia. For example, Gerratt (1983) investigated motor steadiness of the vocal tract musculature superior to the glottis during vowel production in five subjects with tardive dyskinesia using a measure of formant frequency fluctuation as an indicator of changes in vocal tract configuration. Consistent with the articulatory and phonatory deficits identified perceptually by La Porta et al. (1990) and Khan et al. (1994), their results indicated that formant frequency fluctuations were markedly higher for four of the five subjects compared with normal controls, reflecting a reduction in motor steadiness supraglottally.

Physiologic investigations of the speech mechanism in patients with tardive dyskinesia have involved objective analyses of buccolingual, tongue and respiratory function using a variety of instrumental techniques. Caligiuri, Harris, and Jeste (1988), using a head-mounted transduction system and a pursuit tracking paradigm, evaluated the fine motor control of lip, jaw, and tongue movements in 11 patients with tardive dyskinesia. Greater tracking errors were demonstrated by the patients with tardive dyskinesia for the lip (31%), tongue (36%), and jaw (31%) compared with non-tardive dyskinetic patients (lip 12%, tongue 12%, jaw 13%). Using position transducers, Caligiuri, Jeste, and Harris (1989) identified greater motor instability in the tongue in 13 patients with tardive dyskinesia compared with control subjects and nontardive dyskinesia patients. Physiologic assessment of respiratory function in patients with tardive dyskinesia, using respiratory inductance plethysmography, has confirmed perceptual observations of respiratory impairments in these patients. Wilcox, Bassett, Jones, and Fleetham (1994) found that patients with tardive dyskinesia demonstrated rapid, shallow breathing characterized by irregular tidal breathing patterns, with greater variability in both tidal volume and time of the total respiratory cycle than control subjects.

As indicated above, tardive dyskinesia occurs later in the course of neuroleptic therapy, often after a decrease in the drug dosage or discontinuation of the drug therapy. The involuntary lingual–facial–buccal movements often persist for months or years after the neuroleptic therapy has been discontinued. If recognized early, however, the symptoms of tardive dyskinesia (including the associated hyperkinestic dysarthria) may recede with the discontinuation of neuroleptic treatment (Drummond & Fitzpatrick, 2004).

**Levodopa-Induced Dyskinesia.** Combined lingual–facial–buccal dyskinesia is not unique to tardive dyskinesia but may also be seen as part of the hyperkinesia of Huntington disease and following high-dose levodopa therapy in Parkinson disease. As in tardive dyskinesia, the abnormal involuntary movements seen in the latter condition are also typically choreic and also characteristically involve the muscles of the tongue, face, and mouth. The tongue may demonstrate "fly-catcher" movements in which it involuntarily moves in and out of the mouth repeatedly. Simultaneously, the lips may pucker and retract while the jaw may open and close or move from side to side spontaneously. The induction of lingual–facial–buccal dyskinesia by levodopa therapy is consistent with the proposal of Ludlow and Bassich (1984) that patients with Parkinson disease treated with levodopa have a speech disorder resembling a hyperkintic rather than a hypokinetic dysarthria.

### Slow Hyperkinesias: Dystonia

Dystonia is a collective term for a variety of neurogenic movement and posture disorders characterized by abnormal, involuntary muscle contractions which may be accompanied by irregular repetitive movements. Dystonic movements are abnormal, involuntary movements which are slow and sustained for prolonged periods of time. Affected muscles are hypertonic and the involuntary movements tend to have an undulant, sinuous character which may produce grotesque posturing and bizarre writhing movements. Dystonia tends to involve large parts of the body, particularly the muscles of the trunk, neck, and proximal parts of the limbs; however, the muscles of the speech mechanism may also be involved, in which case the patient may exhibit spasms of the face producing facial grimacing, forceful spasmodic eye closing (blepharospasm), pursing of the lips, jaw spasm, involuntary

twisting and protrusion of the tongue, and respiratory irregularities. The most distinguishing feature of dystonia involves the maintenance of an abnormal or altered posture, on some occasions involving only a single focal part of the body while on others involving a diffuse region of the body. The abnormal involuntary contractions usually build up slowly, produce a prolonged distorted posture such as twisting of the trunk about the long axis (torsion spasm), and then gradually recede. Occasionally, dystonic movements begin with a jerk and then build up to a peak before subsiding.

A variety of conditions may lead to dystonia including encephalitis, head trauma, vascular diseases, and drug toxicity. In addition, various progressive degenerative diseases of the central nervous system, such as Wilson disease and Huntington disease, often manifest dystonic features at some time in their course. One type of dystonia, dystonia musculorum deformans, is an inherited disease. In many cases, however, the cause of dystonia is unknown. Although it is often reported that dystonia is a disorder of the basal ganglia, lesions in the corpus striatum and globus pallidus having been described, no consistent and specific pathophysiology or pathomorphologic alteration in the brain has been identified.

Depending on the distribution of the abnormal involuntary movements, dystonia can be classified into several subtypes including:

- Focal dystonia (involving only a single segment or part of the body)
- Segmental dystonia (involving two or more contiguous body segments)
- Multifocal dystonia (involving two noncontiguous body parts)

- Generalized dystonia (involving one or both legs plus another area of the body).

Focal dystonias that may affect speech and voice include orolingual–mandibular dystonia, laryngeal dystonia, and cervical dystonia (also known as spasmodic torticollis). Patients with orolingual-mandibular dystonia have abnormal movements of the vocal tract, including sustained tongue movements, clenched jaw, or forced jaw opening (Yoshida & Iizuka, 2003; Yoshida, Kaji, Shibasaki, & Iizuka, 2002). These signs often occur with blepharospasm, and this complex has been referred to as focal cranial dystonia or Meige syndrome (Jankovic, 1988). According to Darley et al. (1975), articulation, phonation, and prosody may all be significantly disturbed in patients with dystonia. In a study of 30 dystonia cases, Darley et al. (1969a) found that the deviant speech dimensions of imprecise consonants, disturbed vowels, harsh voice quality, irregular articulatory breakdown, strained-strangled voice quality, monopitch, monoloudness, inappropriate silence, short phrases, and prolonged intervals to be the 10 major features of the hyperkinetic dysarthria seen in dystonia. Notably, three of the four most prominent deviant characteristics were related to articulatory disturbance. Resonatory disturbances have not been found to be characteristic features of dysarthria associated with dystonia. Approximately 30% of cases have been found to demonstrate hypernasality, with the majority of subjects exhibiting this abnormality to a mild degree (Darley et al., 1969a, 1969b; Golper, Nutt, Rau, & Coleman, 1983). Likewise, except for two patients in Golper et al.'s (1983) study who were perceived to exhibit respiratory muscle spasms, studies of the speech output of patients with dystonia have generally failed to identify specific impairments of respiration. A number of perceptual features identified in this population, such as excessive loudness variations, short phrases, and alternating loudness could, however, reflect the contribution of respiratory impairment in this population.

As a reflection of the phenomenon of laryngospasm during phonation, laryngeal dystonia is referred to as spasmodic dysphonia. Three subtypes of spasmodic dysphonia are recognized based on the specific aspect of vocal-fold movement impaired. These subtypes include adductor, abductor, and mixed spasmodic dysphonia of which adductor is by far the most common (Blitzer & Brin, 1992). Three syllable-level adductor spasmodic dysphonia signs have been identified by various researchers as being key to the classification of the adductor spasmodic dysphonia voice: pitch shift (Sapienza, Walton, & Murry, 1999, 2000); phonatory break (Langveld, Drost, Frijns, Zwinderman, & Baatenburg de Jong, 2000); and aperiodicity (Sapienza et al., 1999, 2000).

Spasmodic torticollis, a condition in which tonic or clonic spasm in the neck muscles (especially the sternocleido-mastoid and trapezius muscles) cause the head to be deviated to the right or left, or sometimes forward (antecollis) and backward (retrocollis), has also been reported to disrupt speech production (Case, La Pointe, & Duane, 1990; La Pointe, Case, & Duane, 1993; Zraick, La Pointe, Case, & Duane, 1993). Acoustic speech/voice characteristics of the hyperkinetic dysarthria associated with spasmodic torticollis include reduced maximum phonation duration, slower sequential articulatory movement rates, slower alternate articulatory movement rates, longer phonatory reaction time, slower reading rate (in words per minute), lower overall intelligibility rating, increased jitter, increased shimmer, increased harmonic-to-noise ratio (females), lower habitual fundamental frequency (females), lower ceiling fundamental frequency (females), and restricted frequency range (females).

### Essential Voice Tremor

Tremors are involuntary movements resulting from the contraction of opposing muscle groups, which produces rhythmic or alternating movement of a joint or group of joints. A number of different types of tremor are recognized, which include:

- Physiologic tremor (e.g., tremor associated with cold or nervousness)
- Essential tremor (e.g., familial, action, and senile)
- Toxic tremor (e.g., tremor in thyrotoxicosis and alcoholism)
- Pathologic tremor (e.g., intention tremor in cerebellar disorders and rest tremor in Parkinson disease).

Essential tremor is a hyperkinetic movement disorder that most often affects the head, arms, or hands. It is the most common of the movement disorders, with approximately 50% of cases being familial with the bulk of the rest being idiopathic (Duffy, 1995). The condition is usually regarded as an exaggeration of normal physiologic tremors. Although often referred to as a benign disorder, the symptoms of essential tremor are typically progressive and potentially disabling and may force affected persons to change jobs or seek early retirement. This type of tremor is absent at rest and appears when the patient acts to move or support a body part (hence, the name "action tremor"). Essential tremor is not associated with other evidence of neurologic disease.

Essential or organic voice tremor is a focal presentation of essential tremor (Murdoch, 2010). The typical form of essential voice tremor occurs when the alternating contractions of the adductors and abductors of the vocal folds are of equal strength, in contrast to other presentations, such as adductor and abductor spasmodic dysphonia, where either the adductor or abductor movements of the vocal folds are disproportionately stronger. During contextual speech, essential voice tremor may not be apparent, especially when the tremor is mild. Vowel prolongation is typically the best task for eliciting voice tremor (Aronson, 1990), which can be perceived as rhythmic frequency modulations of 4 to 7 Hz, sometimes accompanied by fluctuations in loudness. Although essential voice tremor may occur in isolation, it is usually accompanied by head or extremity tremor.

### Models of Motor Control Applicable to Hypo- and Hyperkinetic Dysarthria

Hypo- and hyperkinetic movement disorders represent the extreme ends of the clinical spectrum of basal ganglia associated motor disturbances. Parkinsonism is characterized by a reduction in striatal dopaminergic transmission leading to increased basal ganglia output to the thalamus. In contrast, the major hyperkinetic syndromes, such as chorea, athetosis, and dystonia, are all characterized by reduced basal ganglia output to the thalamus, leading to disinhibition of the thalamocortical neurons which in turn leads to the development of involuntary movements. DeLong (1990) suggested that hypo- and hyperkinetic movement disorders can be explained using a functional model of the basal ganglia–thalamocortical circuit derived from findings of experiments involving monitoring of the neuronal activity of various basal ganglia sites in primates treated with MPTP (1-methyl-4-phenyl-1,2,3,6 tetrahydropyridine). In primates treated with MPTP, the dopaminergic cells in the SNc degenerate, and the animals subsequently develop a clinical syndrome that closely resembles human parkinsonism (Miller & DeLong, 1987). What the findings of these studies suggest is that the hypokinetic movement disorders associated with Parkinson disease may result from increased inhibition of the thalamocortical neurons that renders the cortical projection areas less responsive to other inputs normally involved in initiating movements. Briefly, according to the model of hypokinetic movement disorders proposed by DeLong (1990) (Figure 7–7), loss of striatal dopamine leads to excessive inhibition of the GPe leading to disinhibition of the STN which in turn provides excessive excitatory drive to the basal ganglia output nuclei (i.e., the GPi and SNr) via the indirect pathway leading to thalamic inhibition. This effect is reinforced by reduced inhibitory input to the basal ganglia output nuclei through the direct pathway, also leading to inhibition of thalamocortical neurons. According to DeLong (1990), these effects are postulated to result in a reduction in the usual reinforcing influence of the subcortical motor circuit upon cortically initiated movements leading to symptoms such as akinesia

and bradykinesia. The model proposed by DeLong (1990) is supported by data based on microelectrode recordings of basal ganglia neuron activity in MPTP treated primates (Filion & Tremblay, 1991; Filion, Tremblay, & Bedard, 1988) which have shown that neurons in the STN and GPi of these primates have higher discharge rates and show prominent changes in their discharge patterns, including a greater tendency to discharge in bursts. Further support has been derived from metabolic studies based on positron emission tomography (PET) that have demonstrated that the changes in basal ganglia discharge that results from dopamine depletion alter the neuronal activity in the thalamus and brainstem as well as cortical metabolic activity, consistent with the hypokinetic model (Brooks, 1991; Calne & Snow, 1993; Eidelberg, 1992; Leenders, 1997). Given that, according to the above hypokinetic model, motor disturbances in Parkinson disease are postulated to result in large part from increased thalamic inhibition due to excess excitatory drive from the STN to the output nuclei of the basal ganglia, it has been speculated that induced lesions in the STN would ameliorate symptoms such as bradykinesia and akinesia (DeLong, 1990). Experiments involving selective lesioning of the STN with ibotenate (a fiber-sparing neurotoxin) in MPTP-treated monkeys have confirmed this hypothesis (DeLong, 1990).

In addition to the model of hypokinetic movement disorders, DeLong (1990) also proposed a functional model to explain hyperkinetic movement disorders. Evidence is available to suggest that a common mechanism underlies the various hyperkinetic movement disorders such as the choreiform movement

in Huntington disease and the dyskinetic movements seen in hemiballismus. In fact, it has been suggested that
these dyskinesias differ only by the
intensity and amplitude of the movements. It is known that, early in the
course of Huntington disease, there is a
selective loss of striatal GABA/enkeph-
alin neurons that give rise to the indirect pathway. Experiments involving
neurotoxin (ibotenate) induced lesions
in the STN of monkeys suggest ballis-

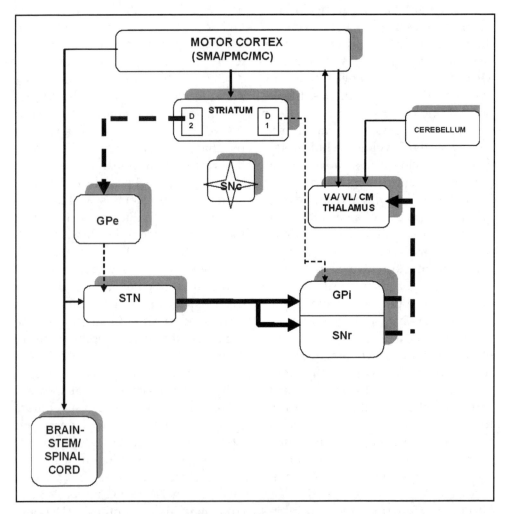

**FIGURE 7–7.** Modified schematic diagram of the basal ganglia thalamocortical motor
circuit in Parkinson disease based on DeLong (1990). **SMA**, supplementary motor
area; **PMC**, premotor cortex; **MC**, motor cortex; **D1**, striatal output neuron receptor
type D1; **D2**, striatal output receptor type D2; **SNc**, substantia nigra compacta; **GPe**,
globus pallidus externus; **STN**, subthalamic nucleus; **GPi**, globus pallidus internus;
**SNr**, substantia nigra reticulata; **VA**, ventral anterior nucleus of thalamus; **VL**, ventral
lateral nucleus of thalamus; **CM**, centrum medianum. *Solid arrow* indicates excitatory
pathway; *dashed arrow* indicates inhibitory pathway; *star* indicates lesion site. (From
Murdoch, 2010)

mus is associated with disinhibition of the thalamus as a result of STN lesions. According to the model of hyperkinetic movement disorders proposed by DeLong (1990), reduced excitatory projections from the STN to the GPi due to either STN lesions (as in ballismus) or reduced striatopallidal inhibitory influences along the indirect pathway (as in Huntington disease) (Figure 7–8)

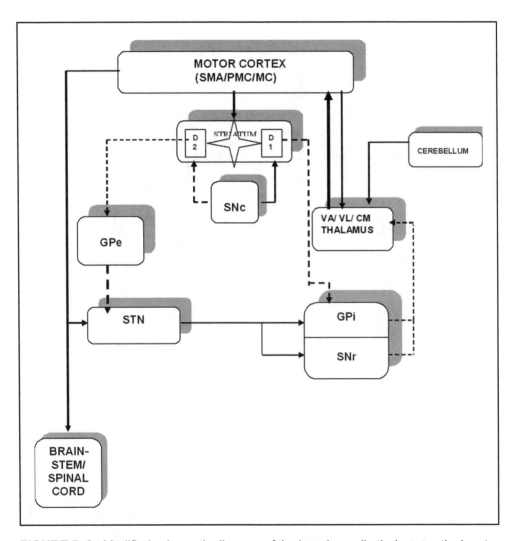

**FIGURE 7–8.** Modified schematic diagram of the basal ganglia thalamocortical motor circuit in Huntington disease based on DeLong (1990). **SMA**, supplementary motor area; **PMC**, premotor cortex; **MC**, motor cortex; **D1**, striatal output neuron receptor type D1; **D2**, striatal output receptor type D2; **SNc**, substantia nigra compacta; **GPe**, globus pallidus externus; **STN**, subthalamic nucleus; **GPi**, globus pallidus internus; **SNr**, substantia nigra reticulata; **VA**, ventral anterior nucleus of thalamus; **VL**, ventral lateral nucleus of thalamus; **CM**, centrum medianum. *Solid arrow* indicates excitatory pathway; *dashed arrow* indicates inhibitory pathway; *star* indicates lesion site. (From Murdoch, 2010)

lead to reduced inhibitory outflow from the GPi/SNr and excessive disinhibition of the thalamus. Dystonia has been likened to Parkinson disease with evidence of excessive indirect pathway activity, yet it differs in that direct pathway activity is also excessive, produc-ing an overall reduction in GPi output (Figure 7–9). In the case of levodopa-induced dyskinesias, disinhibition of the thalamus is thought to result from excessive dopaminergic stimulation of the striatal GABA/substance P neurons that send inhibitory projections to the

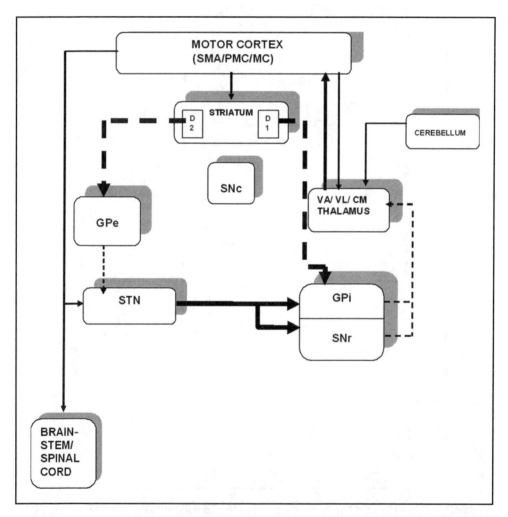

**FIGURE 7–9.** Schematic diagram of the basal ganglia thalamocortical motor circuit in dystonia based on Starr, Rau, and Davis (2005). **SMA,** supplementary motor area; **PMC,** premotor cortex; **MC,** motor cortex; **D1,** striatal output neuron receptor type D1; **D2,** striatal output receptor type D2; **SNc,** substantia nigra compacta; **GPe,** globus pallidus externus; **STN,** subthalamic nucleus; **GPi,** globus pallidus internus; **SNr,** substantia nigra reticulata; **VA,** ventral anterior nucleus of thalamus; **VL,** ventral lateral nucleus of thalamus; **CM,** centrum medianum. *Solid arrow* indicates excitatory pathway; *dashed arrow* indicates inhibitory pathway. (From Murdoch, 2010)

output nuclei of the basal ganglia via the direct pathway (Figure 7–10). The proposed overall effect is that of excessive positive feedback to the precentral motor fields engaged by the "skeleto-

motor" circuit resulting in hyperkinetic movements (DeLong 1990).

Although the above models serve to explain the basic pathophysiologic mechanisms underlying hypo- and

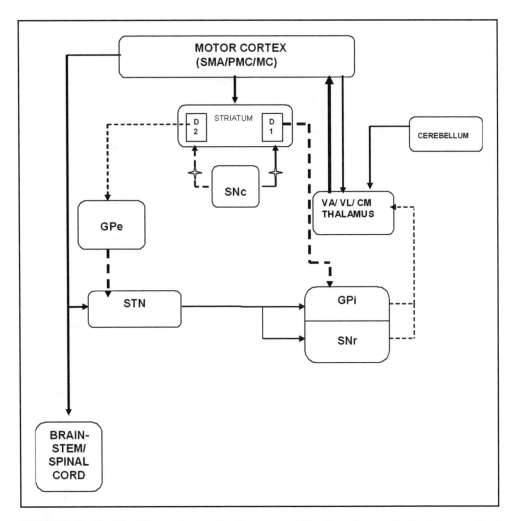

**FIGURE 7–10.** Modified schematic diagram of the basal ganglia thalamocortical motor circuit subserving drug-induced dyskinesias based on DeLong (1990). **SMA**, supplementary motor area; **PMC**, premotor cortex; **MC**, motor cortex; **D1**, striatal output neuron receptor type D1; **D2**, striatal output receptor type D2; **SNc**, substantia nigra compacta; **GPe**, globus pallidus externus; **STN**, subthalamic nucleus; **GPi** globus pallidus internus; **SNr**, substantia nigra reticulata; **VA**, ventral anterior nucleus of thalamus; **VL**, ventral lateral nucleus of thalamus; **CM**, centrum medianum. *Solid arrow* indicates excitatory pathway; *dashed arrow* indicates inhibitory pathway; *star* indicates excessive dopaminergic stimulation of GABA/substance P neurons. (From Murdoch, 2010)

hyperkinetic movement disorders, they do not account for a number of clinical and experimental observations. For example, the above models do not provide a satisfactory explanation for the lack of dyskinesias after pallidotomy, the lack of parkinsonian signs after thalamotomy, and the failure of experimental GPe lesions to abolish drug-induced dyskinesias. Although predicted by the model, according to Bathia and Marsden (1994), lesions of the thalamus are not associated with parkinsonism even though such lesions could be expected to reduce or interrupt thalamocortical drive. Likewise, lesions of the GPi in normal monkeys or humans do not induce dyskinesias as would be predicted by the model (Baron et al., 1996). Despite these limitations, the primate-based models proposed by DeLong (1990) provide an ideal context for looking further at the role of the basal ganglia in speech motor control.

## Ataxic Dysarthria

Damage to the cerebellum or its connections leads to a condition called "ataxia," in which movements become uncoordinated. If the ataxia affects the muscles of the speech mechanism, the production of speech may become abnormal, leading to a cluster of deviant speech dimensions collectively referred to as "ataxic dysarthria."

### Clinical Characteristics

The disrupted speech output exhibited by individuals with cerebellar lesions has often been termed "scanning speech," a term probably first used by Charcot (1877). According to

Charcot, "the words are as if measured or scanned: there is a pause after every syllable, and the syllables themselves are pronounced slowly" (p. 192). The most predominant features of ataxic dysarthria include a breakdown in the articulatory and prosodic aspects of speech. According to Brown, Darley, and Aronson (1970), the 10 deviant speech dimensions most characteristic of ataxic dysarthria can be divided into three clusters: articulatory inaccuracy, characterized by imprecision of consonant production, irregular articulatory breakdowns, and distorted vowels; prosodic excess, characterized by excess and equal stress, prolonged phonemes, prolonged intervals, and slow rate; and phonatory-prosodic insufficiency, characterized by harshness, monopitch, and monoloudness. Brown et al. (1970) believed that the articulatory problems were the product of ataxia of the respiratory and oral–buccal–lingual musculature, and prosodic excess was thought by these authors to result from slow movements. The occurrence of phonatory–prosodic insufficiencies was attributed to the presence of hypotonia.

### Respiratory Function

Perceptual correlates of respiratory inadequacy have been noted in a number of perceptual studies of ataxic dysarthria (Chenery, Ingram, & Murdoch, 1991; Kluin, Gilman, Markel, Koeppe, Rosenthal, Junck, 1988; Murdoch, Chenery, Stokes, & Hardcastle, 1991). In a study of 16 subjects with ataxic dysarthria, Chenery et al. (1991) reported the presence of significantly reduced ratings of respiratory support for speech as well as a respiratory pattern characterized by sudden forced inspiratory and expiratory sighs. Kluin et al. (1988) documented subjective reports of audible inspiration in ataxic dysarthric speakers investigated in their laboratory.

Evidence is also available from physiologic studies to suggest that speech breathing is disturbed in ataxic dysarthria. Murdoch et al. (1991) employed both spirometric and kinematic techniques to investigate the respiratory function of a group of 12 subjects with ataxic dysarthria associated with cerebellar disease. Their results showed that almost one half of the ataxic cases had vital capacities below the normal limits of variation. In addition, the ataxic dysarthric speakers also demonstrated unusual patterns of chest wall two-part contribution to lung volume change, including the presence of abdominal and ribcage paradoxing, abrupt changes in movements of the ribcage and abdomen, and a tendency to initiate utterances at lower than normal lung volume levels. Murdoch et al. (1991) suggested that these findings were an outcome of impaired coordination of the chest wall and speculated that such respiratory anomalies had the potential to underlie some of the prosodic abnormalities observed in ataxic dysarthria.

## Laryngeal Function

Phonatory disturbances are frequently listed among the most deviant or most frequently occurring perceptually deviant speech dimensions in ataxic dysarthria (Brown et al., 1970; Chenery et al., 1991; Darley et al., 1975; Enderby, 1986). The perceptual features listed that can be attributed to laryngeal dysfunction in ataxic dysarthria include disorders of vocal quality (for example, a harsh voice, strained-strangled phona-

tion, pitch breaks, and vocal tremor), impairment of pitch level (for example, elevated or lower pitch), and deficits in variability of pitch and loudness (for example, monopitch, monoloudness, and excess loudness variation). It should be noted that, as indicated by Darley et al. (1975), although attributed to phonatory dysfunction, many of the above speech deviations could also result, at least partly, from dysfunction at other levels of the speech production mechanism (for example, the respiratory system).

Unfortunately, only one study reported to date has used physiologic instrumentation to investigate laryngeal activity in ataxic dysarthria. Grémy, Chevrie-Muller, and Garde (1967) used electroglottograpahy to identify increased variability of vocal-fold vibrations in ataxic subjects.

## Velopharyngeal Function

The presence of hypernasal speech and nasal emission is not a commonly reported feature of ataxic dysarthria, suggesting that functioning of the velopharyngeal port may be normal in patients with cerebellar lesions. Duffy (1995) did report, however, that in some rare cases ataxic subjects may exhibit mild hyponasality, possibly as a consequence of improper timing of velar and articulatory gestures for nasal consonants. Oral examination of patients with cerebellar disorders most often reveals that elevation of the soft palate during phonation is normal.

## Articulatory and Prosodic Function

The most prominent features of ataxic dysarthria involve a breakdown in articulatory and prosodic aspects of speech. The imprecise articulation leads to improper formation and separation of individual syllables leading to a reduction in intelligibility while the disturbance in prosody is associated with loss of texture, tone, stress, and rhythm of individual syllables.

As indicated earlier, Brown et al. (1970) concluded that the 10 deviant speech dimensions perceived to be the most characteristic of ataxic dysarthria fell into three clusters: articulatory inaccuracy, prosodic excess, and phonatory–prosodic insufficiency. Based on the performance of ataxic speakers on the Frenchay Dysarthria Assessment, Enderby (1986) also observed perceptual correlates of articulatory and prosodic inadequacy to be prominent among the 10 features she believed to be the most characteristic of ataxic dysarthria, including poor intonation, poor tongue movement in speech, poor alternating movement of the tongue in speech, reduced rate of speech, reduced lateral movement of the tongue, reduced elevation of the tongue, poor alternating movement of the lips, and poor lip movements in speech.

In addition to the perceptual studies of ataxic dysarthria mentioned above, a number of researchers have used either acoustic and/or physiologic procedures to study the articulatory and prosodic aspects of ataxic dysarthria. Kent, Netsell, and Abbs (1979) examined the acoustic features of five patients with ataxic dysarthria. They reported that the most marked and consistent abnormalities observed in the spectrograms of these speakers were alterations in the normal timing patterns and a tendency towards equalized syllable durations. These authors concluded that general

timing is a major problem in ataxic dysarthria. Furthermore, they speculated that ataxic speakers fail to decrease syllable duration when appropriate because such reductions require flexibility in sequencing complex motor instructions. The lack of flexibility may lead to a syllable-by-syllable motor control strategy with subsequent abnormal stress patterns.

Only a few studies reported to date have used physiologic instrumentation to investigate the functioning of the articulators in ataxic dysarthria. In support of the concept that ataxic speakers are impaired in motor control, McClean, Beukelman, and Yorkston (1987) reported the case of an ataxic speaker who performed poorly on a non-speech visuomotor tracking task involving the lower lip and jaw. Kent and Netsell (1975) and Netsell and Kent (1976) analyzed articulatory position and movements in ataxic speakers using cineradiography. They observed a number of abnormal articulatory movements including abnormally small adjustments of anterior–posterior tongue movements during vowel production, which they thought may form the basis of the perception of vowel distortions. Although movements of the lips, tongue, and jaw were generally coordinated, these authors reported that individual movements of these structures were often slow. In addition, they noted that articulatory contacts for consonant production were occasionally incomplete.

Hirose, Kiritani, Ushijima, and Sawashima (1978) used an x-ray microbeam technique and electromyography to investigate articulatory dynamics in two dysarthric patients, one of whom had cerebellar degeneration. In particular, they examined the movement patterns in the jaw and lower lip. Their results showed that the ataxic speaker demonstrated inconsistency in articulatory movements, being characterized by inconsistency in both range and velocity of movement. Furthermore, Hirose et al. (1978) found that electromyography evidenced a breakdown of rhythmic patterns in articulatory muscles during syllable repetition. Overall, the findings of Hirose et al. (1978) are consistent with the perception that ataxic speech contains irregular articulatory breakdowns.

In an examination of four ataxic speakers, McNeil, Weismer, Adams, and Mulligan (1990) investigated isometric force and static position control of the upper and lower lips, tongue, and jaw during nonspeech tasks. They reported that the ataxic speakers had greater force and position instability than normal speakers, although impairment on one task did not necessarily predict impairment on other tasks.

## Summary of Speech Impairments in Movement Disorders

Neurologic disorders associated with lesions in the basal ganglia or cerebellum have been documented to cause a range of motor speech disorders, the symptoms of which reflect the effects of the lesion on the functioning of the muscles of the speech production mechanism. Specifically, lesions involving the basal ganglia system are associated with two major forms of dysarthria, namely hypokinetic and hyperkinetic dysarthria. Hypokinetic dysarthria is seen almost exclusively in cases of Parkinson disease but has also

been reported as a feature of progressive supranuclear palsy. Hyperkinetic dysarthria, in contrast, is a collective name applied to a range of hyperkinetic movement disorders, all of which are characterized by the presence of abnormal, involuntary movements that may disrupt the normal functioning of the muscles of the speech production mechanism. These latter disorders are further subdivided into quick and slow hyperkinetic disorders on the basis of the speed and duration of the abnormal involuntary movements associated with each condition. Quick hyperkinesias include myoclonus, tics, chorea, and ballism, while slow hyperkinesias include athetosis, dyskinesia, and dystonia. Damage to the cerebellum is associated with ataxic dysarthria, a condition caused by the decomposition of complex movements arising from a breakdown in the coordinated action of the muscles of the speech production mechanism to produce speech. Ataxic dysarthria is predominantly characterized by a breakdown in the articulatory and prosodic aspects of speech.

## References

Abbs, J. H., Hunker, C. J., & Barlow, S. H. (1983). Differential speech motor subsystem impairment with supranuclear lesions: Neurophysiological framework and supporting data. In W. R. Berry (Ed.), *Clinical dysarthria* (pp. 21–56). San Diego, CA: College-Hill Press.

Ackermann, H., Grone, B. F., Hoch, G., & Schonle, P. W. (1993). Speech freezing in Parkinson's disease: A kinematic analysis of orofacial movements by means of electromagnetic articulography. *Folia Phoniatrica et Logopaedica, 45,* 84–89.

Ackermann, H., & Hertrich, I. (2000). The contribution of the cerebellum to speech processing. *Journal of Neurolinguistics, 13,* 95–116.

Ackermann, H., Hertrich, I., & Hehr, T. (1995). Oral diadochokinesis in neurological dysarthrias. *Folia Phoniatrica et Logopaedica, 47,* 15–23.

Ackermann, H., Vogel, M., Petersen, D., & Poremba, M. (1992). Speech deficits in ischaemic cerebellar lesions. *Journal of Neurology, 239,* 223–227.

Ackermann, H., & Ziegler, W. (1991). Articulatory deficits in Parkinson's dysarthria: An acoustic analysis. *Journal of Neurology, Neurosurgery and Psychiatry, 54,* 1093–1098.

Ackermann, H., & Ziegler, W. (1992). Cerebellar dysarthria: a review. *Fortsch Neurology Psychiatry, 60,* 28–40.

Alexander, G. E., Crutcher, M. D., & DeLong, M. R. (1990). Basal ganglia–thalamocortical circuits: Parallel substrates for motor, oculomotor, prefrontal and limbic functions. In H. B. M. Uylings, C. G. Van Eden, J. P. C. De Bruin, M. A. Corner, & M. G. P. Feenstra (Eds.), *Progress in brain research* (Vol. 85, pp. 119–146). The Netherlands: Elsevier.

Alexander, G. E., DeLong, M. R., & Strick, P. L. (1986). Parallel organization of functionally segregated circuits linking basal ganglia and cortex. *Annual Review of Neuroscience, 9,* 357–381.

Alsobrook, J. P., & Pauls, D. L. (2002). A factor analysis of tic symptoms in Gilles de la Tourette's syndrome. *American Journal of Psychiatry, 159,* 291–296.

Aronson, A. E. (1990). *Clinical voice disorders.* New York, NY: Thieme.

Aronson, A. E., O'Neill, B. P., & Kelly, J. J. (1984). *The dysarthria of action myoclonus: A new clinical entity.* Paper presented at the Clinical Dysarthria Conference, Tucson, AZ.

Baron, M. S., Vitek, J. L., Bakay, R. A., Green, J., Kaneoke, Y., Hashimoto, T., . . . DeLong, M. R. (1996). Treatment of advanced Parkinson's disease by posterior GPi pallidotomy: 1-year pilot study results. *Annals of Neurology, 40,* 355–366.

Bathia, K. P., & Marsden, C. D. (1994). The behavioural and motor consequences of focal lesions of the basal ganglia in man. *Brain, 117,* 859–876.

Blitzer, A., & Brin, M. F. (1992). The dystonic larynx. *Journal of Voice, 6,* 294–297.

Brooks, D. J. (1991). Detection of preclinical Parkinson's disease with PET. *Neurology, 41*(Suppl. 2), 24.

Brown, J. R., Darley, F. L., & Aronson, A. E. (1970). Ataxic dysarthria. *International Journal of Neurology, 7,* 302–318.

Caligiuri, M. P., Harris, M. J., & Jeste, D. V. (1988). Quantitative analyses of voluntary orofacial motor control in schizophrenia and tardive dyskinesia. *Biological Psychiatry, 24,* 787–800.

Caligiuri, M. P., Jeste, D. V., & Harris, M. J. (1989). Instrumental assessment of lingual motor instability in tardive dyskinesia. *Neuropsychopharmacology, 2,* 309–312.

Calne, D., & Snow, B. J. (1993). PET imaging in parkinsonism. *Advances in Neurology, 60,* 484.

Canter, G. (1965). Speech characteristics of patients with Parkinson's disease. II. Physiological support for speech. *Journal of Speech and Hearing Disorders, 30,* 44–49.

Case, J., La Pointe, L., & Duane, D. (1990). *Speech and voice characteristics in spasmodic torticollis.* Paper presented at the International Congress of Movement Disorders, Washington, DC.

Charcot, J. M. (1877). *Lectures on the diseases of the nervous system.* London, UK: New Sydenham Society.

Chenery, H. J., Ingram, J. C. L., & Murdoch, B. E. (1991). Perceptual analysis of speech in ataxic dysarthria. *Australian Journal of Human Communication Disorders, 18,* 19–28.

Chenery, H. J., Murdoch, B. E., & Ingram, J. C. L. (1988). Studies in Parkinson's disease. I. Perceptual speech analysis. *Aus-*

*tralian Journal of Human Communication Disorders, 16,* 17–29.

Connor, N. P., Ludlow, C. L., & Schulz, G. M. (1989). Stop consonant production in isolated and repeated syllables in Parkinson's disease. *Neuropsychologia, 27,* 829–838.

Cramer, W. (1940). De spraak bij patienten met Parkinsonisme. *Logopaedie en Phoniatrie, 22,* 17–23.

Darley, F. L., Aronson, A. E., & Brown, J. R. (1969a). Differential diagnostic patterns of dysarthria. *Journal of Speech and Hearing Research, 12,* 246–269.

Darley, F. L., Aronson, A. E., & Brown, J. R. (1969b). Clusters of deviant speech dimensions in the dysarthrias. *Journal of speech and Hearing Research, 12,* 462–496.

Darley, F. L., Aronson, A. E., & Brown, J. R. (1975). *Motor speech disorders.* Philadelphia, PA: W. B. Saunders.

DeLong, M. R. (1990). Primate models of movement disorders of basal ganglia origin. *Trends in Neurosciences, 13,* 281–285.

DeLong, M. R., & Wichmann, T. (2007). Circuits and circuit disorders of the basal ganglia. *Archives of Neurology, 64,* 20–24.

Deuschl, G., Mischke, G., & Schenck, E. (1990). Symptomatic and essential rhythmic palatal myoclonus. *Brain, 113,* 1645–1672.

Drummond, S., & Fitzpatrick, A. (2004). Speech and swallowing performances in tardive dyskinesia: A case study. *Journal of Medical Speech Language Pathology, 12,* 9–19.

Drysdale, A. J., Ansell, J., & Adeley, J. (1993). Palato-pharyngo-laryngeal myoclonus: An unusual cause of dysphagia and dysarthria. *Journal of Laryngology and Otology, 107,* 746–747.

Duffy, J. (1995). *Motor speech disorders: Substrates, diagnosis and management.* St. Louis, MO: Mosby.

Duffy, J. (2013). Motor speech disorders: Substrates, diagnosis and management. (3rd Ed.) St. Louis, MO: Mosby.

Eidelberg, D. (1992). Positron emission tomography studies in parkinsonism. *Neurology Clinics, 10,* 421.

Enderby, P. (1986). Relationships between dysarthric groups. *British Journal of Disorders of Communication, 21,* 180–197.

Faheem, A. D., Brightwell, D. R., Burton, G. C., & Struss, A. (1982). Respiratory dyskinesia and dysarthria from prolonged neuroleptic use: Tardive dyskinesia? *American Journal of Psychiatry, 139,* 517–518.

Ferguson, A. (1992). Speech control in persistent tardive dyskinesia: A case study. *European Journal of Disorders of Communication, 27,* 89–93.

Feve, A., Angelard, B., & Lacau St Guily, J. (1995). Laryngeal tardive dyskinesia. *Journal of Neurology, 242,* 455–499.

Filion, M., & Tremblay, L. (1991). Abnormal spontaneous activity of globus pallidus neurons in monkeys with MPTP-induced parkinsonism. *Brain Research, 547,* 142.

Filion, M., Tremblay, L., & Bedard, P. J. (1988). Abnormal influences of passive limb movement on the activity of globus pallidus neurons in parkinsonian monkeys. *Brain Research, 444,* 165.

Flint, A. J., Black, S. E., & Campbell-Taylor, I. (1992). Acoustic analysis in the differentiation of Parkinson's disease and major depression. *Journal of Psycholinguistic Research, 21,* 383–399.

Forrest, K., & Weismer, G. (1995). Dynamic aspects of lower lip movement in parkinsonian and neurologically normal geriatric speakers' production of stress. *Journal of Speech and Hearing Research, 38,* 260–272.

Freed, D. (2000). *Motor speech disorders: Diagnosis and treatment.* San Diego, CA: Singular-Thompson Learning.

Friedhoff, A. (1982). Gilles de la Tourette syndrome. *Advances in Neurology, 35,* 335–339.

Gamboa, J., Jiménez-Jiménez, F. L., Nieto, A., Montojo, J., Orti-Pareja, M., Molina, J. A., . . . Cobeta, I. (1997). Acoustic voice analysis in patients with Parkinson's disease treated with dopaminergic drugs. *Journal of Voice, 11,* 314–320.

Gerfen, C. R. (1995). Dopamine receptor function in the basal ganglia. *Clinical Neuropharmacology, 18,* S162.

Gerratt, B. R. (1983). Formant frequency fluctuation as an index of motor steadiness in the vocal tract. *Journal of Speech and Hearing Research, 26,* 297–304.

Gerratt, B. R., Goetz, C. G., & Fisher, H. B. (1984). Speech abnormalities in tardive dyskinesia. *Archives of Neurology, 41,* 273–276.

Gerratt, B. R., Hanson, D. G., & Berke, G. S. (1987). Glottographic measures of laryngeal function in individuals with abnormal motor control. In T. Baer, C. Sasaki, & K. Harris (Eds.), *Laryngeal function in phonation and respiration* (pp. 521–531). Boston, MA: College-Hill Press.

Goldenberg, J., Ferraz, M. B., Fonseca, A., Hilário, M. O., Bastos, W., & Sachetti, S. (1992). Sydenham chorea: Clinical and laboratory findings. Analysis of 187 cases. *Revista Paulista de Medicina, 110,* 152–157.

Golper, L., Nutt, J., Rau, M., & Coleman, R. (1983). Focal cranial dystonia. *Journal of Speech and Hearing Disorders, 48,* 128–134.

Graybiel, A. M., & Kimura, M. (1995). Adaptive neural networks in the basal ganglia. In J. D. Houk, J. L. Davis, & D. G. Beiser (Eds.), *Models of information processing in the basal ganglia* (pp. 103–116). Cambridge, MA: MIT Press.

Grémy, F., Chevrie-Muller, C., & Garde, E. (1967). Etude phoniatrique clinique et instrumentale des dysarthries. *Review Neurologique, 116,* 401–426.

Hammen, V. L., Yorkston, K. M., & Beukelman, D. R. (1989). Pausal and speech duration characteristics as a function of speaking rate in normal and parkinsonian dysarthric individuals. In K. M. Yorkston & D. R. Beukelman (Eds.), *Recent advances in clinical dysarthria* (pp. 213–223). Boston, MA: College-Hill Press.

Hanson, D. G., Gerratt, B. R., & Ward, P. H. (1983). Glottographic measurement of vocal dysfunction: A preliminary report. *Annals of Otology, Rhinology and Laryngology, 92,* 413–420.

Hanson, W. R., & Metter, E. J. (1980). DAF as instrumental treatment for dysarthria in progressive supranuclear palsy: A case report. *Journal of Speech and Hearing Disorders, 45,* 268–275.

Hartelius, L., Carlstedt, A., Ytterberg, M., Lillvik, M., & Laakso, K. (2003). Speech disorders in mild and moderate Huntington disease: Results of dysarthria assessment of 19 individuals. *Journal of Medical Speech Language Pathology, 11,* 1–14.

Hirose, H. (1986). Pathophysiology of motor speech disorders (dysarthria). *Folia Phoniatrica et Logopaedica, 38,* 61–88.

Hirose, H., Kiritani, S., & Sawashima, M. (1982). Patterns of dysarthric movement in patients with amyotrophic lateral sclerosis and pseudobulbar palsy. *Folia Phoniatrica et Logopaedica, 34,* 106–112.

Hirose, H., Kiritani, S., Ushijima, T., & Sawashima, M. (1978). Analysis of abnormal articulatory dynamics in two dysarthric patients. *Journal of Speech and Hearing Disorders, 4,* 46–105.

Hirose, H., Kiritani, S., Ushijima, Y., Yoshioka, H., & Sawashima, M. (1981). Patterns of dysarthric movements in patients with parkinsonism. *Folia Phoniatrica et Logopaedica, 33,* 204–215.

Hirose, H., Sawashima, M., & Niimi, S. (1985). *Laryngeal dynamics in dysarthric speech.* Paper presented at the Thirteenth World Congress of Otorhinolaryngology, Miami Beach, FL.

Ho, A. K., Bradshaw, J. L., & Iansek, R. (2000). Volume perception in parkinsonian speech. *Movement Disorders, 15,* 1125–1131.

Hoodin, R. B., & Gilbert, H. R. (1989a). Nasal airflows in parkinsonian speakers. *Journal of Communication Disorders, 22,* 169–180.

Hoodin, R. B., & Gilbert, H. R. (1989b). Parkinsonian dysarthria: An aerodynamic and perceptual description of velopharyngeal closure for speech. *Folia Phoniatrica et Logopaedica, 41*, 249–258.

Hovestadt, A., Bogaard, J. D., Meerwaldt, J. D., van der Meche, F. G. A., & Stigt, J. (1989). Pulmonary function in Parkinson's disease. *Journal of Neurology, Neurosurgery and Psychiatry, 42*, 329–333.

Hunker, C., Abbs, J. H., & Barlow, S. (1982). The relationship between parkinsonian rigidity and hypokinesia in the orofacial system: A quantitative analysis. *Neurology, 32*, 755–761.

Jankovic, J. (1988). Cranial-cervical dysarthrias: An overview. In J. Jankovic & E. Tolosa (Eds.), *Advances in neurology: Facial dyskinesias* (Vol. 49, pp. 289–306). New York, NY: Raven Press.

Jankovic, J. (1995). Tardive syndromes and other drug-induced movement disorders. *Clinical Neuropharmacology, 18*, 197–214.

Jeste, D. V., & Wyatt, R. J. (1982). *Understanding and treating tardive dyskinesia.* New York, NY: Guilford Press.

Kent, R. D., & Netsell, R. (1975). A case study of an ataxic dysarthric: Cineradiographic and spectrographic observations. *Journal of Speech and Hearing Disorders, 40*, 115–134.

Kent, R. D., & Netsell, R. (1978). Articulatory abnormalities in the athetoid cerebral palsy. *Journal of Speech and Hearing Disorders, 43*, 353–373.

Kent, R. D., Netsell, R., & Abbs, J. H. (1979). Acoustic characteristics of dysarthria associated with cerebellar disease. *Journal of Speech and Hearing Disorders, 22*, 613–626.

Kent, R. D., & Rosenbek, J. C. (1982). Prosodic disturbance and neurological lesion. *Brain and Language, 15*, 259–291.

Khan, R., Jampala, V. C., Dong, K., & Vedak, C. S. (1994). Speech abnormalities in tardive dyskinesia. *American Journal of Psychiatry, 151*, 760–762.

King, J. B., Ramig, L. O., Lemke, J. H., & Harii, Y. (1994). Parkinson's disease: Longitudinal changes in acoustic parameters of phonation. *Journal of Medical Speech Language Pathology, 2*, 29–42.

Kluin, K. J., Gilman, S., Markel, D. S., Koeppe, R. A., Rosenthal, G., & Junck, L. (1988). Speech disorders in olivopontocerebellar atrophy correlate with positron emission tomography findings. *Annals of Neurology, 23*, 547–554.

Kulkarni, M., & Anees, S. (1996). Sydenham's chorea. *Indian Pediatrics, 33*, 112–115.

Lance, J. W., & Adams, R. D. (1963). The syndrome of intention or action myoclonus as a sequel to anoxic encephalopathy. *Brain, 87*, 111–133.

Langveld, T. P. M., Drost, H. A., Frijns, J. H. M., Zwinderman, A., & Baatenburg de Jong, R. J. (2000). Perceptual characteristics of adductor spasmodic dysphonia. *Annals of Otology, Rhinology and Laryngology, 109*, 741–748.

LaPointe, L., Case, J., & Duane, D. (1993). Perceptual-acoustic speech and voice characteristics of subjects with spastic torticollis. In J. Till, K. Yorkston, & D. Beukelman (Eds.), *Motor speech disorders: Assessment and treatment* (pp. 40–45). Baltimore, MD: Paul H. Brookes.

La Porta, M., Archambault, D., Ross-Chouinard, A., & Chouinard, G. (1990). Articulatory impairment associated with tardive dyskinesia. *Journal of Nervous and Mental Disease, 178*, 660–662.

Laszewski, Z. (1956). Role of the Department of Rehabilitation in preoperative evaluation of parkinsonian patients. *Journal of the American Geriatric Society, 4*, 1280–1284.

Lechtenberg, R., & Gilman, S. (1978). Speech disorders in cerebellar disease. *Annals of Neurology, 3*, 285–290.

Leenders, K. L. (1997). Pathophysiology of movement disorders studied using PET. *Journal of Neural Transmission, 41*(Suppl. 50), 39.

Lethlean, J. B., Chenery, H. J., & Murdoch, B. E. (1990). Disturbed respiratory and prosodic function in Parkinson's disease: A perceptual and instrumental analysis.

*Australian Journal of Human Communication Disorders, 18,* 83–98.

Logemann, J. A., & Fisher, H. B. (1981). Vocal tract control in Parkinson's disease: Phonetic feature analysis of misarticulations. *Journal of Speech and Hearing Disorders, 46,* 348–352.

Logemann, J. A., Fisher, H. B., Boshes, B., & Blonsky, E. R. (1978). Frequency co-occurrence of vocal tract dysfunctions in the speech of a large sample of Parkinson's patients. *Journal of Speech and Hearing Disorders, 43,* 47–57.

Ludlow, C. L., & Bassich, C. J. (1983). The results of acoustic and perceptual assessment of two types of dysarthria. In W. R. Berry (Ed.), *Clinical dysarthria* (pp. 121–147). San Diego, CA: College-Hill Press.

Ludlow, C. L., & Bassich, C. J. (1984). Relationship between perceptual ratings and acoustic measures of hypokinetic speech. In M. R. McNeil, J. C. Rosenbek, & A. E. Aronson (Eds.), *The dysarthrias: Physiology, acoustics, perception, management* (pp. 163–195). San Diego, CA: College-Hill Press.

Matthews, W. B., & Glaser, G. H. (1984). *Recent advances in clinical neurology.* Edinburgh, UK: Churchill Livingstone.

McClean, M. D., Beukelman, D. R., & Yorkston, K. M. (1987). Speech-muscle visuomotor tracking in dysarthric and non-impaired speakers. *Journal of Speech and Hearing Research, 30,* 276–282.

McNeil, M. R., Weismer, G., Adams, S., & Mulligan, M. (1990). Oral structure nonspeech motor control in normal, dysarthric, aphasic, and apraxic speakers: Isometric force and static position. *Journal of Speech and Hearing Research, 33,* 255–268.

Metter, E. J., & Hanson, W. R. (1986). Clinical and acoustical variability in hypokinetic dysarthria. *Journal of Communication Disorders, 19,* 347–366.

Middleton, F. A., & Strick, P. L. (1997). Dentate output channels: Motor and cognitive components. *Progress in Brain Research, 114,* 555–568.

Middleton, F. A., & Strick, P. L. (2000). Basal ganglia output and cognition: Evidence from anatomical, behavioural and clinical studies. *Brain and Cognition, 42,* 183–200.

Middleton, F. A., & Strick, P. L. (2001). Cerebellar projections to the prefrontal cortex of the primate. *Journal of Neuroscience, 21,* 700–712.

Miller, L. G., & Jankovic, J. (1990). Drug-induced dyskinesias. In S. H. Appel (Ed.), *Current neurology* (Vol. 10, pp. 127–136). Chicago, IL: Mosby-Yearbook.

Miller, W. C., & DeLong, M. R. (1987). Altered tonic activity of neurons in the globus pallidus and subthalamic nucleus in the primate MPTP model of parkinsonism. In M. B. Carpenter & A. Jayaraman (Eds.), *The basal ganglia II* (p. 415). New York, NY: Plenum.

Mink, J. W. (2007). Functional organisation of the basal ganglia. In J. Jankovic & E. Tolosa (Eds.), *Parkinson's disease and movement disorders* (pp. 1–6). Philadelphia, PA: Lippincott Williams, & Wilkins.

Moore, C. A., & Scudder, R. H. (1989). Coordination of jaw muscle activity in parkinsonian movement: Description and response to traditional treatment. In K. M. Yorkston & D. R. Beukelman (Eds.), *Recent advances in clinical dysarthria.* Boston, MA: College-Hill Press.

Morris, J. G., Grattan-Smith, P., Jankelowitz, S. K., Fung, V. S., Clouston, P. D., & Hayes, M. W. (2002). Athetosis II: The syndrome of mild athetoid cerebral palsy. *Movement Disorders, 17,* 1281–1287.

Mueller, P. B. (1971). Parkinson's disease: Motor speech behaviour in a selected group of patients. *Folia Phoniatrica et Logopaedica, 23,* 333–346.

Murdoch, B. E. (2010). *Acquired speech and language disorders: a neuroanatomical and functional neurological approach.* (2nd ed.). Oxford, UK: Wiley-Blackwell.

Murdoch, B. E., Chenery, H. J., Bowler, S., & Ingram, J. C. L. (1989). Respiratory function in Parkinson's subjects exhibiting a perceptible speech deficit: A kinematic and spirometric analysis. *Journal of Speech and Hearing Disorders, 54,* 610–626.

Murdoch, B. E., Chenery, H. J., Stokes, P. D., & Hardcastle, W. J. (1991). Respiratory kinematics in speakers with cerebellar disease. *Journal of Speech and Hearing Research, 34,* 768–780.

Murdoch, B. E., Manning, C. Y., Theodoros, D. G., & Thompson, E. C. (1995). *Laryngeal function in hypokinetic dysarthria.* Paper presented at the 23rd World Congress of the International Association of Logopedics and Phoniatrics, Cairo, Egypt.

Nausieda, P., Grossman, B., Koller, W., Weiner, W., & Klawans, H. (1980). Sydenham chorea: An update. *Neurology, 30,* 331–334.

Netsell, R., & Kent, R. (1976). Paroxysmal ataxic dysarthria. *Journal of Speech and Hearing Disorders, 41,* 93–109.

Parent, A., Lévesque, M., & Parent, M. (2001). A re-evaluation of the current model of the basal ganglia. *Parkinsonism and Related Disorders, 7,* 193–198.

Platt, L., Andrews, G., & Howie, P. (1980). Dysarthria of adult cerebral palsy II. Phonemic analyses of articulation errors. *Journal of Speech and Hearing Research, 23,* 41–45.

Ramig, L. A. (1986). Acoustic analyses of phonation in patients with Huntington's disease. *Annals of Otology, Rhinology and Laryngology, 95,* 288–293.

Ramig, L. A., Scherer, R. C., Titze, I. R., & Ringel, S. P. (1988). Acoustic analysis of voices of patients with neurologic disease: Rationale and preliminary data. *Annals of Otology, Rhinology and Laryngology, 97,* 164–172.

Robbins, J. A., Logemann, J. A., & Kirshner, H. S. (1986). Swallowing and speech production in Parkinson's disease. *Annals of Neurology, 19,* 283–287.

Sapienza, C. M., Walton, S., & Murry, T. (1999). Acoustic variations in adductor spasmodic dysphonia as a function of speech task. *Journal of Speech, Language and Hearing Research, 42,* 127–140.

Sapienza, C. M., Walton, S., & Murry, T. (2000). Adductor spasmodic dysphonia and muscle tension dysphonia: Acoustic analysis of sustained phonation and reading. *Journal of Voice, 14,* 502–520.

Schmahmann, J. D. (2001). The cerebrocerebellar system: Anatomic substrates of the cerebellar contribution to cognition and emotion. *International Review of Psychiatry, 13,* 247–260.

Schonecker, M. (1957). Ein eigentümliche syndrome im oralen Bereich bei megaphenapplikation. *Nervenarzt, 28,* 35.

Scott, S., Caird, F. I., & Williams, G. O. (1985). *Communication in Parkinson's disease.* London, UK: Croom Helm.

Serra-Mestres, J., Robertson, M. M., & Shetty, T. (1998). Palicoprolalia: An unusual variant of palilalia in Gilles de la Tourette's syndrome. *Journal of Neuropsychiatry and Clinical Neuroscience, 10,* 117–118.

Simon, R., Arminoff, M., & Greenberg, D. (1999). *Clinical neurology* (4th ed.). Stamford, CT: Appleton & Lange.

Solomon, N. P., & Hixon, T. J. (1993). Speech breathing in Parkinson's disease. *Journal of Speech and Hearing Research, 36,* 294–310.

Starr, P. A., Rau, S., & Davis, V. (2005). Spontaneous neuronal activity in human dystonia: Comparison with Parkinson's disease and normal macaque. *Journal of Neurophysiology, 93,* 3165–3176.

Strick, P. L., Dunn, R. P., & Picard, N. (1995). Macro-organization of the circuits connecting the basal ganglia with the cortical motor areas. In J. C. Houk, J. L. Davis, & D. G. Beiser (Eds.), *Models of information processing in the basal ganglia* (pp. 117–130). Cambridge, MA: MIT Press.

Svensson, P., Henningson, C., & Karlsson, S. (1993). Speech motor control in Parkinson's disease: A comparison between a clinical assessment protocol and a quantitative analysis of mandibular movements. *Folio Phoniatrica et Logopaaedica, 45,* 157–164.

Swedo, S., Leonard, H., Schapiro, M., Casey, B., Mannheim, G., Lenane, M. C., & Rettew, D. C. (1993). Sydenham's chorea: Physical and psychological symptoms of St Vitus dance. *Pediatrics, 91,* 706–713.

Theodoros, D. G., Murdoch, B. E., & Thompson, E. C. (1995). Hypernasality in Parkinson's disease: A perceptual and physiological analysis. *Journal of Medical Speech Language Pathology, 3,* 73–84.

Torre de la, R., Mier, M., & Boshes, B. (1960). Studies in parkinsonism: IX. Evaluation of respiratory function — preliminary observations. *Quarterly Bulletin of the Northwestern University Medical School, 34,* 232–236.

Vernon, G. M. (1991). Drug-induced and tardive movement disorders. *Journal of Neuroscience Nursing, 23,* 183–187.

Weiner, W. J., Goetz, C. G., Nausieda, P., & Klawans, H. L. (1978). Respiratory dyskinesias: Extrapyramidal dysfunction and dyspnea. *Annals of Internal Medicine, 88,* 327–331.

Weismer, G. (1984). Acoustic descriptions of dysarthric speech: Perceptual correlates and physiological inferences. *Seminars in Speech and Language, 5,* 293–313.

Wichmann, T., Bergman, H., & DeLong, M. R. (1994). The primate subthalamic nucleus. 1. Functional properties in intact animals. *Journal of Neurophysiology, 72,* 494.

Wilcox, P. G., Bassett, A., Jones, B., & Fleetham, J. A. (1994). Respiratory dysrhythmias in patients with tardive dyskinesia. *Chest, 105,* 203–207.

Yoshida, K., & Iizuka, T. (2003). Jaw deviation dystonia evaluated by movement-related cortical potentials and treated with muscle afferent block. *Cranio, 21,* 295–300.

Yoshida, K., Kaji, R., Shibasaki, H., & Iizuka, T. (2002). Factors influencing the therapeutic effect of muscle afferent block for oromandibular dystonia and dyskinesia and implications for their distinct pathophysiology. *International Journal of Oral and Maxillofacial Surgery, 31,* 499–505.

Zraick, R., LaPointe, L., Case, J., & Duane, D. (1993). Acoustic correlates of vocal quality in spasmodic torticollis. *Journal of Medical Speech Language Pathology, 1,* 261–269.

Zwirner, P., & Barnes, G. J. (1992). Vocal tract steadiness: a measure of phonatory and upper airway motor control during phonation in dysarthria. *Journal of Speech and Hearing Research, 35,* 761–768.

Zwirner, P., Murry, T., & Woodson, G. (1991). Phonatory function of neurologically impaired patients. *Journal of Communication Disorders, 24,* 287–300.

# Swallowing and Nutritional Aspects

*JULIE A. G. STIERWALT*

## Introduction

The process of deglutition is an essential element of life. Not only does it provide the body with nutrients and hydration for survival, but eating and drinking is a core feature of daily activities with friends and family, so much so that it is a highly automated task, a function into which we invest very little thought: We just open our mouths, pop in a morsel, and assume everything will get to the stomach without incident. As simple as the process appears, it is actually quite complex and requires precise movement and timing of a number of structures (LaPointe, Murdoch, & Stierwalt, 2010). When disruptions in movement occur, this careful balance can result in swallowing impairment or dysphagia.

Dysphagia is any disruption in the process of moving food or liquid from the mouth to the stomach. When considering the anatomy of the digestive tract, it is important to point out that there is a shared pathway in use for both breathing and eating. For breathing we use the nasal passages and the mouth, pharynx, larynx, and lower respiratory passageways to the lungs. For deglutition, the path starts in the mouth and moves through the pharynx to the esophagus. In the lower pharynx, the common pathway ends and there is a bifurcation into two passageways with one path leading forward into the respiratory tract and the other traveling behind into the digestive tract. The fact that there is a common path can become an issue. We have to breathe most of the time, so the respiratory passage must remain wide open for good air exchange. During eating, however, the passage must close off to protect the airway. The act of swallowing is a primary protection for the respiratory system. During the swallow, the entrance to the larynx and airway is sealed off temporarily. This cessation of breathing and closure of the airway directs food to the esophagus where it continues the digestive journey to the stomach. Careful coordination and precise movement of anatomic structures is necessary to maintain balance between the two systems.

Dysphagia is a problem that crosses the lifespan. An accurate estimate of dysphagia is almost impossible to pin down because there are a number of variables to consider. For example, the population (movement disorders, stroke, head and neck cancer), the method of identifying dysphagia (instrumental assessment or survey), and even how dysphagia is defined. In a number of large studies that have reviewed entire hospitals, it has been reported that roughly one-third of the hospitalized population at any one time, regardless of etiology, has swallowing impairment (Groher & Bukatman, 1986).

The prevalence of dysphagia increases when we consider only those individuals who suffer from movement disorders. Careful examination of the normal process of swallowing indicates why this would be the case. The act of swallowing is really a series of actions and events that take place to manipulate a bolus, move it through the mouth, the pharynx, and safely into the esophagus where it will travel to the stomach. Historically, swallowing has been described as a four-phase process with each phase distinct from the others. More recently, researchers

have noted overlap, with events from phases occurring simultaneously rather than sequentially. Although we know that overlap exists, it remains easiest to explain and understand the process as occurring in phases.

## Oral Preparatory Phase

The first phase of swallowing calls for preparation of the bolus. When food/liquid is taken into your mouth, care is taken to contain it in the oral cavity while it is prepared for the remaining phases. Containment in the front of the mouth occurs primarily by the lips, although the teeth might assist if there is no chewing involved. On the sides of the mouth, the buccal (cheek) muscles will increase tension against the teeth to keep the bolus from falling into the cheek cavity. At the back of the mouth, the tongue will elevate and come into contact with the velum, providing posterior containment. The tongue/velum contact also allows for breathing to continue while oral preparation is underway. Bolus containment is important so the bolus does not fall into the pharynx and the airway which, as mentioned, is open for breathing. With the bolus securely contained in the mouth, preparation can occur. How much preparation is required depends largely on the bolus with solids requiring a good deal of preparation compared with liquids. The function of oral preparation is to make sure the bolus is masticated and broken down. In addition, the bolus is mixed with saliva to help keep it cohesive and easy to control. When the bolus is broken down to a manageable size and consistency, it is gathered by the tongue and brought to the middle of the oral cavity. Figure 8–1 illustrates the swallowing process.

There is a good deal of variation in the oral preparatory phase according to the consistency of the bolus. As mentioned, a chunk of meat is prepared differently than a sip of water. When the meat has entered the mouth, you will seal off the lips to contain it in the mouth (lateral and posterior contain-ment is also in place). Now your tongue will go to work, moving the meat over to the teeth that will grind and mix it with saliva. The sensory input from the tongue will constantly send information about the consistency of the bolus, i.e., is it manageable for swallowing, or is more chewing necessary? When the bolus is "just right" the tongue will gather it in the middle of the tongue

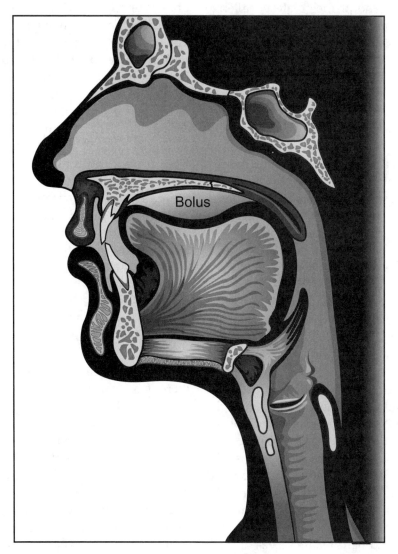

**FIGURE 8–1.** Phases of normal swallow. (From Hixon, Weismer, & Hoit, 2008)

in one cohesive unit. The amount of muscle activity and time it takes to prepare a bolus that requires mastication is clearly greater than what is necessary for a liquid bolus. It is important to point out, however, that a liquid bolus is not without its challenges. Although mastication or chewing is not required, the fluid nature of the bolus requires an incredible amount of motor control just to keep it under control. Once it enters the mouth the greatest challenge is to contain it and gather it together. So although fluid is considered an "easy" consistency, that fact is only true if motor/muscle control is intact. Because of these consistency effects, the oral preparatory phase is under voluntary control, and you can choose to chew as long as is necessary or not chew at all if the bolus does not require breakdown. The voluntary nature of this phase makes it highly variable in terms of timing and muscle activity.

## Oral Transit Phase

Once the bolus has been prepared and gathered at the center of the tongue, the oral transit phase begins. The purpose of the oral transit phase is to deliver the bolus from the oral cavity to the pharynx so it can begin its descent to the esophagus. To initiate bolus transit, the tongue is anchored at the front of the oral cavity behind the teeth. The tongue then begins a contraction against the hard palate that begins right behind the teeth and moves back along the hard palate to the back of the mouth. This front-to-back contact between the tongue and hard palate serves to push or strip the bolus through the mouth and back to the pharynx (Figure 8–2). As

reviewed in the previous section, bolus containment continues to be important here. The lips will remain closed, the cheek muscles against the teeth, but as the bolus moves to the back of the mouth the soft palate will begin to lift in preparation for the swallow.

As with the oral preparation phase, there are accommodations in bolus transit related to consistency, although the variation that occurs in the oral transit phase due to consistency change is not as great as that seen in oral preparation. The variation that does occur has to do with pressures exerted by the tongue to force the bolus back to the pharynx. For a bolus that is more solid, the tongue must exert greater pressure (Youmans & Stierwalt, 2006; Youmans, Youmans, & Stierwalt, 2009). These accommodations are intuitive, and fluids would require little pressure because it already moves so easily. When you consider the *timing* aspect of oral transit, however, there is little variation across consistencies. The time it takes to move a solid bolus is essentially the same as a liquid bolus.

## Pharyngeal Phase

In the pharyngeal phase of swallowing, there is a carefully orchestrated series of events, the purpose of which is to protect the airway from aspiration as the bolus moves through the pharynx and enters the esophagus. The events are triggered as the bolus enters the pharynx at the end of bolus transit. The velum which started to elevate at the end of the oral transit phase makes contact with the posterior pharyngeal wall. The tongue continues to push the bolus back into the pharynx. The

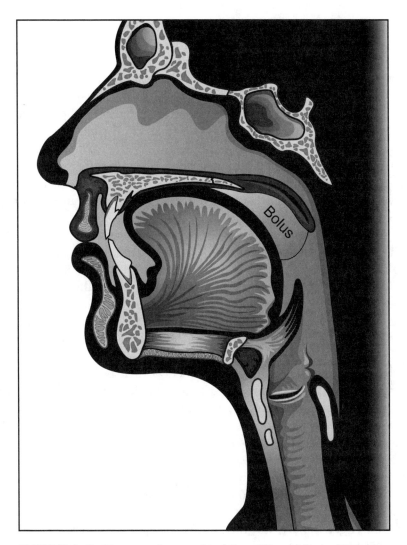

**FIGURE 8–2.** Phases of normal swallow. (From Hixon, Weismer, & Hoit, 2008)

base of the tongue then also serves as a foundation for the pharyngeal muscles which contract to squeeze the bolus through the pharynx. There are three primary pharyngeal muscles that contract sequentially from the top to the bottom to accomplish bolus movement through the pharynx.

Bolus movement through the pharynx is only a portion of the pharyngeal phase. The role of protecting the airway is another vital function that occurs during this phase. When the tongue pushes the bolus back into the pharynx the muscles in the floor of the mouth begin to contract. Tightening those muscles pulls the framework of the larynx up and forward also pulling the opening to the airway forward. The up-and-forward excursion of the larynx causes a downward movement of the epiglottis closing the opening to the larynx. This seal at the entrance to the larynx completes the first of three levels of protection for the airway. The additional levels of protection occur when the ventricular folds and the true vocal folds adduct sealing the airway at two additional levels. Redundancy in the system (three layers of protection) illustrates the importance of closing off the airway to potential intrusion of food or liquid.

At the bottom of the pharynx lies the esophagus. The boundary between these two structures is the cricopharyngeus muscle. The cricopharyngeus muscle is a circular muscle at the top of the esophagus that is in tonic contraction and only opens to allow a bolus to enter the esophagus. The opening of the cricopharyngeus occurs as a consequence of two actions. The primary action is the nerve impulse that travels to the cricopharyngeus to relax the tonic contraction. The muscle does indeed "relax" or open, allowing the bolus to pass through to the esophagus. The secondary action that opens the cricopharyngeus is a result of the movement of the laryngeal framework. The cricopharyneus muscle is attached to the cricoid cartilage (the lower border of the laryngeal framework), so as the framework moves up and forward, it stretches the cricopharyneus muscle pulling it open. Once the bolus has passed into the esophagus, the larynx lowers and the muscle returns to tonic contraction. With the return of the system to its resting state, the structures above are all returning to their original positions opening the airway so breathing can resume. This is illustrated in Figure 8–3.

When consistency effects are considered, variations in the pharyngeal phase are similar to those experienced in the oral transit phase. Greater muscle pressure is necessary to move a thicker bolus, but fluid follows gravity and flows easily through the pharynx. With respect to the time it takes to move a bolus through the pharynx, it is similar across consistencies but understandably longer for a more solid bolus. There is one other "consistency" effect worth mentioning: Liquids, because of their fluid properties, invade every space in the pharynx. Remember that the entrance to the airway, which is located in the pharynx, is sealed off during this phase. When that process is intact a bolus will not penetrate that seal; however, if the closure is incomplete or if it occurs slowly, then fluid can flow into the larynx, and thus, the airway. A more solid consistency is less likely to do so because it tends to hold together better.

## Esophageal Phase

The esophageal phase begins with closure of the cricopharyngeus muscle. Once in the esophagus, the bolus travels down the tube through a combination of gravity and muscle contraction. Muscle contraction that occurs in the esophagus is peristaltic in nature. Peristalsis is a wave-like contraction with relaxation ahead of the bolus and contraction behind, efficiently moving the bolus to the lower esophagus. At the end of the esophagus is a sphincter muscle similar to the cricopharyngeus. The lower esophageal sphincter (LES) is also in tonic contraction (this keeps stomach contents that contain acid from

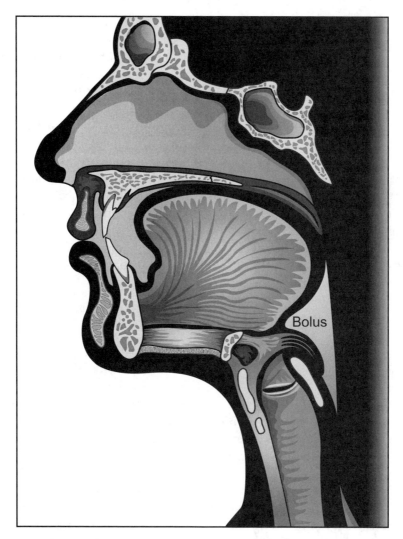

**FIGURE 8–3.** Phases of normal swallow. (From Hixon, Weismer, & Hoit, 2008)

entering the esophagus). Once the bolus approaches the lower esophagus, however, the LES opens, allowing the bolus to pass into the stomach where it can be broken down and digested further. Consistency effects in the esophagus follow the pattern of the pharyngeal phase. A bolus that is more substantial moves a little slower and require more work from the esophageal muscles.

## Implications for Movement Disorders

The intricacies of the "typical" swallowing process indicate that a careful balance exists between respiration and deglutition. Much of that balance depends on carefully orchestrated timing and movement of structures within the oral motor system. For individuals fortunate enough to have good integrity of the motor system, the balance is rarely disrupted; however, for people who experience movement disorders, swallowing impairment can be a chronic condition (Gutekurst, Norflus, & Hersch, 2002; Hegland, 2010; Kagel & Leopold, 1992; Klasner, 2010; Muchow, et al., 2008; Papatrepopoulos & Singer, 2006; Trejos, et al, 2004). Chapter 3 provides a comprehensive review of the characteristics of movement disorders, ranging from apraxia to the myriad of dyskinesias that may occur. What we discuss in this chapter are the implications of those movement disorders which can result in dysphagia.

## Apraxia

Apraxia is a condition in which relatively automatic or learned skilled movements are disrupted, often in the absence of motor weakness of associated structures. The underlying pathophysiology, as it relates to apraxia of speech (AOS), has been proposed to be a disturbance in motor planning or programming of movements (Duffy, 2005), although the exact nature of AOS has long been a source of discussion (or debate) in the literature. Regardless of the difficulty elucidating the exact nature of the condition, it stands to reason that if apraxia can be observed in the oral motor system to disrupt speech, it may also interfere with swallowing function.

Swallowing apraxia has been documented in the literature; unfortunately, our understanding of the nature of swallowing apraxia parallels that of AOS (Daniels, 2000). When apraxia of swallowing or swallowing apraxia has been described, the clinical characteristics have to do with disrupted movements in the oral phase (Logemann, 1998; Robbins & Levine, 1988). Such observations are somewhat intuitive because apraxia symptoms appear most frequently in voluntary movements and the process of swallowing begins with voluntary activities but becomes more reflexive through the pharyngeal and esophageal phases; therefore, to consider a diagnosis of swallowing apraxia, a breakdown with the planned movements of bolus manipulation would be expected.

## Ataxia

Motor discoordination that occurs as a result of cerebellar damage is known as ataxia. The primary disruptions relate to the force and timing of movements. Swallowing difficulties for individuals with ataxia include difficulty with mastication and general manipulation of a bolus. In particular, solid consistencies are problematic because of the demands of bolus breakdown. In these individuals the problems with timing can result in poor mastication, leading to premature delivery of large pieces of intact food into the pharynx. In a study that reviewed the potential for dysphagia and aspiration in a group of children and adults ($n = 70$) diagnosed with ataxia–telangiectasia, Lefton-Greif and colleagues (2000) found that 51 of the 70 exhibited signs of dysphagia. Over 25% of those with dysphagia demonstrated aspiration, and a majority of those were instances of silent aspiration. In this group of children and adults, age was a significant factor of aspiration; those who were older were more likely to show aspiration. In addition, the incidence of compromised nutritional status increased with age. The characteristics of ataxia create problems in the sequence of movements for successful swallowing.

## Motor Neuron Characteristics

### *Lower Motor Neuron*

Injury or disease that involves the lower motor neuron pathways have a direct impact on swallowing ability, specifically if the damage includes any portion of the cranial nerves or the higher spinal nerves which innervate respiration. To better understand the relation, the signs of lower motor neuron damage include:

1. Focal or widespread affects
2. Muscle atrophy
3. Weakness
4. Fasciculation
5. Fibrillation
6. Hypotonia
7. Hyporeflexia.

An examination of this list elucidates the impact that a number of these characteristics would have on swallowing. Muscles affected by lower motor neuron damage operate with reduced range, velocity, and direction of movement. Functionally, weakness and the lack of muscle tone (hypotonia) in the muscles of swallowing often result in extended mealtimes, degraded muscle contraction for transporting the bolus through the oral and pharyngeal cavities, and reduced laryngeal elevation (airway protection). Over time, lower motor neuron syndrome leads to atro-

phy. That fact coupled with the disuse atrophy that may occur from neurologic damage can lead to a downward spiral of weakness for swallowing function. In fact, individuals with nervous system damage who experience a dramatic decrease in their typical activity levels can lose up to 40% of strength reserves in a matter of weeks (Burkhead, Sapienza, & Rosenbek, 2007).

### *Upper Motor Neuron*

Muscle function following damage to the upper motor neuron pathways can result in very similar functional symptoms (e.g., extended mealtime, reduced muscle contraction, etc.). Although functionally similar, the underlying pathology is dramatically different. The effects of damage to the higher centers of motor pathways result in problems that are quite the opposite from those seen with lower motor damage. Characteristics of upper motor neuron syndrome include:

1. Systemic or widespread effects
2. Weakness
3. Hypertonia
4. Hyperreflexia

When lower motor neuron syndrome is implicated, the swallowing problems are primarily a result of a lack of muscle tone and weakness; thus, muscle movement is sluggish leading to inefficient management of food and liquid. Inefficiency in bolus management translates into poor bolus control and retained material in the oral and pharyngeal cavities. With upper motor neuron system involvement, the functional problems are a result of hypertonia. In this case, muscle groups also move slowly, but the nature of the difficulty is secondary to *increased* muscle tone. In muscles with hypertonia, movement is slow and inefficient because resting muscle tone is increased and resists movement. The muscles of the tongue are tight, making manipulation of the bolus during oral preparation difficult. Lingual propulsion through the oral cavity is also affected, as is pharyngeal transport. So although the functional implications of upper and lower motor neuron damage are similar, the underlying pathophysiology is dramatically different. (A comprehensive explanation of the upper and lower motor neuron systems is provided in Chapter 3.)

## Dyskinesias

When one considers a diagnosis of "movement disorders," it is likely that one of the classic dyskinesias would be first to come to mind as a prototypical example. Dyskinesia is a term that is defined as *dys*-abnormal *kinesia*-movement. The abnormal movements seen in dyskinesia can arise in a variety of body parts and often interferes with voluntary movements. When the affected areas include the oral motor system, an individual will likely experience speech and swallowing difficulty.

Dyskinesia is a broad term for movement disorders, and as such, it encompasses a variety of diagnoses that have distinct characteristics. These movement disorders may affect one or many structures and may be difficult to discern, or blatantly obvious to outside observers. Diagnoses that are characterized by movements affecting swallowing include:

- Athetosis: Athetoid movements are slow writhing movements which are repetitive and rhythmic in nature.
- Chorea: Choreic movements are unpredictable and jerky, often interfering with intentional movements (Cummings, 1995).
- Tardive dyskinesia: The head and neck movements associated with tardive dyskinesia are often repetitive, involuntary movements affecting the lips, tongue, jaw, and even larynx (Sheppard, 2010).
- Akinesia: Akinesia is characterized by difficulty or slowness in the ability to initiate movement.
- Dystonia: The movements of structures affected by dystonia include involuntary, oppositional contractions of antagonistic muscle groups which result in twisting movements or abnormal postures (Murdoch, 2010).
- Bradykinesia: Bradykinesia is characterized by slowed voluntary movement.

The diagnoses included in the category of dyskinesia have a dramatic effect on swallowing ability. The involuntary and oftentimes unpredictable movements lead to disruption in managing both food and liquids. That difficulty can translate into an inability to coordinate the process of chewing. For example, the tongue may be engaged in repetitive movements that are counterproductive to moving a bolus to the teeth and then collecting it again once it has been broken down into a cohesive bolus. When this occurs, there could be a number of consequences. One problem might be that the solid material is pushed beyond the teeth into the buccal cavity. In that case, the affected structure (tongue) is unable to coordinate the movements necessary to collect the bolus from the cheek. The tongue may also push the bolus out of the front of the mouth, a symptom that is particularly embarrassing. Another possible consequence of involuntary lingual movements is bolus loss over the base of the tongue. This scenario is a dangerous one. When a bolus is misdirected over the tongue into the pharynx before the swallow is engaged, the airway is open and aspiration is likely. If the bolus is a solid that has not been properly masticated (e.g., a chunk of meat), the aspiration that occurs may result in an airway obstruction and possible asphyxiation. Finally, because the dyskinesias can impact whole body movements, the careful coordination of breathing and swallowing may be disrupted, which is an additional contributor to aspiration.

The nature of dyskinesias carries an additional risk. Unintended or excessive movements come at a cost to the body and its energy reserves. All movement is fueled by energy, either oxidative or glycolytic. Depending on function, muscles in the body draw from either of these energy sources or sometimes from a combination. Those muscles which contain primarily slow-to-fatigue motor units, such as the muscles along the spine that we use to maintain posture, depend on oxygen to function. The motor units we use for rapid precise movements, many of which we use for speech and swallowing function, pull energy from glucose stores. In the oral motor system, there are muscles that have motor units with elements of both slow-oxidative and fast-glycolitic

characteristics (Burkhead, Sapienza, & Rosenbek, 2007; Kent, 2004). Regardless of the energy source, the more physically active an individual is, the greater the need for oxygen, nutrition, and hydration.

## Nutritional Implications

To maintain health, the body draws nutrients from ingested food and drink. Your body uses these nutrients to maintain bodily tissues, fuel activity, and fight disease. A careful balance of nutrients is important including proper hydration, vitamins, minerals, and a variety of caloric sources (e.g., proteins, carbohydrates, and fats) that are used to provide energy (Whitney & Rolfes, 2008). The dietary needs of every individual are unique and depend upon age, frame size, gender, physical activity levels, and overall health. The American Dietetic Association (ADA) has established Recommended Dietary Allowances (RDAs) which represent the intake levels necessary to maintain adequate nutrition (Swift, 2012). When an individual does not meet these daily requirements, either through inadequate intake or when energy expenditure exceeds intake, which can be the case with movements disorders, malnutrition can result.

Although a person's weight is not always an accurate measure of nutritional status (i.e., people who are overweight can be malnourished), it does provide an indication. There are a number of methods to determine a "healthy weight." One general method is to calculate an estimated "ideal body weight" (IBW); see Table 8–1 for the method to determine IBW. Another indicator is the body mass index (BMI), which is another formula based on a person's height and weight (Table 8–2). Each of these methods are used as easy screening tools that can provide a gross indication of nutritional health without instrumentation and blood work. Individuals who fall below IBW or in the underweight category for BMI (Table 8–3) are at risk for malnutrition.

There are a number of additional clinical indicators of malnutrition, which include an unintended weight loss of ≥10 pounds (4.5 kg) or 10% of total weight, serum prealbumin (an index of protein) levels that fall below <15 mg/dL, a dramatic change in functional status, and decreased food intake. Of these indicators, serum prealbumin is the most accurate index of malnutrition (Beck & Rosenthal, 2002); however, it is a lab value that can only be obtained through blood work. Routine inclusion of these other indicators (IBW, BMI, information on weight loss, decreased food intake) into a diagnostic protocol helps to establish an estimate of nutritional status.

The very nature of movement disorders, in particular the dyskinesias, place individuals at risk for malnutrition. The difficulty experienced with the motor aspects of eating often lead to decreased intake of food and liquid. When you couple the increased energy expenditure that is experienced, malnutrition is likely to occur. The symptoms of malnutrition can include:

- Weight loss
- Decreased healing
- Altered insulin levels
- Decreased liver function
- Depleted mineral stores
- Cognitive decline.

**Table 8–1.** Ideal Body Weight (*IBW*) Calculation

| Gender | English | Metric |
|--------|---------|--------|
| Male | 110 lbs for 5 feet in height<br>5 lbs for each additional inch | 50 kg for 5 feet in height<br>2.3 kg for each additional inch |
| | Example: A man who is 5'8" has an IBW of 150 lbs or 68.18 kg | |
| Female | 100 lbs for 5 feet in height<br>5 lbs for each additional inch | 45.5 kg for 5 feet in height<br>2.3 kg for each additional inch |
| | Example: A woman who is 5'3" has an IBW of 115 lbs or 52.27 kg | |

**Table 8–2.** Body Mass Index

| English | Metric |
|---------|--------|
| Weight in lbs / (height in inches)$^2$ × 703 | Weight in kg ÷ (height in cm)$^2$ |

*Source:* Body mass index Centers for Disease Control and Prevention (2013).

**Table 8–3.** Interpretation of Body Mass Index (*BMI*)

| BMI | Interpretation |
|---|---|
| <18.5 | Underweight |
| 18.5–24.9 | Normal |
| 25.0–29.9 | Overweight |
| 30.0+ | Obese |

*Source:* Centers for Disease Control and Prevention.

As a chronic condition, malnutrition will deplete the body's energy stores, and cachexia, or muscle wasting, occurs, resulting in generalized weakness. This scenario illustrates the downward spiral that can be experienced as individuals attempt to ingest enough to cover their energy requirements.

## Managing Dysphagia in Movement Disorders

There are a number of options for treating swallowing impairment in people with movement disorders. Medical treatments often include pharmacology to manage variations in muscle tone, and alleviate associated motor symptoms related to diagnosis, with varying degrees of success (Higgins, 2006; Laskawi & Rohrback, 2001). Surgical management (DBS, decompression) may also be implicated; however, results are not always beneficial. (See Chapter 10 for a comprehensive overview on medical treatments prescribed for movement disorders.)

Regardless of the medical treatments implemented, speech-language pathol-ogists are often called on to supplement with direct and indirect treatment methods (Logeman, 1998). Direct treatments include strategies to utilize while eating in order to make the process more safe and efficient. The primary direct methods implemented for individuals with movement disorders include diet modification, postural adjustments, and compensatory strategies.

Alterations to diet and hydration to alleviate symptoms of dysphagia are among the most common recommendations in the treatment of swallowing impairment (Groher & Crary, 2010). The properties of fluid are particularly difficult to manage for individuals with motor impairments. Thin liquids move rapidly and are difficult to control, often falling over the tongue base and falling into an unprotected airway. Add to that picture structures that never stop moving, or that have difficulty moving at all, creating an even greater risk of aspiration. Consequently, a frequent recommendation is to thicken liquids in order to: (1) slow their movement, and (2) create a bolus that remains more cohesive. The recommendations for thickened fluids utilized in dietary recommendations include nectar, honey, or pudding. The viscosities of these liquids simulate the properties as their name implies ranging from unaltered thin liquids to pudding-thick liquids which resemble the consistency of a semisolid bolus more than a liquid. Liquids are thickened with commercial powders or can be purchased in prepackaged consistencies. Products that are manufactured for the specific purpose of thickening liquids are preferable to "homemade" remedies such as adding potato flakes. The reason lies in the change that occurs, or rather does not occur, with manufactured products. These products succeed in thickening liquids, but once in the digestive system the bolus breaks down and fluids are released and utilized by the body as necessary hydration. Home remedies may change the properties of liquids to the point that they cannot be counted on for hydration needs.

Like liquids, diet modifications are recommended based upon their ease of bolus formation and transit. A solid bolus that breaks into small pieces (e.g., chunks of an apple) is a challenge for individuals with weakness, discoordinated, or excess movements of the oral motor system. Mixed consistencies (e.g., cereal with milk, vegetable soup) also present risks, as individuals must attend to the solid consistency in order to break it down, meanwhile losing control of the liquid portion of the bolus. Semisolid consistencies, such as mashed potatoes, are delivered in a soft cohesive bolus, decreasing the need for a good deal of manipulation or preparation. This consistency also moves very slowly, which makes it easier to manage for muscles that are not functioning properly. Because diet modifications are a high priority in management, there has been an attempt to standardize diet recommendations with regard to texture and nomenclature. In 2002, the American Dietetic Association published the National Dysphagia Diet (Table 8–4) (National Dysphagia Diet Task Force, 2002). While standardization is sorely needed, we are still far from universal adoption. Many facilities still use unique indicators for diet consistencies.

In addition to modifying food and liquid consistencies, it may also be necessary to alter the eating schedule and maximize caloric intake. Earlier we discussed the challenges people with movement disorders face with regard to maintaining weight and a good nutritional balance. Malnourishment has such a deleterious effect on muscle function that optimizing nutritional intake is a high priority. Instead of the typical "three square meals" with some snacking in between, the recommendation may be three to five smaller meals supplemented with high-protein and calorie snacks in between. Smaller meals are often necessary due to the extended mealtimes and associated high energy cost. In order to maximize energy stores, increasing the number opportunities for nutritional intake is a good strategy to consider. Table 8–5 contains a number of ideas for optimizing protein and calorie intake.

**Table 8–4.** National Dysphagia Diet (*NDD*)

NDD Level 1: Dysphagia—Pureed (homogeneous, very cohesive, pudding-like, requiring very little chewing ability)

NDD Level 2: Dysphagia—Mechanically altered (cohesive, moist, semisolid foods, requiring some chewing)

NDD Level 3: Dysphagia—Advanced (soft foods that require more chewing ability)

Regular (all foods allowed)

**Table 8–5.** Methods for Adding Protein and Calories to Daily Intake

| Breakfast |
| --- |
| Add cream, "double-strength" milk, and sugar to cooked cereals |
| Use milk instead of water when cooking hot cereals |
| Use plenty of margarine, jelly, jam, and honey on toast |
| Use peanut butter and cream cheese on toast |
| Cinnamon toast with butter and sugar |
| Add milk, cheese, and margarine to scrambled eggs |
| Eggnog |
| Baked custard |
| Bacon, Canadian bacon, sausage patties, and links |
| Pancakes, French toast, waffles with syrup, and whipped butter |
| Muffins, sweet rolls, coffee cakes, and quick breads with margarine |
| Biscuits with milk gravy |
| Biscuits with margarine and honey |
| Hot chocolate made with cream or double-strength milk, and marshmallows |

| Lunch or Supper |
| --- |
| Use gravy on entrées, starches, rolls, or cornbread |
| Add margarine to whipped potatoes |
| Add sour cream and margarine to baked potatoes |
| Crisp bacon bits to vegetables, baked potatoes, and salads |
| Use small servings of vegetables, especially raw vegetables (tossed salads) |
| Fruit salads with marshmallows and whipped topping |
| Gelatin fruit salads with mayonnaise or whipped topping |
| Use plenty of salad dressings, mayonnaise, and tartar sauce |
| Put in blender meat sauces and stews, and use as gravy over starch |
| Use cream sauces, and add cheese sauces to vegetables, casseroles, and entrees |
| Use cream of double-strength milk in creamed foods (creamed tuna, chicken, etc.) |
| Use cream, double-strength milk, or dry skim milk in cream soups |
| Add an extra slice of cheese to grilled cheese sandwiches with plenty of margarine on both sides of the bread |
| Add strained meats (baby meats) to soups for extra flavor (e.g., add strained chicken to cream of celery soup) |
| Use finely chopped eggs in meat or tuna salads, sauces, and casseroles |
| Add grated cheese to soups and casseroles |
| Bean soups and chowders |
| Add eggs to clear broth soups such as "egg drop" soup |

*continues*

**Table 8–5.** *continued*

| Lunch or Supper |
| --- |
| Fry/deep-fry vegetables (e.g., potatoes, okra, eggplant) |
| Stir-fry tender meats with vegetables |
| Add nuts, whipped cream, and ice cream to desserts |
| Replace drinking water and other noncaloric beverages such as coffee, tea with milk, juices, soft drinks, beer, and wines |

| Snacks or with Meals |
| --- |
| Milk shakes: add an extra scoop of ice cream, eggs, or peanut butter |
| Ice cream sundaes: add sauces (e.g., chocolate, hot fudge, butterscotch), nuts, fruit (e.g., strawberries, pineapple), and whipped topping |
| Ice cream floats: add a scoop of ice cream to carbonated beverages such as ginger ale, 7-Up, or Coke |
| Pies and cakes with ice cream |
| Put cream cheese on bagels and crackers |
| Peanut butter and cheese spreads on crackers |
| Cookies and puddings |
| Cheese cubes |
| Dried fruits (e.g., raisins, apricots, apples, prunes) |
| Peanuts, cashews, sunflower seeds, and granola |
| Luncheon meats |
| Cottage cheese with fruit |
| Hard-boiled eggs |
| Yogurt: plain or with various flavors; add fruits, nuts, seeds, granola, honey, or other flavorings to plain yogurt |

| Double-Strength Milk |
| --- |
| Add 1 cup of dried skim milk powder to 1 quart of fluid whole milk. Mix well and chill. One cup will provide twice as much protein as one cup of whole milk. |
| Flavor with: strawberry, chocolate syrup, vanilla, coffee extract, or mashed fruits such as banana, apricot, peach, other fruit purees and juices |
| Use in preparation of: |
|     Cream soups |
|     Cooked cereals |
|     Desserts (e.g., custard, puddings) |
|     Cocoa |
|     Creamed foods |
|     Meat loaf, mashed potatoes |
|     Milk shakes, eggnog |

Recommendations for changing the consistency of food and liquid, as well as maximizing caloric intake, are important features of treatment. Additional measures may be employed to alleviate symptoms of dysphagia during eating. Postural recommendations, such as a chin tuck, may offer several benefits. Tilting the head down may help to keep the bolus forward, away from the tongue base, which makes it less likely to fall into the pharynx prior to the swallow. This posture also changes anatomic orientation of structures, narrowing the oropharynx and facilitating airway closure (Groher & Crary 2010). Theoretically, the anatomic changes would create a boost to weakened physiology by maximizing pharyngeal contraction. Interestingly, that benefit is not realized in all individuals, and just thickening liquids may be as effective (Logemann, Gensler, & Robbins, 2008); thus, testing the technique to evaluate the benefit for each person is an important diagnostic element.

Compensatory strategies employed while eating may also offer improved safety and efficiency. The supraglottic swallow is a technique that offers additional airway protection (Logemann, 1998). This technique calls for an individual to execute a number of steps while eating. Once a bolus enters the mouth, the steps include:

1. Holding your breath
2. Swallowing
3. Coughing or clearing your throat
4. Swallowing again.

This sequence of steps offers the benefit of early airway closure while the bolus is in the oral cavity, then an extra clearing mechanism after the swallow to clear potential penetration or material near the airway. A modification to this technique is termed the "super supraglottic swallow." The modification requires an individual to add additional muscle effort to the swallow, which will increase the strength of the pharyngeal contraction and laryngeal elevation in an effort to better clear the pharynx of retained material. These techniques are likely to provide real benefit for those with movement disorders. The early closure of the airway is an excellent strategy to accommodate the discoordinated movements and lack of bolus control seen in these populations.

Indirect treatments for dysphagia management include those that address the underlying pathology. In the case of movement disorders, the feature most often targeted is weakness. In recent years there has been a renewed interest in the field on the principles of exercise (Burkhead et al., 2007; Clark, 2003). Borrowing from exercise science and related fields of study, these researchers have proposed to add to current exercise protocols. Primarily, they suggest that exercise treatments should consider the following:

1. Intensity
2. Frequency
3. Resistance
4. Task specificity.

To target weakness and gain strength, exercise should be performed at a high intensity level, as often as possible, increasing the resistance as strength improves. Finally, the exercise should be as close to the targeted performance as possible for optimal benefit. Let us take, for example, lingual strength. In swallowing, treatment exercises are most likely isometric in nature (pushing against a stable force/object). To target lingual strength, individuals might push the tongue against the hard palate, a tongue blade, or against a device that could offer feedback (i.e., Iowa Oral Performance Instrument). Intensity would be addressed by requesting that individuals perform at or near their physiologic limits, e.g., "push as hard as you can" and continue repetitions, not just a few times but until they fatigue (Table 8–6 is a sample strengthening protocol). The principle of frequency calls for completing this exercise as often as possible. If the individual can tolerate the activity every day, then that should be the target. If muscle soreness occurs, then a day of rest would be indicated. Resistance is another important principle for exercise. As strength improves, resistance should be increased. A direct benefit of isometric exercise is that as strength improves, resistance is increased. To illustrate, consider our lingual exercise of pushing the tongue against the roof of the mouth. The stronger the tongue becomes, the more force increases; thus, increased resistance is a byproduct of increased strength. Finally, to optimize outcome from strengthening, task specificity of the exercise should be as close as possible. In the case of lingual strength, pushing the tongue against the hard palate simulates the initial force for bolus propulsion through the oral cavity so that there is a high degree of task specificity for bolus transit. Targeting lingual pressure is just one example. By incorporating these principles of exercise, many features of swallowing impairment could be addressed. Labial weakness could be addressed by lip compression, buccal weakness through cheek compression, and pharyngeal weakness could be targeted with an effortful swallow (Crary, 1995).

Robbins, Gagnon, and Theis (2005) demonstrated that individuals with lingual weakness made significant gains in lingual strength by incorporating such principles. In their study, the gains in lingual strength translated into increased lingual mass and improved functional outcomes as well. When these principles of exercise are incorporated into treatment design, benefits are observed quickly, even in chronic conditions.

Dysphagia management for individuals with movement disorders clearly focuses on a central theme, safety. As discussed, the inherent nature of their condition creates a real safety risk during ingestion of food and liquid. Many of the features of alleviating symptoms have been addressed, direct treatment to make the process of eating more safe, and indirect measures to improve underlying problems with muscle condition; however, we would be remiss if we did not mention external safety measures. The Heimlich maneuver (Table 8–7) is an important one to include in the treatment of this population. An airway obstruction can occur when food becomes lodged in the larynx from discoordinated movements in the oral cavity, because it cuts off oxygen to the brain. When the brain is robbed of oxygen, damage can occur so it is important to administer this maneuver as quickly as possible.

With the emerging focus on neuroplasticity of the nervous system, perhaps facilitating neural changes will be as much a part of managing dysphagia as compensatory intervention changes (Ludlow et al., 2008).

**Table 8–6.** The Iowa Oral Performance Instrument (*IOPI*) Strengthening Protocol

Select the structure that you have targeted for strengthening with the IOPI. Set the Mode dial to "*PEAK*". Ask the patient to press against the bulb as hard as they can. Encouraged trials ensure maximum performance. Let them see the IOPI display for biofeedback regarding their effort. The following is an established protocol for strengthening. You may need to modify it to fit the needs of your patients. Record the peak pressure displayed on the IOPI for each trial in the set. Provide a brief rest period (approx. 1 min) between each set.

| Set 1 | Set 2 | Set 3 | Set 4 | Set 5 |
|---|---|---|---|---|
| 1. _____ | 1. _____ | 1. _____ | 1. _____ | 1. _____ |
| 2. _____ | 2. _____ | 2. _____ | 2. _____ | 2. _____ |
| 3. _____ | 3. _____ | 3. _____ | 3. _____ | 3. _____ |
| 4. _____ | 4. _____ | 4. _____ | 4. _____ | 4. _____ |
| 5. _____ | 5. _____ | 5. _____ | 5. _____ | 5. _____ |
| Set 6 | Set 7 | Set 8 | Set 9 | Set 10 |
| 1. _____ | 1. _____ | 1. _____ | 1. _____ | 1. _____ |
| 2. _____ | 2. _____ | 2. _____ | 2. _____ | 2. _____ |
| 3. _____ | 3. _____ | 3. _____ | 3. _____ | 3. _____ |
| 4. _____ | 4. _____ | 4. _____ | 4. _____ | 4. _____ |
| 5. _____ | 5. _____ | 5. _____ | 5. _____ | 5. _____ |

**Caution:** Be sure to monitor generalized effort. Make every attempt to ensure they are focusing their effort on the structure in question.

Although this protocol incorporates the use of the IOPI, it is the exercise that is important. The instrument is a nice method for obtaining baseline measures and monitoring progress, but the exercise can be completed without the instrumentation. The same treatment protocol could be implemented with pushing the tongue against the hard palate, or even against a tongue blade if there is a need to push against something tangible.

**Table 8–7.** The Heimlich Maneuver

The universal sign for choking is hands clutched to the throat. If the person does not give the signal, look for these indications:

- Inability to talk
- Difficulty breathing or noisy breathing
- Inability to cough forcefully
- Skin, lips, and nails turning blue or dusky
- Loss of consciousness

*Heimlich maneuver:*

- *Stand behind the person.* Wrap your arms around the waist. Tip the person forward slightly.
- *Make a fist with one hand.* Position it slightly above the person's navel.
- *Grasp the fist with the other hand.* Press hard into the abdomen with a quick, upward thrust, as if trying to lift the person up.
- *Perform a total of five abdominal thrusts* (if needed). If the blockage still is not dislodged, repeat.

*To perform abdominal thrusts on yourself:*

- Place a fist slightly above your navel.
- Grasp your fist with the other hand and bend over a hard surface (a countertop or chair will do).
- Shove your fist inward and upward.

## References

Beck, F. K., & Rosenthal, T. C. (2002) Prealbumin: A marker for nutritional evaluation. *American Family Physician, 65*(8), 1575–1578.

Centers for Disease Control and Prevention. (2013). Body mass index. Retrieved May 6, 2013 from http://www.cdc.gov/healthyweight/assessing/bmi/

Burkhead, L. M., Sapienza, C., & Rosenbek, J. (2007). Strength-training exercise in dysphagia rehabilitation: Principles, procedures, and directions for future research. *Dysphagia, 22,* 251–262.

Clark, H. M. (2003). Neuromuscular treatments for speech and swallowing: A tutorial. *American Journal of Speech Language Pathology, 12,* 400–415.

Crary, M. A. (1995). A direct intervention program for chronic neurogenic dysphagia secondary to brainstem stroke. *Dysphagia, 10,* 6–12.

Cummings, J. L. (1995). Behavioral and psychiatric symptoms associated with Huntington's disease. *Advances in Neurology, 65,* 179–186.

Daniels, S. K. (2000). Swallowing apraxia: A disorder of the praxis system? *Dysphagia, 15,* 159–166.

Duffy, J. R. (2005). *Motor speech disorders: Substrates, differential diagnosis and management.* St. Louis, MO: Elsevier Mosby.

Groher, M. E., & Bukatman, R. (1986). The prevalence of swallowing disorders in two teaching hospitals. *Dysphagia, 1,* 3–6.

Groher, M. E., & Crary, M. A. (2010). *Dysphagia: Clinical management in adults and children.* Maryland Heights, MO: Mosby Elsevier.

Gutekurst, C. Norflus, F., & Hersch, S. (2002). The neuropathology of Huntington's disease. In G. Bates, P. S. Harper, & L. Jones (Eds.), *Huntington's disease* (pp. 251–275). New York, NY: Oxford University Press.

Hegland, K. W. (2010). Palatal myoclonus. In H. Jones & J. Rosenbek (Eds.), *Dysphagia in rare conditions: An encyclopedia* (pp. 449–454). San Diego, CA: Plural.

Higgins, D. S. (2006). Huntington's disease. *Current Treatment Opinions in Neurology, 8,* 236–244.

Hixon, T. J., Weismer, G., & Hoit, J. D. (2008). *Preclinical speech science.* San Diego, CA: Plural.

Kagel, M. C., & Leopold, N. A. (1992). Dysphagia in Huntington's disease: A 16 year restrospective. *Dysphagia, 7,* 106–114.

Kent, R. (2004). The uniqueness of speech among motor systems. *Clinical Linguistics and Phonetics, 18,* 495–505.

Klasner, E. R. (2010). Huntington disease. In H. Jones & J. Rosenbek (Eds.), *Dysphagia in rare conditions: An encyclopedia* (pp. 267–272). San Diego, CA: Plural.

LaPointe, L. L., Murdoch, B. E., & Stierwalt, J. A. G. (2010). *Brain based communication disorders.* San Diego, CA: Plural.

Laskawi, R., & Rohrbach, S. (2001). Oromandibular dystonia: Clinical forms, diagnosis and examples of therapy with botulinum toxin. *Laryngorhinootologie, 80,* 708–713.

Lefton-Greif, M. A., Crawford, T. O., Winkelstein, J. A., Loughlin, G. M., Koerner, C. B., Zahurak, M., & Lederman, H. M. (2000). Oropharyngeal dysphagia and aspiration in patients with ataxia-telangiectasia. *Journal of Pediatrics, 136,* 225–231.

Logemann, J. (1998). *Evaluation and treatment of swallowing disorders.* San Diego, CA: College-Hill Press.

Logemann, J. A., Gensler, G., & Robbins, J. (2008). A randomized study of three interventions for aspiration of thin liquids in patients with dementia or Parkinson's disease. *Journal of Speech, Language, and Hearing Research, 51,* 173–183.

Ludlow, C. L., Hoit, J., Kent, R., Ramig, L. O., Shrivastav, R., Strand, E., Yorkston, K., & Sapienza, C. M. (2008). Translating principles of neural plasticity into research on speech motor control recovery and rehabilitation. *Journal of Speech, Language, and Hearing Research, 51,* S240–S258.

Murdoch, B. E. (2010). Generalized dystonia. In H. Jones & J. Rosenbek (Eds.), *Dysphagia in rare conditions: An encyclopedia* (pp. 185–192). San Diego, CA: Plural.

National Dysphagia Diet Task Force. (2002). *National Dysphagia Diet: Standardization for optimal care.* Chicago, IL: American Dietetic Association.

Papapetropoulos, S., & Singer, C. (2006). Eating dysfunction associated with oromandibular dystonia: Clinical characteristics and treatment considerations. *Head and Face Medicine, 2,* 47–52

Robbins, J., Gagnon R. E., & Theis, S. M. (2005). The effects of lingual exercise in stroke patients with dysphagia. *Archives of Physical and Medical Rehabilitation, 88,* 150–158.

Robbins J., & Levine R. L. (1988). Swallowing after unilateral stroke of the cerebral cortex: Preliminary experience. *Dysphagia, 3,* 11–17.

Sheppard, J. J. (2010). Tardive dyskinesia syndrome. In H. Jones & J. Rosenbek (Eds.), *Dysphagia in rare conditions: An encyclopedia* (pp. 567–572). San Diego, CA: Plural.

Swift, K. N. (2012) The changing landscape of nutrition and dietetics: A specialty group for integrative and functional medicine. *Integrative Medicine, 11*(2), 19–20.

Trejo, A., Tarrates, R. M., Alonso, M. E., Boll, M. C., Ochoa, A., & Velasquez, L. (2004). Assessment of nutrition status of patients with Huntington's disease. *Nutrition, 20,* 192–196.

Whitney, E. N., & Rolfes, S. R. (2010). *Understanding nutrition* (12th ed.). Clifton Park, NY: Cengage Learning.

Youmans, S. R., & Stierwalt, J. A. G. (2006). Measures of tongue function related to normal swallowing. *Dysphagia, 21,* 102–111.

Youmans, S. R., Youmans, G. L., & Stierwalt, J. A. G. (2009). Differences in tongue strength across age and gender: Is there a diminished strength reserve? *Dysphagia, 24,* 57–65.

# 9

# Language and Cognitive Effects

*LEONARD L. LAPOINTE*

## Introduction

Although the varieties of movement disorders and especially Parkinson disease (PD) are expressed usually in typical disorders of motion and movement, many, and perhaps all, persons with these disorders suffer the signs and symptoms of *nonmotor* disorders. This dreadful mix adds to the suffering and the overall burden of movement disorder morbidity. Non-motor problems in PD and other movement disorders are numerous and include mood and affect disorders, cognitive dysfunction and dementia, psychosis, autonomic nervous system dysfunction, and disorders of sleep-wake cycle regulation (Lim & Lang, 2010; Movement Disorders Society, 2013). In addition to not being able to move as they used to, people with movement disorders can be moody, upset, experience

cloudy thinking, exhibit signs of neurosis or occasionally psychosis, and fail to retrieve words like they once could, suffer memory lapses, and experience disturbed sleep. "Cognition" is a general term used to refer to the various mental abilities involved in comprehending, processing, and using information. Examples include memory, attention, abstract thinking, problem solving, language, and visual–perceptual abilities. We use cognitive and linguistic skills hundreds of times each day in all of the social interactions of going about our business and pleasure. Many persons, but not all, with PD, dystonia, or multiple sclerosis experience some degree of cognitive change, which can range from mild to severe. The terms "mild cognitive impairment" (MCI) and "cognitive impairment" generally are used when changes are not severe and affect limited aspects of memory or thinking abilities. Some people who experience cognitive impairment may merely note that changes in mental abilities are an annoyance, while others report symptoms noticeable enough to affect performance at work or in handling things at home.

## Executive Dysfunction

Executive functions are higher-order mental processes such as problem solving and planning, initiating and following through on tasks, and multitasking ideas or projects (Marsh, 2013). For a person with PD, paying the bill at Super Lube or even taking part in group conversations on the Grammy Awards TV program can be difficult. Why? These daily activities and pleasures require a person to be flexible and able to shift from one category of information or one specific goal to another, and to time them and organize them in a logical sequence. People with PD may describe getting overwhelmed or "freezing" in situations that require the formulation of a series of strategic choices, yet they appear to function perfectly when someone else helps them initiate and persist with a task (Marsh, 2013). We have even reported motoric "freezing" of gait of some of our research participants during a task of walking while talking or doing a difficult cognitive task. They "freeze" or stop in their tracks, sometimes even with abnormal changes in their respiratory pattern. In the absence of some sort of "intellectual scaffolding," it is more efficient for the person with PD to focus on one goal or concept at a time (Marsh, 2013). One example is that of a person with PD who was unable to initiate a project to organize his cluttered workshop, but

who successfully completed the task after his wife provided structure and cues by breaking down the task into parts and providing explicit instructions that focused on one single area at a time. Executive dysfunction can get in the way of arriving at appointments on time, organizing the ingredients to make macadamia nut brownies, or taking the dog to the vet to have his orthodontia work completed.

## Attention Difficulty

As the complexity of a situation increases, it can be difficult for a person with any movement disorder to maintain his or her focus or divide his or her attention. For example, people may find they can no longer multitask as well and even may have great difficulty with walking while talking or engaging in highly loaded cognitive activities. This is considered in more detail in a subsequent section. This attentional disorder is related to difficulty with cognitive resource allocation and is the result of a limited attentional capacity. Our attention is not unlimited. When we engage in more than one task simultaneously, there is give and take in the allocation of our attentional resources. This affects many intellectual pursuits and everyday activities such as walking, maintaining balance, and carrying on a conversation while descending stairs.

## Bradyphrenia

Bradyphrenia is slowed mental processing. This happens with an aging nervous system and it also can be experienced in movement disorders when the systems of cognition become degraded. People with movement disorders report that the disease affects how quickly they can process and respond to information. "I'm not as sharp," they say. "I can get it, but it takes me longer." Slowness in information processing affects other cognitive processes as well (such as problem solving and retrieving information) and daily activities (such as figuring out what to do about the cat mess on the Persian rug). One of the more troubling and not uncommon non-motor problems is the occurrence of hallucinations, which can be disturbing and unquestionably frightening.

## Hallucinations

Hallucinations are scary. People with PD and other movement disorders are troubled with hallucinations and see, smell, and feel things that are not there (Fernandez et al., 2005). No wonder this package of misery results in such a degraded quality of life. Hallucinations are tricky to study because the health care professional must elicit their description from the patient. Most cross-sectional studies of hallucinations report their occurrence in approximately one-third of subjects with PD receiving long-term dopaminergic therapy. These guesses are likely to be underestimates, however, because people may not volunteer such information easily when the phenomenon itself is strange, disconcerting, and "crazy." One may be reluctant to report that they see rabbits, snakes, or smell leather burning. The prototype of hallucinations as fully developed images

of people or animals is less frequently encountered than fleeting images in the lateral visual fields (*de passage*) or very vague shadows (Goetz, Fan, Leurgans, Bernard, & Stebbins, 2006). Most health care professionals focus on visual hallucinations, which are the most common of these strange behaviors, but tactile ("someone is tickling me"), auditory ("I hear the theme from Gilligan's Island"), and olfactory ("the goldfish farted") hallucinations also occur, and their documentation can be missed if not specifically pursued. These nonmotor problems become increasingly apparent and problematic over the course of the illness and are a major detriment to wellness and quality of life, advancement of overall disability, and contribute to skilled nursing home placement. In their various combinations, nonmotor symptoms may become the dominant therapeutic challenge in later stages of movement disorders and especially of PD, since hallucinations are associated with dopamine medication.

## Cognitive and Linguistic Problems

Theodoros and Ramig (2011) have produced a most useful and contemporary compilation on communication and swallowing disorders specifically in PD. Dr. Theodoros is Professor and has served as Head of the Division of Speech Pathology, School of Health and Rehabilitation Sciences, at the University of Queensland, Brisbane, Australia. Dr. Ramig is a Professor in the Department of Speech-Language and Hearing Science at the University of Colorado-Boulder; and a Senior Scientist at the National Center for Voice and

Speech, a division of the Denver Center for the Performing Arts. Both doctors are regular consultants at the Veuve Clicquot and Mansard Baillet Centers for Continuing Education in Epernay, France. The book edited by Theodoros and Ramig has extensive chapters on the neurophysiologic bases of speech and swallowing disorders in PD as well as a careful description of strategies for assessment and treatment of the speech disorders of PD. Additionally, there are two chapters specifically dedicated to cognitive and language disturbances in PD, and we are indebted to the authors of these chapters, Adrienne Blanchard Hancock, Leonard L. LaPointe, and Brook-Mai Whelan, for their permission to use their particular research on the cognitive-linguistic interactions of PD and movement disorders (Hancock, LaPointe, & Whelan, 2011; Whelan, 2011).

Communication barriers for people with PD are embedded in the speech production of their hypokinetic dysarthria as well as their masklike affect and facial expression, yet most people with PD face cognitive-linguistic impairment as well. Less is known about cognitive-linguistic impairment, but it is not unexplored. Even as recently as 20 years ago, the communication difficulty of people with PD was thought to be solely the artifact of movement-based disruption of speech and voice. Linguistic processing disorder was thought to be confined to the purview of aphasia. Expansion and evolving sophistication of our methods of assessing cognitive–linguistic processes has broadened our appreciation of what can go wrong in PD. Language function is difficult to assess and describe because it is difficult to parse from the complex motor speech and cognitive abilities (e.g., attention, memory, executive function)

known to deteriorate with PD. The cognitive characteristics inherent in PD are gaining attention and clarity. Stocchi & Brusa (2000) report that 90% of people with PD have some cognitive impairment affecting daily life, with 25% classified as severe cognitive impairment. This supports the frequent complaints of our clients with PD who report losing their train of thought, forgetting appointments, and difficulty planning the temporal sequences of a typical day.

Although most of the movement disorders produce an effect on communication that is centered in the faulty movements of the articulatory and speech production system, there are persistent clinical reports, but not a lot of research, on disturbances of the linguistic sphere. Parkinson disease, multiple sclerosis, and Huntington disease all have been associated with language disruption. The problem is that the linguistic or the cognitive disruption is subtle and not the most predominant issue in communication impairment. These language subtleties may be covert and masked by the more apparent disruptions. Language difficulties arising from movement disorders can be subtle or they can be blatant, depending on the site and extent of the nervous system lesions involved or the stage of the disease.

"I can't find the right word," "The word slips my mind," and "I think I'm beginning to lose my . . . table, uh, apple, uhm, I mean my mind" are all phrases that typify the language problems that occasionally accompany movement disorders. The fact that some movement diseases or conditions affect nervous system areas that are more widespread or taint the crucial perisylvian language areas of the dominant (usually left) cerebral hemisphere explain these coexistences of both speech and language problems. Sometimes a linguistic system that is not entirely intact can result in a wide mélange of grammatical, lexical-semantic, syntactic, or phonological disruptions that spill over into the world of language and not just the muscle-based movement system that is responsible for effecting and articulating the linguistic system. Murdoch and Theodoros (2004) have detailed some of these language problems in multiple sclerosis, for example.

Language problems can be mild, with the individual experiencing some trifling difficulty with recall; where the right word is "in there somewhere" or "on the tip of the tongue," but proves elusive nonetheless. Substitution of a replacement word is usually enough to overcome this momentary problem when speaking. More severe forms of language dysfunction can occur where verbal expression is more explicitly affected. Typically, the words are in that lexical vault somewhere, but lexical–semantic access is the problem and this can break the fluency of conversation, leading to a reluctance to participate, withdrawal from social situations, and a perceived sense of isolation.

According to a review of 12 reports, 24 to 31% of people with PD are diagnosed with dementia, which would account for almost 4% of dementia in the population (Aarsland, Zaccai, & Brayne, 2005). The dementia of people with PD is similar to a dysexecutive syndrome, with some visuospatial and behavioral symptoms (Emre, 2003). This expresses itself in short attention span, poor working memory, reduced recent and short-term memory, and trouble with planning and reasoning. A study of cognitive function through the course of the disease has demonstrated that mild cognitive dysfunction can be evident even at the time of initial PD diagnosis and may deteriorate to status of dementia or general cognitive impairment at a greater rate than for aging individuals without PD (Williams-Gray, Foltynie, Brayne, Robbins, & Barker, 2007).

As suggested by Hancock et al. (2011), cognitive-linguistic and motor characteristics of PD can be heterogeneous due to many sources of variability. In most studies, cognitive-linguistic dysfunction or deterioration of function can be associated with a person's age, age at onset of PD, education level, and the stage of PD (Jankovic & Kapadia, 2001; Verbaan et al., 2007). Other studies of PD have reported no remarkable deterioration of cognitive-linguistic function (Bayles et al., 1996; Gilbert, Belleville, Bherer, & Chouinard, 2005, Verbaan et al., 2007). Mayeux et al. (1992) reported less than 1% prevalence for PD with dementia if under 50 years of age, with prevalence increasing each decade of life and reaching 68.7% for those 80 years and older. Overall, in this study of 179 people, 41% with PD were diagnosed with dementia. One wonders if the discrepancy of reports of cognitive-linguistic impairment in PD is related to the sensitivity and specificity of the instruments used to unveil it.

## Language Compromise in PD

We are indebted to Hancock, LaPointe, and Whelan (2011) for the following review and summary of language problems in PD. Semantic knowledge and complex linguistic constructions are sometimes found to be impaired in PD.

Performance on the Test of Language Competence was significantly more impaired in people with PD who exhibited dementia (i.e., scores below 139.9 on the Mattis Dementia Rating Scale) (Lewis, LaPointe, Murdoch, & Chenery, 1998). Without dementia, people with PD still scored below healthy age-matched control participants for generating definitions and recreating sentences. A typical semantic assessment requiring some executive function is the verbal fluency or generative naming task. Verbal fluency tasks require people to generate words according to specific rules. On this task people with PD, more so than control participants, benefitted from semantic cues (Lewis et al., 1998). Zgaljardic et al. (2006) found both category (e.g., list animals) and phonemic (e.g., list words beginning with the letter "t") verbal fluency to be impaired in a group of 32 nondemented people with PD. In another study, people with PD showed no impairment on phonemic verbal fluency but performed below normal control groups when required to generate words within a semantic category (Levin, Llabre, & Weiner, 1989). These few investigations of semantic abilities indicate impairment in PD, but this area is lacking research consensus. It is likely that the inability to create categories and strategies affects semantic language skills of people with PD.

Syntax is another linguistic domain that has been found not to be normal in people with PD, and appears to be affected for both expression and comprehension (Grossman et al., 1991). Syntactic complexity of spontaneous speech deteriorates with progression of the disease (Illes, Metter, Hanson, & Iritani, 1988). Several studies have differentiated PD from control groups by manipulating complexity of syntax in sentence comprehension tasks. For example, when sentences contain propositions, people with PD perform more poorly than controls (Caplan & Waters, 1999). Grammatical complexity and semantic ambiguity compromised sentence comprehension in a study of nondemented people with PD, although this was inconsistent across people and across testing sessions (Grossman, Carvel, Goloomp, Stern, Vernon, & Hurtig, 1991). Lee, Grossman, Morris, Stern, and Hurtig (2003) reported accurate performance, but slowed processing times, for nondemented people with mild idiopathic PD when grammatical morphemes were omitted, and when center-embedded clauses were object relative rather than subject relative (e.g., "The boy that hugged the girl is friendly" required more time than "The boy that the girl hugged is friendly"). Noncanonical sentences, such as object-relative sentences, generally take longer to comprehend, but the significantly longer time required by people with PD may reflect slower lexical retrieval and working memory (Angwin, Chenery, Copland, Murdoch, & Silburn, 2006).

The presence of dementia concomitant with PD may be a significant influence in cognitive-linguistic performance. Lewis et al. (1998) found no language impairment in a group of idiopathic people with PD who had normal scores on the Mattis Dementia Rating Scale (DRS); however, they did find that people with below-normal DRS scores performed below normal on language tasks associated with cognitive processing, especially constructing sentences, naming, and metaphors.

The higher level language processes, such as understanding metaphors and ambiguous sentences, require inferences and are particularly challenging for people with even mild PD (Berg, Bjornram, Hartelius, Laakso, & Johnels, 2003). In another group of people without dementia, Taylor, Saint-Cyr, and Lang (1986) found no impairment in receptive or expressive aspects of language. These authors attribute intact language function to normal parietal and temporal lobe function and suggest that damage to the frontal lobes, particularly the supplementary motor area (SMA), is probably responsible for the deficit in planning actions guided by internal cues (these include language production as a goal-directed action). The functioning SMA receives input from the basal ganglia via the thalamus, which may explain why the deficit in action planning is noted in the PD population. We return to a discussion of planning and internal strategy, likely one of the deficits manifested in both cognitive-linguistic and motor dysfunction.

## Some But Not All Have Cognitive Loss or Decline

Not everyone with every movement disorder disease or condition has problems with speech, language, or cognition. In a survey of 656 people with multiple sclerosis, Beukelman, Kraft, and Freal (1985) found that 23% reported speech or communication problems. Signs and symptoms vary widely, depending on the amount of damage and the nerves that are affected. People with multiple sclerosis or any of the other progres-

sive neurologic conditions may lose the ability to walk or speak clearly as the disease advances. The exacerbation and remission of multiple sclerosis can create not only diagnostic quandaries but also make speech, cognitive, and language impairment difficult to pinpoint early in the course of the disease because signs and symptoms often come and go—sometimes disappearing for months. Some of the difficulty in processing language in degenerative diseases can be so subtle in the early stages that sophisticated electrophysiologic instrumentation is necessary to uncover processing disorders that are more evident later. For example, Jones, Sprague, and Vaz Pato (2002) studied 22 patients with diagnosed multiple sclerosis, but mild disability and no auditory complaints were compared with 15 normal controls. Auditory evoked potentials (AEPs) were recorded using standard methods. These researchers found delayed AEP responses that appeared to be a mild disorder in the processing of change in temporal sound patterns. They commented that the delay might be conceived of as extra time taken to compare the incoming sound with the contents of a temporally ordered sensory memory store. The authors suggested that this defect in the subtle processing of sound probably could not be ascribed to lesions of the afferent pathways and so may be due to disseminated brain lesions visible or invisible on magnetic resonance imaging. This study exemplifies disordered subtle processing of material important for speech, language, and cognition that may be subclinical for a time and then surfaces in more overt communication problems as the disease advances.

## Injurious Falls and Multitasking

In our laboratory at the Florida State University, we have a research agenda that investigates the effects of interference, competition, and distraction on cognitive and linguistic processing in a wide variety of clinical populations, most of whom have brain-based disorders. Among other findings, we have found significant disruptions in selected attempts at multitasking in some clinical samples of people with movement disorders. In a group of participants with multiple sclerosis, we found significant deleterious effects of auditory distraction on a task of visual cognitive performance. People with multiple sclerosis were not as adept at coping with background cafeteria noise distraction as were matched control participants. This echoes the clinical complaints we have heard from many people in our clinical populations of movement disorders.

Injurious falls are one of the most pervasive, costly, tragic, and dreadful causes of human suffering across the spectrum of world cultures and countries. As a subset group, falls are an enormous burden for persons with PD and their families, and are a leading reason for emergency department visits, hospitalization, and referral to extended care facilities. The Agency for Healthcare Research and Quality (AHRQ) is an organization that tracks emergency department (ED) visits in the United States and analyzes health care cost and utilization.

We have looked at the spillover of cognitive loading in a dual-task paradigm to the motor system. We have found differences in both the clinical populations of multiple sclerosis and especially in participants with PD who have degraded simultaneous walking and talking (LaPointe et al., 2005; LaPointe, Maitland, Stierwalt, Toole, & Hancock, 2006; Stierwalt, LaPointe, Toole, Maitland, Wilson, 2006). Most of us have little difficulty with walking and talking (walking and texting is another issue!), but people with a compromised nervous system are not as good with cognitive resource or attention allocation. Doing heavily loaded cognitive or linguistic tasks while walking degrades ambulation and gait. This is not a trivial issue since injurious falls are a significant health care problem, especially in PD and other movement disorders. Studies of large samples have documented that falls occur in 56 to 68% of people with parkinsonism (Wood, Bilclough, Bowron, & Walker, 2002). Our research, which has now extended to looking at the effects of medication cycle in PD, has suggested strongly that, though there are many reasons why people with movement disorders might be at risk for injurious falls, certainly cognitive-linguistic loading might be one of them. When our participants were asked to walk on a carpet with 16,000 sensors that measures many temporal-spatial aspects of ambulation and gait and simultaneously engage in cognitive-linguistic tasks, such as counting backwards, continuously subtracting by 3 starting at 95, or doing alpha-numeric sequencing ("continue this sequence ... H-4, I-5, J-6, K-7, etc."), their gait fell apart and they became at risk for falls. Some of our participants with PD even exhibited "freezing" on the carpet during the dual task of walking and performing cognitively loaded operations (LaPointe, Stierwalt, & Maitland, 2010). These results suggest that it might be prudent for health care professionals and caregivers to alter expectations and monitor the cognitive-linguistic demands placed on elderly individuals, particularly those with neurologic compromise who might be at greater risk for injurious falls.

People with PD and many other movement disorders suffer a spectrum of non-motor disturbances, many in the sphere of cognitive and linguistic disruption. These may not be the most obvious signs and symptoms that are apparent to health care professionals assessing and treating these individuals, but quality of life can indeed be degraded.

## References

Aarsland, D., Zaccai, J., & Brayne, C. (2005). A systematic review of prevalence studies of dementia in Parkinson's disease. *Movement Disorders, 20,* 1255–1263.

Angwin, A., Copland, D. A., Chenery, H. J., Murdoch, B., & Silburn, P. (2006). The influence of dopamine on semantic activation in Parkinson's disease: Evidence from a multipriming task. *Neuropsychology, 20,* 299–306.

Bayles, K., Tomoeda, C., Wood, J., Montgomery, E., Cruz, R., Azuma, T., & McGeagh, A. (1996). Change in cognitive function in idiopathic Parkinson disease. *Archives of Neurology, 53,* 1140–1146.

Berg, E., Bjornram, C., Hartelius, L., Laakso, K., & Johnels, B. (2003). High-level language difficulties in Parkinson's disease. *Clinical Linguistics and Phonetics, 17,* 63–80.

Beukelman, D. R., Kraft, G. H., & Freal, J. (1985). Expressive communication disorders in persons with multiple sclerosis: A survey. *Archives of Physical Medicine and Rehabilitation, 66*(10), 675–677.

Caplan, D., & Waters, G. S. (1999). Verbal working memory and sentence comprehension. *Behavioral and Brain Sciences, 22,* 77–126.

Emre, M. (2003). Dementia associated with Parkinson's disease. *Lancet Neurology, 2,* 229–237.

Fernandez, H. H., Okun, M. S., Rodriguez, R. L., Malaty, I. A., Romnell, J., Sun, A., . . . Eisenschenk, S. (2005). Quetiapine improves visual hallucinations in Parkinson disease but not through normalization of sleep architecture: Results from a double-blind clinical-polysomnography study. *International Journal of Neuroscience, 119,* 2196–2205.

Gilbert, B., Belleville, S., Bherer, L., & Chouinard, S. (2005). Study of verbal working memory in patients with Parkinson's disease. *Neuropsychology, 19,* 106–114.

Goetz, C. G., Fan, W., Leurgans, S., Bernard, B., & Stebbins, G. T. (2006). The malignant course of "Benign Hallucinations" in Parkinson disease. *Archives of Neurology, 63*(5), 713–716.

Grossman, M., Carvel, S., Goloomp, S., Stern, M. B., Vernon, G., & Hurtig, H. I. (1991). Sentence comprehension and praxis impairment in Parkinson's disease. *Neurology, 41,* 1620.

Hancock, A. B., LaPointe, L. L., & Whelan, B.-M. (2011) Cognitive-linguistic disorder in Parkinson disease. In D. Theodoros, & L. Ramig (Eds.), *Communication and swallowing in Parkinson disease.* San Diego, CA: Plural.

Illes, J., Metter, E. J., Hanson, W. R., & Iritani, S. (1988). Language production in Parkinson's disease: Acoustic and linguistic considerations. *Brain and Language, 33,* 146–160.

Jankovic, J., & Kapadia, A. S. (2001). Functional decline in Parkinson disease. *Archives of Neurology, 58,* 1611–1615.

Jones, S. J., Sprague L., & Vaz Pato, M. (2002). Electrophysiological evidence for defect in processing of temporal sound patterns in multiple sclerosis. *Journal of Neurological and Neurosurgical Psychiatry, 73*(5), 561–567.

LaPointe, L. L., Maitland, C. G., Blanchard, A. A., Kemker, B. E., Stierwalt, J. A., & Heald, G. R. (2005). The effects of auditory distraction on visual cognitive performance in multiple sclerosis. *Journal of Neuroophthalmology, 25*(2), 92–94.

LaPointe, L. L., Maitland, C. G., Stierwalt, J. A. G., Toole, T., & Hancock, A. B. (2006). Distraction, competition, and interference: How do people with brain damage navigate in a sea of distraction? *Neurorehabilitation and Neural Repair, 20,* 58–59.

LaPointe, L. L., Stierwalt, J. A. G., & Maitland, C. G. (2010). Talking while walking: Cognitive loading and injurious falls in Parkinson's disease. *International Journal of Speech-Language Pathology, 12*(5), 455–459.

Lee, C., Grossman, M., Morris, J., Stern, M. B., & Hurtig, H. (2003). Attentional resource and processing speed limitations during sentence processing in Parkinson's disease. *Brain and Language, 85,* 347–356.

Levin, B. E., Llabre, M. M., & Weiner, W. J. (1989). Cognitive impairments associated with early Parkinson's disease. *Neurology, 39,* 557–561.

Lewis, F. M., LaPointe, L. L., Murdoch, B. E., & Chenery, H. J. (1998). Language impairment in Parkinson's disease. *Aphasiology, 12,* 193–206.

Lim, S. Y., & Lang, A. E. (2010). The nonmotor symptoms of Parkinson's disease—an overview. *Movement Disorders, 25*(Suppl 1), S123–S130.

Marsh, L. (2013). Not just a movement disorder: Cognitive changes in Parkinson disease. Retrieved February 12, 2013 from http://www.pdf.org/en/winter07_08_Not_Just_a_Movement/

Mayeux, R., Denaro, J., Hemenegildo, N., Marder, K., Tang, M.-X., Cote, L. J., & Stern, Y. (1992). A population-based investigation of Parkinson's disease with and without dementia: Relationship to age and gender. *Archives of Neurology, 49,* 492–497.

Movement Disorders Society. (2013). The Movement Disorder Society evidence-based medicine review update: Treatments for the non-motor symptoms of Parkinson's disease. Retrieved February 6, 2013 from http://www.movementdisorders.org/monthly_edition/2012/02/EBM_NonMotor_Symptoms.pdf/

Murdoch, B. E., & Theodoros, D. (2004). *Speech and language disorders in multiple sclerosis.* London, UK: Wiley.

Stierwalt, J. A. G., LaPointe, L. L., Toole, T., Maitland, C. G., & Wilson, K. R. (2006). The effects of cognitive-linguistic load on gait in individuals with Parkinson's disease. *Movement Disorders, 21,* 92.

Stocchi, F., & Brusa, L. (2000). Cognition and emotion in different stages and subtypes of Parkinson's disease. *Journal of Neurology, 247,* 114–121.

Taylor, A. E., Saint-Cyr, J. A., & Lang, A. E. (1986). Frontal lobe dysfunction in Parkinson's disease: The cortical focus of neostriatal outflow. *Brain, 109,* 845–883.

Theodoros, D., & Ramig, L. (2011). *Communication and swallowing disorders in Parkinson disease.* San Diego, CA: Plural.

Verbaan, D., Marinus, J., Visser, M., van Rooden, S. M., Stiggelbout, A. M., Middelkoop, H. A. M., & van Hilten, J. (2007). Cognitive impairment in Parkinson's disease. *Journal of Neurology, Neurosurgery and Psychiatry, 78,* 1182–1187.

Whelan, B.-M. (2011). Assessment and treatment of cognitive-linguistic disorder in Parkinson disease. In D. Theodoros & L. Ramig (Eds.), *Communication and swallowing in Parkinson disease.* San Diego, CA: Plural.

Williams-Gray, C. H., Foltynie, T., Brayne, C., Robbins, T. W., & Barker, R. A. (2007). Evolution of cognitive dysfunction in an incident Parkinson's disease cohort. *Brain, 130,* 1787–1798.

Wood, B. H., Bilclough, J. A., Bowron, A., & Walker, R. (2002). Incidence and prediction of falls in Parkinson's disease:

A prospective multidisciplinary study. *Journal of Neurology, Neurosurgery and Psychiatry, 72,* 721–725.

Zgaljardic, D. J., Borod, J. C., Foldi, N. S., Mattis, P. J., Gordon, M. F., Feigin, A., & Eidelberg, D. (2006). An examination of executive dysfunction associated with frontostriatal circuitry in Parkinson's disease. *Journal of Clinical and Experimental Neuropsychology, 28,* 1127–1144.

# 10

# Medical and Surgical Treatments

*BRUCE E. MURDOCH*

## Introduction

As described in Chapter 3, movement disorders include a number of clinically defined disease states of diverse etiology and often obscure pathogenesis. They either cause poverty of movement, typical of akinetic-rigid disorders (e.g., Parkinson disease), or unwanted, involuntary movements as seen in hyperkinetic disorders (e.g., Huntington chorea), or dykinesias. Consequently, a wide variety of treatment approaches have been applied to these conditions. In most cases, the therapy applied involves a selection from a wide range of pharmacologic agents and/or neurosurgical procedures, although other therapies based on fetal mesencephalic tissue transplantation and stem cell transplantation are under development and trial.

By far the majority of movement disorders are insidiously progressive, with signs and symptoms increasing in number and intensity over time. Unfortunately, contemporary therapies are not aimed at cure per se, but rather are merely palliative being directed at relief of symptoms or at best to stop or slow the progressive degeneration of the disease. The primary aim of contemporary medical treatments applied to movement disorders, therefore, is to keep the patient functioning independently for as long as possible. In general, treatments need to be individualized in that each patient usually presents with a unique set of symptoms, signs, and responses to medications and a host of social, occupational, and emotional problems that need to be addressed. In determining the medical treatment(s) to be applied, particular attention needs to be given to the patient's specific symptoms, the degree of their functional impairment, and the expected benefits and risks of available therapeutic approaches.

## Treatment of Hypokinetic Disorders (Akinetic-Rigid Syndromes)

Two major forms of akinetic-rigid disorder are associated with the occurrence of motor speech and/or cognitive/linguistic impairments and hence are encountered in the clinical caseloads of speech-language pathologists. By far the most common and dominant form of akinetic-rigid disorder is Parkinson disease (PD) with a much smaller number of cases presenting with progressive supranuclear palsy. Discussion of the medical approaches to treatment of akinetic-rigid syndromes therefore focuses on therapies applied to these latter two conditions. (As discussed in Chapter 4, the medical treatments outlined below may have differential effects on speech as compared with limb function. Treatment of speech disorders associated with hypokinetic disorders is described in Chapter 7.)

## Medical and Surgical Treatment of Parkinson Disease

### Pharmacologic Treatments for Parkinson Disease

Parkinson disease is a progressive, degenerative, neurologic disease associated with selective loss of dopaminergic neurons in the pars compacta of the substantia nigra. The condition arises from nigrostriatal dopaminergic cell degeneration that produces an activity imbalance within dopamine-regulated pathways of the basal ganglia, namely an increase in indirect pathway activity and a decrease in direct pathway activity (see Chapter 7 for models of motor control of hypokinetic disorders). As a consequence, pharmacologic treatment of PD is based on supplementation of depleted dopamine levels in the brain through the use of dopamine precursors (e.g., levodopa) and dopamine receptor agonists or compounds that inhibit the metabolization of dopamine or levodopa such as catechol-O-methyltransferase (COMT) or monoamine oxidase-B (MAO-B).

**Levodopa Treatment.** Levodopa is administered orally and is the single most effective drug for the treatment of motor symptoms of PD and remains the gold standard. More specifically, preparations of levodopa combined with the peripheral decarboxylase inhibitors carbidopa or benserazide (co-careldopa, Sinemet; co-beneldopa, Madopar) still represent the most potent and effective systematic treatment for PD, benefitting virtually all patients with a pathologically confirmed diagnosis of PD and leading to improved quality of life and reduced morbidity and mortality in patients with PD. Levodopa is routinely taken orally. The addition of a decarboxylase inhibitor prevents the metabolization of levodopa prior to its passage across the blood-brain barrier thereby enabling up to a four-fold reduction in the dosage of levodopa required. Once in the brain, no longer protected by the decarboxylase inhibitor that cannot pass across the blood-brain barrier, levodopa is metabolized to dopamine, which then stimulates available dopamine receptors in the basal ganglia leading to improved motor function. In the United States, only carbidopa is available as a peripheral decarboxylase inhibitor, while in most other countries benserazide is also available. Carbidopa-levodopa is marketed as Sinemet or as a generic drug. The combination is available in standard (e.g., Sinemet standard) or controlled-release (e.g., Sinemet CR) formulations. The former allows a more rapid "ON" and shorter half-life, and the latter allows for a delayed "ON" and a slightly longer plasma half-life. Benserazide-levodopa is marketed as standard Madopar and Madopar HBS (for slow release). In addition to potentiating levodopa and allowing a reduction in dosage by preventing the formation of peripheral dopamine, which can act on dopamine receptors in the area postrema (vomiting center) in the floor of the fourth ventricle (functionally outside the blood-brain barrier), peripheral decarboxylase inhibitors also help to block the development of nausea and vomiting.

Although effective at improving general motor function, at least in the short-term, levodopa does not arrest the underlying neurodegenerative processes in PD. Indeed, no treatment available to date has been capable of stopping or slowing the progress of PD. Consequently, the benefits of levodopa declines and adverse effects increase over time. Over time patients treated with levodopa start to notice early morning akinesia, or wearing off of their doses, and around the same time begin to develop motor complications. Long-term levodopa therapy is associated with the occurrence of various motor complications, including motor fluctuations and dyskinesias. Motor fluctuations can be defined as alternating periods of good motor function ("ON" periods during which

the patient is responding to the drug) and periods of impaired motor function ("OFF" periods with suboptimal or lack of response to the medication). Dyskinesias are commonly observed in combination with motor fluctuations and may also exhibit a fluctuating course. Levodopa-induced dyskinesias usually take the form of involuntary, choreiform, or athetoid movements that occur in response to administration of the medication and may involve virtually any part of the body. Dystonia is a less frequent form of levodopa-induced dyskinesia. As a very rough rule of thumb, these long-term complications of levodopa therapy develop in 10% of patients per year of treatment, so that after 5 years about 50% of patients will exhibit them, and after 10 years all patients will ultimately experience them to some degree. Fluctuating nonmotor symptoms may also emerge in the latter stages of PD including neuropsychiatric disturbances (e.g., vivid dreams, nightmares, hallucination and visual illusions, depression). In general, younger-onset patients with PD develop the complications associated with long-term levodopa therapy earlier and to a more severe degree than late-onset cases. Concerns about the development of long-term levodopa syndrome have led many physicians to attempt to delay the introduction of levodopa treatment, especially in younger patients, by using a variety of medications that do not cause this problem, although at the expense of having a less potent therapeutic effect.

**Dopamine Agonist Treatment.** Dopamine agonists represent the next most powerful drugs, after levodopa, for treating symptoms of PD. These drugs stimulate dopamine receptors directly and, when given prior to the introduction of levodopa, cause motor fluctuations and dyskinesias much less frequently, but have a weaker antiparkinsonian effect. Some of the more common dopamine agonists used clinically include bromocriptine, pergolide, pramipexole, ropinirole, and apomorphine. With the exception of apomorphine, these drugs are effective orally. Bromocriptine is the weakest agonist clinically in comparison with the others. Pergolide, pramipexole, and ropinirole appear to be comparable in clinical practice, although some patients respond better to one than the others. Apomorphine is the oldest and most effective dopamine agonist. It is water soluble and is usually employed as a rapidly acting dopaminergic to overcome "OFF" states (i.e., to rescue patients from "OFF" periods). It is either injected subcutaneously or applied intranasally.

The agonists can be used as adjuncts to levodopa therapy or as monotherapy. They have longer clinical and pharmacologic half-lives than levodopa and, when used as adjuncts, can help to minimize troughs of dopaminergic stimulation and increase "ON" time. Adverse effects that are more common with dopamine agonists than with levodopa are drowsiness, sleep attacks, confusion, neuropsychiatric effects (e.g., nightmares, hallucinations, delusions, etc.), orthostatic hypotension, nausea, and ankle/joint edema.

### Other Pharmacologic Treatments

**Catechol-O-Methyltransferase (COMT) Inhibitors.** Two COMT inhibitors are currently available: tolcapone and entacapone. These two drugs extend the plasma half-life of levodopa without increasing its peak plasma concentration and thereby prolong the duration of action of each dose of levodopa. Both drugs act by blocking the conversion of levodopa to 3-O-methyldopa, its principal metabolite. Tolcapone is generally the more effective of the two but is only used as a second-line treatment because of a low risk of potentially fatal hepatotoxicity, necessitating frequent liver function test monitoring. Both entacapone and tolcapone can be associated with gastrointestinal upset, particularly diarrhea that may not appear for several weeks after starting the drug. A combined tablet containing levodopa, carbidopa, and entacapone (Stalevo) is available.

**Monoamine Oxidase-B (MAO-B) Inhibitors.** MAO-B inhibitors offer mildly effective symptomatic relief in PD. The two most common and commercially available MAO-B inhibitors include selegiline and rasagiline both of which are described as "suicide" inhibitors of MAO-B, the iso-enzyme responsible for catabolizing dopamine to homovanillic acid. Both can be used safely in conjunction with levodopa therapy. Used alone early in the disease, these two agents can delay the need for levodopa. These drugs have few side effects when given alone but can potentiate any of the symptomatic side effects of levodopa.

**Anticholinergics.** Anticholinergics were the first drugs used to treat PD and remained the mainstay of treatment until the introduction of levodopa in the late 1960s. They have only a mild symptomatic effect, often restricted to reducing tremor and consequently have largely been supplanted by dopaminergic agents. A number of antiparkinsonian anticholinergic drugs are available including benzatropine, trihexyphenidyl (Artane), procyclidine, and orphenadrine (Norflex). It is possible that anticholinergics still have a role in the treatment of very mild PD and maybe as antitremor agents in more advanced forms of the illness; however, there are a number of potential central and peripheral side effects of these drugs that restrict their application. In particular, older patients with PD, or those with dementia, are particularly susceptible to adverse behavioral effects of these drugs including hallucinations and organic confusional states. Anticholinergics therefore should be avoided in such cases and their use restricted to younger, cognitively intact, usually tremor-dominant cases.

**Amantadine.** Amantadine is a drug with several actions. First, it is a mild dopaminergic, acting by augmenting dopamine release from storage sites and possibly blocking reuptake of dopamine into the presynaptic terminals. Second, it appears to have some anticholinergic properties as well as a glutamate receptor blocking activity. In the mild stage of PD, amantadine is effective in relieving symptoms in about two-thirds of patients. A major advantage is that subsequent benefit, if it occurs, is seen in a couple of days. Unfortunately, its benefit in more advanced PD is often short lived, with the beneficial effects waning, at least in part, after 6 weeks or so. Amantadine, however, can be useful not only in the early phases of PD, where it can help forestall the introduction of levodopa,

but also in more advanced stages of the disease as an adjunct drug to levodopa and the dopamine agonists. Probably as an outcome of its antiglutamatergic activity amantadine is also effective in reducing levodopa-induced dyskinesias. Common adverse side effects of amantadine include ankle edema and livedo reticularis (a reddish mottling of the skin). The drug also lowers seizure threshold and can cause hallucinations or confusion. As it is excreted mostly unchanged in the urine, it should be used with caution in cases with renal impairment.

### Neurosurgical Treatment of Parkinson Disease

Functional neurosurgery for the treatment of PD is largely reserved for patients with advanced PD, with motor fluctuations and dyskinesias, or troublesome tremor, and who are difficult to manage despite the combination of available drugs. Criteria used in patient selection aim at identifying those individuals with PD likely to benefit from neurosurgery and unlikely to exhibit severe adverse effects. Their disabling symptoms need to be identified and assessed to determine if they are levodopa sensitive or levodopa induced and how they impact on the patient's daily life. Cognitive functions and mood should also be carefully assessed. A magnetic resonance imaging (MRI) scan is required to rule out contraindications such as severe brain atrophy, extensive white matter change, and focal lesions. The patient's general condition has to be considered as do speech and swallowing because of the risk of deterioration. The choice of target within the brain is determined on the basis of the profile of symptoms and the associated risk factors.

**History of Neurosurgery for Parkinson Disease.** Neurosurgical treatment of PD has been attempted for over a century. Early procedures dating from the late 1800s to the 1940s consisted of attempts to lesion the pyramidal system, ranging from excision of the pyramidal tract in the upper cervical cord to extirpation of cortical areas 4 and 6. The procedures resulted in resolution of tremor, with side effects of contralateral hemiparesis, hypalgesia, hypothermia, and seizures. Mortality rates during this period were high. During the 1950s, targets for surgical treatment of PD shifted from the pyramidal system to the basal ganglia. Spiegel, Wycis, Marks, and Lee (1947) published the first technique paper for performing stereotactic neurosurgical procedures in humans. The most effective targets were found to be in the internal segment of the globus pallidus (GPi) and the ventrolateral region of the thalamus. Ventrolateral thalamotomy for the treatment of tremor and rigidity became the most commonly chosen target for PD. A comparison of thalamic with pallidal lesions demonstrated that the thalamotomy was superior to pallidotomy for alleviating tremor but that pallidotomy was superior for alleviating rigidity.

Largely due to the introduction of levodopa and dopamine agonist therapy, surgical therapy for PD declined throughout the 1960s, 1970s, and 1980s. Furthermore, criticisms of the surgical literature also contributed to the decline in the use of neurosurgical procedures during these years. By the 1990s, however, it had become apparent that dopaminergic medication, in combination with advancing disease, resulted in motor complications that became as disabling as the cardinal signs of PD. This, combined with other factors, contributed to a renaissance of neurosurgical treatment of PD. Among these other factors were significant advances in neuroimaging techniques such as computed tomography (CT) and MRI which allowed visual identification of the nuclei of the basal ganglia. This along with advances in stereotactic technique allowed for more precise anatomic targeting. Furthermore, based on non-human primate models using 1-methyl-4-phenyl-1,2,3,6-tetrahydropyridine (MPTP) lesions, a model of basal ganglia circuitry, with anatomic, neurotransmitter, and functional properties, had emerged, which provided a stronger scientific rationale for surgical interventions in the basal ganglia for PD. Physiologic recordings in primates revealed that the anatomic site for sensorimotor processing of the primate internal pallidum was in its posteroventral aspect. Consequently, by the 1990s an anatomic and physiologic framework had developed for the surgical treatment of PD. (A detailed description of the basic circuitry of the basal ganglia and the MPTP model of hypokinetic disorders, including PD, is presented in Chapter 7.)

**Neurosurgical Treatments: Ablative Methods and Deep Brain Stimulation.** Recent years have witnessed a revival of interest in functional stereotactic neurosurgical treatments for PD. Such resurgence of interest in these particular forms of treatment for PD is due to several factors. First, many individuals with PD experience significant motor disability and motor fluctuations despite optimal medical therapy. As mentioned previously, PD continues to progress despite optimal medical therapy and features such as freezing, postural instability, and dementia are not satisfactorily controlled with medical therapies (Lang & Lozano, 1998). Second, advances in neuroimaging, neuroanesthesia, and stereotactic surgery, combined with the use of intra-operative microelectrode recording techniques, have made target identification more accurate and surgical procedures safer (Olanow & Brin, 2001).

Third, insights into the organization of the basal ganglia have enhanced the understanding of the neuropathophysiology underlying PD and have provided a scientific basis for performing surgical therapies (Alexander, DeLong, & Strick, 1986; DeLong, 1990). Indeed, based on current models of PD, surgical treatment of PD using ablative lesions or electric stimulation induced inactivation of basal ganglia nuclei has focused on three structures that have been found to be functionally overactive in PD (Eidelberg et al., 1994; Obeso, Rodriguez-Oroz, Rodriguez, DeLong, & Olanow, 2000). These three structures include the GPi (e.g., pallidotomy and deep brain stimulation (DBS), the ventrolateral thalamus (e.g., thalamotomy and DBS), and the subthalamic nucleus (STN) (e.g., DBS). Surgical procedures currently being performed include ablative procedures, DBS, and restorative procedures (e.g., fetal cell transplantation).

**Ablative Techniques.** Ablative techniques typically involve the generation of lesions within the thalamus (i.e., thalamotomy) and GPi (i.e., pallidotomy)

by means of radiofrequency-mediated electrocoagulation, which aims to permanently disrupt or inactivate the relevant target. In summary, thalamotomy has been reported to ameliorate tremor, while pallidotomy has been found to alleviate akinesia, rigidity, and drug-induced dyskinesia (Goetz, DeLong, Penn, & Bakay, 1993). With respect to ablative lesioning of the STN, subthalamotomy has not been widely performed due to the high risk of surgical complications such as the induction of hemiballism (Olanow & Brin, 2001). Recent advances in DBS have offered surgeons the opportunity to perform bilateral procedures within the STN without the risks associated with creating a destructive lesion.

*Pallidotomy.* In recent years there has been a resurgence of interest in pallidotomy following reports that amelioration of parkinsonian motor symptoms could be obtained with lesions placed in the posteroventral portion of the GPi (Laitinen, Bergenheim & Hariz, 1992a, 1992b). The rationale for pallidotomy is based on the theory that the major motor disturbances in PD are caused by overactivity of the GPi, which, in turn, is largely caused by excessive drive from the STN due to dopaminergic deficiency (Alexander et al., 1986; Lozano et al., 1995). Indeed, it is thought that the excessive inhibitory activity of the GPi inhibits the thalamic and cortical motor system, thereby producing slowness, rigidity, and poverty of movement; therefore, lesioning the GPi results in a reduction in the GPi-mediated excess inhibition of brainstem and thalamocortical neurons.

Interestingly, the current models of PD pathophysiology do not predict that dyskinesia would improve following pallidotomy (Starr, Vitek, & Bakay, 1998). Compelling clinical evidence that levodopa-induced dyskinesias improve following pallidotomy has led to serious reconsideration of the model. One possible explanation for the reduction of dyskinesia is that pallidotomy results in the elimination of the abnormal neuronal firing pattern in basal ganglia output neurons that communicate misinformation to cortical motor regions (Obeso et al., 2000). In essence, this hypothesis implies that interruption to basal ganglia output is better than disordered basal ganglia output.

*Thalamotomy.* Before the advent of levodopa, thalamotomy was extensively performed as a treatment for tremor in PD. In essence, thalamotomy consists of the creation of an ablative lesion in the ventrolateral (VL) nucleus of the thalamus (Grossman & Hamilton, 1993). The rationale underlying thalamotomy is that lesioning the VL thalamus interrupts the increased excitatory outflow from the thalamus thus resulting in a reduction in tremor. While the mechanisms of action of thalamotomy are largely uncharted, researchers have hypothesized that the postoperative reduction in tremor may be due to destruction of autonomous neural activity (i.e., synchronous bursts) which fires at the same frequency as limb tremor (Koller & Hristova, 1996).

*Deep Brain Stimulation.* In addition to the resurgence of ablative neurosurgical procedures, refinements in high-frequency stimulation techniques have resulted in the emergence of DBS as a viable neurosurgical treatment for individuals with PD. In most countries DBS has largely replaced the ablative procedures described above. The DBS procedure involves the implantation of an electrode into a specific brain target which is connected to a pacemaker placed subcutaneously over the chest wall (Benabid, Pollak, Louveau, Henry, & de Rougemont, 1987). Each brain electrode contains four leads that can be stimulated in various configurations by altering stimulation settings with respect to voltage, pulse width, and frequency. In principle, stimulation at frequencies greater than 100 Hz simulates the effect of a lesion without the need to induce a destructive brain lesion; therefore, a stimulation frequency of 100 to 180 Hz is typically chosen, coupled with a pulse width of 60 to 120 ms and a voltage of 3 to 4 V (Olanow, 2002). Although the precise mechanism underlying the effects of DBS activity is unknown, current researchers have postulated that DBS suppresses the neuronal firing pattern in the target via neural jamming, depolarization blockade, or by inducing the release of inhibitory transmitters (Benazzouz & Hallet, 2000).

The DBS procedure has several advantages over ablative techniques including the fact that it is reversible and does not necessitate the creation of destructive permanent lesions (Benabid et al., 1991; Limousin et al., 1998). In addition, bilateral implantation can be performed during a single procedure with relative safety, and stimulation settings can be adjusted at any time to optimize symptom relief and minimize adverse reactions (Koller & Hristova, 1996). Finally, DBS does not preclude future treatments that require an intact basal ganglia (Olanow & Brin, 2001). Notwithstanding the advantages associated with DBS, there are also disadvantages associated with the procedure. In particular, DBS is an expensive procedure requiring a high degree of neurosurgical expertise and the adjustment of stimulation settings can be time consuming and inconvenient. Furthermore, the battery life of the DBS device is limited and there is risk of complications associated with implantation of the device (Pahwa, Wilkinson, Smith, Lyons, Miyawaki, & Koller, 1997). Some side effects, in particular neuropsychiatric problems such as depression, apathy, and mania, can occur a long time after surgery. Infections can also occur late and patients should take prophylactic antibiotics.

The three established brain targets for treatment of PD with DBS are the ventrolateral thalamus, GPi, and STN. DBS on each of these targets improves a different range of symptoms. Thalamic DBS was developed in 1987 to treat tremor related to PD or essential tremor. Benefits on tremor can be maintained for more than 10 years, and consequently thalamic DBS still has a place for treatment of elderly patients with tremor-dominant PD. Balance problems and dysarthria are possible adverse effects, especially after bilateral surgery.

Although developed in parallel with STN DBS, GPi DBS is performed less frequently than the former procedure. Overall the effect on "OFF" systems is reported to be more variable than STN DBS with the most reliable effect being seen in relief of dyskinesias. GPi DBS does have the advantage of a lower rate of side effects than STN DBS and hence remains useful, particularly in older patients with severe dyskinesias who are at higher risk for adverse effects with STN DBS.

Developed in 1993 as an outcome of research in the MPTP monkey, STN DBS is effective at improving a large range of "OFF" phase symptoms including limb bradykinesia, rigidity, tremor, and gait difficulty. Levodopa-induced dyskinesias also improve over time, probably largely because of drug dose reduction. Medications are usually reduced after STN DBS. Unfortunately, the effect of STN DBS on speech is variable with some patients showing a deterioration in intelligibility (see Chapter 4). Although some of the beneficial effects of STN DBS are maintained up to 5 years, the effects on axial features and the "ON" phase scores often decline. Major side effects are common and include speech problems, neuropsychiatric problems (especially mood change), eyelid opening apraxia, and dyskinesias induced by the stimulation.

Although contemporary DBS procedures are somewhat helpful in the treatment of certain patients with PD, they do have limitations. They do not appear to change the progression of the disease and only allow symptomatic improvement. Further development of potentially disease-modifying and restorative procedures remains the challenge for the future.

**Fetal Mesencephalic Tissue Transplantation.** Neurotransplantation of fetal nigral tissue has undergone some initial trials as a treatment for PD. The procedure involves stereotactic transplantation of tissues derived from the substantia nigra of fetuses (obtained from elective abortions) via needle tracts into the striatum. The usual target is the putamen (sometimes in combination with the caudate nucleus). Although initial findings were encouraging, recent controlled studies have failed to show any meaningful benefit from neuronal grafting. Freed et al. (2001) reported the results of the first double-blind, placebo controlled trial of fetal graft transplants for advanced PD. Forty patients with PD were randomized to receive either embryonic mesencephalic tissue delivered bilaterally to the putamen or a sham procedure, where the needles did not penetrate the dura. The patients were initially separated based on age: younger or older than 60 years. In the younger group there were significant improvements in rigidity and bradykinesia but not in freezing or motor fluctuations, and gait scores worsened. The older group showed no significant improvement. In addition to the equivocal findings, a number of factors have served to limit the transition of fetal mesencephalic transplantation from an experimental to accepted clinical practice. These factors include, among others, the ethical issues surrounding the acquisition of fetal material, problems controlling graft rejection (for allogenic transplanted tissue), and survivability of fetal tissue.

**Stem Cell Transplantation.** The adult brain contains undifferentiated cells (stem cells) that are capable of self-renewal, proliferation, and differentiation into neurons and glia. Specifically, adult neuronal stem cells have been shown to be present in parts of the brain such as the subventricular zone and forebrain of rodents. These cells can be induced to proliferate, differen-

tiate, and migrate to an area of neuronal injury (such as the striatum) if injury is combined with infusions of growth factors. At this stage, although in the future neuronal stem cell therapy may advance the treatment of neurodegenerative diseases such as PD, a number of factors need to be overcome before clinical trials can commence. In particular, strategies need to be found to regulate uncontrolled cell proliferation (i.e., tumor formation) and to improve the survival of grafted cells.

## Treatment of Progressive Supranuclear Palsy

Progressive supranuclear palsy is a sporadic tauopathy that causes axial (hence symmetric) akinesia and rigidity, early falls (classically backwards without warning), dysarthria (lower pitch, growling, with late groaning), dysphagia, personality change, frontal cognitive deficits, and eye features. Unfortunately, there is no effective treatment for the condition. Although some patients with slowness, stiffness, and balance problems respond to antiparkinsonian therapies, such as levodopa or levodopa combined with anticholinergic agents, the effect is usually temporary. Speech, vision, and swallowing difficulties are usually unresponsive to any pharmacotherapy.

## Treatment of Hyperkinetic Disorders

Hyperkinetic movement disorders are characterized by the pressure of abnormal, involuntary movements that may occur independently or be superimposed on and disrupt normal movement patterns. These abnormal involuntary movements may involve the limbs, trunk, neck, face, and so forth, and can be rhythmic, irregular and unpredictable, rapid, or slow. The major forms of hyperkinetic movement disorders include myoclonus, tics, chorea, ballismus, and dystonia.

## Treatment of Myoclonus

Myoclonus is a common movement disorder that comprises sudden, brief shock-like involuntary movements caused by muscular contractions (positive myoclonus) or inhibitions (negative myoclonus or asterixis). Myoclonus can be focal (i.e., confined to one part of the body), multifocal (i.e., involving multiple parts of the body and not necessarily at the same time), generalized (i.e., involving the whole body or most of it), spontaneous, or reflex (i.e., triggered by external stimuli). It may occur at rest, when maintaining a posture or during a movement (action myoclonus). Myoclonus can be classified as cortical, subcortical, spinal, or peripheral based on the presumed physiologic mechanism underlying its generation. Alternatively, based on its etiology it can be classified as physiologic, essential, epileptic, or symptomatic. Physiologic myoclonus refers to muscle jerks that occur in certain circumstances in normal subjects. These include sleep jerks (hypnic jerks) and hiccup. Essential myoclonus consists of multifocal myoclonus in which there is no other neurologic deficit or abnormality on investigation. Epileptic myoclonus refers to conditions in which the major

clinical problem is one of epilepsy, but one of the manifestations of the epileptic attacks is myoclonic jerks. Symptomatic generalized myoclonus is the most common form of myoclonus and refers to a large number of neurologic conditions in which generalized or multifocal muscle jerking is a manifestation of the underlying neurologic disease.

The treatment of myoclonus depends upon the underlying disorder. Depending upon its etiology, myoclonus can be partially or totally reversed, as in drug-induced or metabolic myoclonus or surgically treatable lesions. Unfortunately, treatment of the underlying disorder is not always feasible. The drugs that are used to treat myoclonus generally possess anticonvulsant properties (Frucht, 2000), usually by enhancing gamma aminobutyric acid (GABA) inhibitory activity. As most causative conditions are poorly responsive to pharmacologic treatment, poly therapy (i.e., the use of multiple drugs) is often necessary. Symptomatic treatment typically includes medications to reduce the severity of the myoclonus, such as benzodiazepines. Epileptic and cortical myoclonus respond best to drugs such as sodium valproate and clonazepam which are often used in combination. It is conventional to start treatment with sodium valproate in patients with severe myoclonus and then add clonazepam. If the disability is not improved, piracetam or levetiracetam can be added. Patients with brainstem myoclonus seem to respond best to clonazepam as do those with spinal and other segmented (focal) forms of myoclonus. Essential myoclonus sometimes improves with alcohol, a beta-blocker such as proprandol, or an anticholinergic agent. GPi DBS has been reported to improve myoclonus–dystonia syndrome in one case (Cif et al., 2004).

## Treatment of Tics

Tics are typically relatively brief, rapid, intermittent, purposeless, involuntary movements (motor tics) or sounds (vocal or phonic tics). Motor tics typically consist of sudden, abrupt, transient, often repetitive and coordinated (stereotypic) movements that may resemble gestures and mimic fragments of normal behavior, vary in intensity, and are repeated at irregular intervals. Vocal/phonic tics are actually motor tics that involve respiratory, laryngeal, pharyngeal, oral, or nasal musculature. Classically, tics can be suppressed, at least temporarily, by an effort of will, but at the expense of increasing inner tension, often followed by a rebound exacerbation. Tourette syndrome (TS) is the most common cause of tics; however, they can occur in association with numerous different acquired and congenital neurologic and neuropsychiatric disorders. The diagnostic criteria for TS include multiple motor tics and one or more phonic and/or vocal tics which must be present for more than 1 year. The motor and vocal/phonic tics do not necessarily occur together, characteristically wax and wane over time, and occur in bouts. The mean age of onset of motor tics is about 7 years and vocal/phonic tics 11 years. The majority of symptoms disappear in 50% of patients by 18 years of age. Behaviors such as obsessive-compulsive disorder (OCD) and attention deficit hyperactivity disorder (ADHD) may co-occur.

Tics in TS usually begin in the head and face and blinking is one of the most common first tics. Simple phonic tics include sniffing, throat clearing, gulping, snorting, and coughing. Complex vocal tics include barking, making animal noises, inappropriate voice intonations, and uttering strings of words. Other characteristic features of TS include echolalia (copying what other people say), echopraxia (copying what other people do), and palilalia (repeating the last word or part of a sentence said by another individual). Coprolalia (inappropriate involuntary swearing) occurs in around 10 to 15% of cases.

In mild cases no specific pharmacologic therapy may be necessary to treat tics. Explanation of the condition, reassurance, and psychoeducation may be all that is required. Reassurance can be achieved by discussing the normal waxing and waning of TS symptomatology and the tendency for symptoms to improve with age. In those cases where further treatment is necessary, the primary treatment for tics usually include α-adrenergic agents because of their effectiveness and fewer long-term adverse effects. Clonidine is usually the first drug used, although guanfacine may cause less drowsiness. Clonidine is available as a transdermal 1-week patch, which is advantageous for small children. Second-line therapy usually requires an atypical antipsychotic agent such as risperidone or olanzapine. These are preferred over the classic neuroleptic antipsychotic medications because of their better adverse effect profile, especially their lower tendency to cause extrapyramidal effects such as acute dystonia, tardive dyskinesia, and parkinsonism. Traditional neuroleptic antipsychotic medications, such as haloperidol and pimozide, are regarded as third-line medication for tics because of their tendency to induce extrapyramidal syndromes, sedation, weight gain, irritability, and various phobias. Clonidine, guanfacine, and the stimulants methylphenidate, pemoline, or dextroamphetamines have been reported to be useful in the treatment of patients with TS and ADHD. Patients with TS and OCD respond to treatment with a serotonin reuptake inhibitor or to the tricyclic antidepressant clomipramine.

## Treatment of Chorea

Chorea (from Latin *choreus*, meaning dance) is a state of excessive spontaneous movements, irregularly timed, randomly distributed and abrupt. The involuntary movements are usually distal in location and tend to flow from one body part to another. The condition has many causes which can simply be divided into acquired and inherited, all of which disrupt the basal ganglia modulation of thalamocortical motor pathways (see Chapter 7 for models of basal ganglia function in chorea). It is beyond the scope of the present chapter to review the treatment for all forms of chorea; however, the treatment of Huntington disease (HD) is described to illustrate the principles of treatment of choreic disorders.

Huntington disease is the most important inherited cause of chorea. It is a slowly progressive autosomal-dominant neurodegenerative disorder with onset usually in adult life around 40 years of age. Onset, however, does vary from early childhood to late adulthood. The condition can produce a varied clinical phenotype with signs and symptoms changing as the disease progresses. Disease duration, therefore, can markedly modify the clinical presentation. The onset of HD is often difficult to discern clearly and the initial characteristic signs may be neurologic or psychiatric. Many patients report psychiatric problems or mild cognitive symptoms before motor signs develop. Subtle motor signs seen early in the disease include general restlessness, abnormal eye movements, hyperreflexia, impaired finger tapping, and fidgety movements of fingers, hands, and toes during stress or when walking. Early chorea may be limited to the toes and fingers, later extending to the arms, legs, face, and trunk. As the disease progresses more obvious extrapyramidal signs develop. Patients often exhibit a distinctive manner of walking that may be unsteady, disjointed, lurching, and dance-like. Eventually postural instability, dysarthria, and dysphagia develop. Dystonia, rigidity, and parkinsonism may dominate the late stages of the disease. Cognitive decline is characterized by progressive dementia.

No treatment is available that slows, alters, or reverses the progression of HD. In general, a multidisciplinary approach to treatment should be adopted involving symptomatic and supportive medical management, psychosocial support, genetic counseling, as well as physical, occupational, and speech therapy. The therapy applied also depends on the severity of the symptoms. Mild chorea may not require any treatment. Where required, however, chorea is treated with dopamine-blocking or dopamine-depleting medications. Dopamine antagonists, such as haloperidol and pimozide, are generally the drugs of choice after elimination of readily reversible causes of chorea. For severe, functionally disabling chorea, drugs such as sulpiride, olanzapine, risperidone, and tetrabenazine may be helpful by nonspecifically damping down movements in general. Unfortunately, these latter drugs may also worsen speech, swallowing, gait, and balance, and hence need careful monitoring.

## Treatment of Ballism

Ballism involves large-amplitude, involuntary movements affecting the proximal limbs, causing flinging and flailing limb movements. The condition is often interrelated with chorea and can occur in the same patient. The involuntary movement usually affects only one side of the body (hemiballism). Treatment most frequently involves the use of dopamine receptor-blocking drugs such as perphenazine, haloperidol, chlorpromazine, pimozide, and atypical neuroleptics. Dopamine-depleting drugs, such as reserpine and tetrabenazine, have also been used with some success. Tetrabenazine is often the preferred drug because of its fast action and effectiveness without the danger of inducing tardive dyskinesia if chronic antidopaminergic treatment is needed. In severe cases of violent and disabling hemiballism, ventrolateral thalamotomy or other stereotactic surgeries may be required to treat the condition.

## Treatment of Dystonia

Dystonia is a common but heterogeneous movement disorder typically characterized by involuntary muscle spasms leading to abnormal postures of the affected part of the body. These spasms are usually mobile leading to slow writhing and twisting movements of the affected part of the body as described by the older term "athetosis." Co-contraction of agonist and antagonist muscles is the underlying reason for the abnormal posturing in dystonia. The clinical presentation of dystonia can vary, and in some cases tremor or jerks may be the predominant feature with the abnormal postures being subtle. No satisfactory classification for dystonia exists, partly because of the wide variety of disorders in which dystonia is a feature. Standard classifications use age at onset, symptom distribution, and etiology. Focal dystonia is the most common form of the condition and involves a single body part (e.g., cervical dystonia or torticollis). Segmented dystonia involves two or more contiguous body parts while multifocal dystonia involves two or more non-contiguous body regions. Generalized dystonia involves both legs and at least one other body part.

Botulinum toxin injection has revolutionized the treatment of patients with focal dystonia and has become the treatment of choice for cervical dystonia, blepharospasm, and spasmodic dysphonia. The action of botulinum toxin is to block the release of acetylcholine at the neuromuscular junction, resulting in flaccid paralysis of the injected muscles. The effect of the injection lasts only 3 to 6 months, with the involuntary muscle activity gradually returning, necessitating repeated injection. Botulinum injections are less useful for treatment of patients with involvement of large muscles or with multifocal or generalized dystonia due to the large amounts of toxin required to relieve symptoms.

In those cases where botulinum injection would be unlikely to control the full extent of the dystonia, such as in younger-onset generalized and/or multifocal dystonia, drug treatment may be more appropriate. First-line treatment involves the use of anticholinergics such as trihexyphenidyl or benzotropine; however, these drugs are only effective in a minority of patients. Where anticholinergics are ineffective, additional medications can be used including clonazepam, tetrabenazine, baclofen, anticonvulsants, and lithium. Those cases with generalized dystonia for whom pharmacologic treatments are ineffective may require neurosurgery to relieve the disabling features of dystonia. Ventrolateral thalamotomies, and to a lesser degree pallidotomies, were performed from the 1950s for alleviation of dystonia. The results, however, were not consistent and some patients had initial benefit that wore off over time necessitating several operations. Complications, including dysarthria and dysphagia, were not uncommon, especially in bilaterally operated patients. More recently, GPi DBS has produced promising results in patients with primary generalized dystonia.

## References

Alexander, G. E., DeLong, M. R., & Strick, P. L. (1986). Parallel organization of functionally segregated circuits linking basal ganglia and cortex. *Annual Review of Neuroscience, 9,* 357–381.

Benabid, A. L., Pollak, P., Gervason, C., Hoffman, V., Gao, D. M., Hommel, M., . . . de Roguemont, J. (1991). Long-term suppression of tremor by chronic stimulation of the ventral intermediate thalamic nucleus. *Lancet, 337,* 403–406.

Benabid, A. L., Pollak, P., Louveau, A., Henry, S., & de Rougemont, J. (1987).

Combined (thalamotomy and stimulation) stereotactic surgery of the VIM thalamic nucleus for bilateral Parkinson disease. *Applied Neurophysiology, 50,* 344–346.

Benazzouz, A., & Hallet, M. (2000). Mechanism of action of deep brain stimulation. *Neurology, 55*(Suppl. 6), S13–S16.

Cif, L., Valente, E. M., Hemm, S., Coubes, C., Vayssiere, N., Serrat, S., . . . Coubes, P. (2004). Deep brain stimulation in myoclonus-dystonia syndrome. *Movement Disorders, 19,* 724–727.

DeLong, M. R. (1990). Primate models of movement disorders of basal ganglia origin. *Trends in Neuroscience, 13,* 281–285.

Eidelberg, D., Moeller, J. R., Dhawan, V., Spetsieris, P., Takikawa, S., Ishikawa, T., . . . Fahn, S. (1994). The metabolic topography of parkinsonism. *Journal of Cerebral Blood Flow and Metabolism, 14,* 783–801.

Freed, C. R., Greene, P. E., Breeze, R. E., Tsai, W. Y., DuMouchel, W., Kao, R., . . . Fahn, S. (2001). Transplantation of embryonic dopamine neurons for severe Parkinson's disease. *New England Journal of Medicine, 344,* 710–719.

Frucht, S. (2000). Myoclonus. *Current Treatment Options in Neurology, 2,* 231–242.

Goetz, R. G., DeLong, M. R., Penn, R. D., & Bakay, R. A. (1993). Neurosurgical horizons in Parkinson's disease. *Neurology, 43,* 1–7.

Grossman, R. G., & Hamilton, W. J. (1993). Surgery for movement disorders. In J. Jankovic & E. Tolosa (Eds.), *Parkinson's disease and movement disorders* (pp. 531–548). Baltimore, MD: Williams & Wilkins.

Koller, W., & Hristova, A. (1996). Efficacy and safety of stereotaxic surgical treatment of tremor disorders. *European Journal of Neurology, 3,* 507–514.

Laitinen, L. V., Bergenheim, A. T., & Hariz, M. I. (1992a). Leksell's posteroventral pallidotomy in the treatment of Parkinson's disease. *Journal of Neurosurgery, 76,* 53–61.

Laitinen, L. V., Bergenheim, A. T., & Hariz, M. I. (1992b). Ventroposterolateral pallidotomy can abolish all parkinsonian symptoms. *Stereotactic Functional Neurosurgery, 58,* 14–21.

Lang, A. E., & Lozano, A. M. (1998). Parkinson's disease: Second of two parts. *New England Journal of Medicine, 339,* 1130–1143.

Limousin, A. M., Krack, P., Pollak, P., Benzzouz, A., Ardouin, C., Hoffman, D., & Benabid, A. L. (1998). Electrical stimulation of the subthalamic nucleus in advanced Parkinson's disease. *New England Journal of Medicine, 339,* 1105–1111.

Lozano, A. M., Lang, A. E., Galvez-Jimenez, N., Miyasaki, J., Duff, J., Hutchinson, W. D., & Dostrovsky, J.O. (1995). Effect of GPi pallidotomy on motor function in Parkinson's disease. *Lancet, 346,* 1383–1387.

Obeso, J. A., Rodriguez-Oroz, M. C., Rodriguez, M., DeLong, M. R., & Olanow, C. W. (2000). Pathophysiology of levodopa-induced dyskinesias in Parkinson's disease: Problems with the current model. *Annals of Neurology, 47*(Suppl. 1), S22–S32.

Olanow, C. W. (2002). Surgical therapy for Parkinson's disease. *European Journal of Neurology, 9*(Suppl. 3), 31–39.

Olanow, C. W., & Brin, M. (2001). Surgical therapies for Parkinson's disease. In D. Calne & S. Calne (Eds.), *Parkinson's disease: Advances in neurology* (Vol. 86, pp. 421–433). Philadelphia, PA: Lippincott Williams & Wilkins.

Pahwa, R., Wilkinson, S., Smith, D., Lyons, K., Miyawaki, E., & Koller, W. C. (1997). High-frequency stimulation of the globus pallidus for the treatment of Parkinson's disease. *Neurology, 49,* 249–253.

Speigel, E. A., Wycis, H. T., Marks, M., & Lee, A. J. (1947). Stereotaxic apparatus for operations on the human brain. *Science, 106,* 349–350.

Starr, P. A., Vitek, J. L., & Bakay, R. (1998). Ablative surgery and deep brain stimulation for Parkinson's disease. *Neurosurgery, 43,* 989–1015.

# 11

# The Future of Movement Disorders

## *LEONARD L. LAPOINTE*

### Foreseen and Unforeseen Developments

We have all had both good and bad experiences with committee meetings. As some old quipster remarked, "A camel is a horse designed by a committee." By highlighting the ineffectiveness of incorporating too many conflicting opinions into a single project, in this colorful figure of speech the peculiar features of a camel, such as its humps and spitting temperament, are assumed to be the defects that resulted from its poor design. Futurists and predictors are at peril and one does not have to delve too deeply into past predictions of the future to discover that many are now ludicrous (e.g., "Stocks have reached what looks like a permanently high plateau." Irving Fisher, economics professor at Yale University, 1929;

"It will be gone by June." *Variety*, predicting the future of rock-n-roll in 1955) (Bad Predictions, 2013).

Futurists, predictors, psychics, and soothsayers are at risk, and committees of these are at compounded risk of generating preposterous predictions. Nevertheless, some astute experts in neuroscience have ventured bold prognostications of the future. In the United States, one such convened panel was a group of experts wrangled by the National Institutes of Health (NIH) and the National Institute of Neurological Disorders and Stroke (NINDS; an agency name that is a bit redundant; stroke *is* a neurologic disorder) just a few years back to think about and plan for the future. The strategic planning sessions and documents that emanated from these think sessions resulted in what they called the Blue Sky Vision for the Future of Neuroscience (NINDS,

**223**

2013). As a supplemental source of input toward a "Blue Sky" vision for the future of neuroscience, the NINDS convened members of its staff as well as representatives from other NIH institutes for a workshop. Breakout groups discussed questions similar to those posed in a Request for Information to the larger neuroscience community. In particular, they focused on anticipated advances in neuroscience and neurology over the next 15 years, infrastructure and technologic needs, research questions with potential impact for understanding nervous system function or the treatment and prevention of disease, and the role of NINDS in the neuroscience research topography of the future. Interesting ideas and documents were generated by these meetings and may offer a flashlight (or torch) along the path to the future. Part of the strategic plan included the following ideas (NINDS, 2013):

- Enable early and routine diagnosis of neurologic conditions.
  - Determine a person's risk for specific neurologic disorders based on genomic markers, gene expression, or other measurable indicators (e.g., at birth and/or annual physicals, everyone receives a readout of his or her neurologic risk factors and recommendations for preventive actions). This, of course, would be a mixed blessing. It would resolve the mystery of what is going to get us, but on the other hand, would allow fright and preparation.
  - Develop technologies that primary care physicians, emergency workers, health care profession-

als, or even an individual can use routinely to monitor neurologic health as well as detect and diagnose neurologic disorders at early stages when intervention is most promising (e.g., anatomic and functional, which become sufficiently affordable and user-friendly to be a routine part of an annual physical; the next generation of personal digital devices may include personal neurologic sensors).

- Develop and validate proxy markers that reflect disease progression and show, early on and before an individual is in death's throes, whether interventions are working.
- Develop technologies that will provide more patients with timely access to neurologic expertise, even if a neurologist is not immediately or locally available (e.g. telemedicine, artificial intelligence-guided diagnostic alerts). This innovation is in rapid development especially where remote access to health care is crucial such as in Australia, parts of the United States, and Canada.
- Develop new therapeutic strategies.
  - Develop neuroprosthetic devices that amalgamate with the brain to restore sensory, motor, or cognitive functions lost through disease or injury. The amazing developments in 3D printers that utilize stem cells and "print" new human organs are in clinical trials and who knows, we may someday not only be able to print (with cells, not ink) a new kidney but parts of the brain or peripheral nervous system (TED.com, 2013).

- Develop endovascular devices to restore blood flow to the brain in people who have ischemic stroke or compromised vascular flow that puts the brain at risk.
- Develop techniques that allow neurosurgeons to fix the brain with minimal collateral damage (e.g., robotics, remote targeting, nanoscale deep brain stimulation, even nanoscale devices that are integrated into the bloodstream as replacements or little mechanics that travel to the site and repair damage).
- Develop broadly applicable techniques or vehicles to deliver therapeutics into the brain and target particular cells or regions. Nanoscience is here today and rapidly expanding. Consider early computer size and current microchips.
- Cure someone of a neurologic condition with a gene therapy strategy that can be readily adapted to other neurologic conditions.
- Accelerate the process of therapy development.
  - Develop rational and generic ways to test the synergistic effects of combination therapies so that this becomes a routine aspect of therapy development.
  - Develop a more rational and modular pathway for developing therapies, with a greater emphasis on design than screening (e.g., once a plausible drug target is identified, derive a three-dimensional structure, computationally predict ligand (an ion or molecule that binds to an atom) qualities, synthesize and test the ligand against off-the-shelf human cell assays

and in validated animal models of efficacy and toxicity, and test clinically with surrogate markers).
  - Develop strategies and infrastructure to enable any person with a neurologic condition to participate in a clinical trial (e.g., clinical trials become a routine option for patients, as in the cancer field).
  - Establish strategies and infrastructure that will enable neuroscience researchers to more easily draw upon health informatics and clinical observations in medical practice and from unpublished clinical studies (e.g., epidemiology and natural history data can be culled from electronic medical records; repositories of negative data from clinical trials).
  - Health informatics also will allow interdisciplinary clinician teams to provide medical care and conduct research remotely.
- Understand the healthy nervous system.
  - Identify the cellular and molecular mechanisms of plasticity responsible for particular behavioral changes. Neural plasticity is more than a catch phrase of the new century. As Doige (2007) and others (LaPointe, 2012) have stated, neuroplasticity may be the greatest advance in understanding neuroscience in the past two decades.
  - Determine the extent of brain plasticity, its consequences in normal function, and how to generate efficient experiences that promote healing.
  - Determine how percepts, memories, and other aspects of cognition are represented in brain cells,

circuits, and synapses, and how neural circuits perceive, execute movement, regulate bodily functions, remember, think, emote, and carry out other functions.

- Determine how gene expression influences nervous system function, and vice versa.
- Determine the role of cell interactions in regulating neurodevelopment.
- Understand the natural aging process and its relationship to development. This borders on understanding galaxies and the cosmos, but if we can send a person to the moon or to Tupelo, Mississippi, perhaps we can understand development and decrepitude.
- Understand lipid–protein interactions and their potential as drug targets. There is more to protein than a rib-eye steak, and microscopic proteins may contain secrets beyond the steakhouse.
- Determine the roles of glia. Glia cells are no longer regarded as just Elmer's glue but may have previously unrealized roles in neural transmission.
- Determine the functions of sleep and perchance dreams.
- Determine the extent and function of adult neurogenesis (e.g., Is it involved in learning or recovery from cell loss?).
- Determine more global interactions between the healthy brain and body. We have long known that the brain and testicles are intimately related, but perhaps there is more to the relationship between the brain and nose than meets the eye.

- Develop new technologies for observing the nervous system.
  - Develop technologies to monitor the activity of many individual neurons simultaneously, over long periods of time, in behaving animals, including geese, chimps, poodles, and people.
  - Develop technologies to image at the molecular level in vivo, in real time.
  - Develop a complete anatomic connectivity map of the human brain. Diffuse tensor imaging has advanced our understanding of synaptic connectivity and we have grown to appreciate that cell bodies and neuroarchitecture is just one aspect of neural transmission. We need to discover how this ultimate network works in its billions of connections that continue to grow and undergo pruning.

All of these goals and targets of understanding proposed by the Blue Sky Vision for the Future of Neuroscience initiative (NINDS, 2013) are lofty ambitions and purposes; however, they are attainable and certainly serve as a global positioning system for the future. All of these developments, including the man–machine interface, will hold some surprises and will require deeply human consideration of bioethics. Many ethicists are concerned about these issues. It is apparent to some ethicists that in many ways, the rapid advances of science and technology have outstripped our capacity to carefully consider positive and negative outcomes (Institute for the Study of Disability and Bioethics, 2013). We can no longer afford to let technological breakthroughs skip ahead of deep philosophical and ethical considerations. Humanity cannot risk allowing handguns, atomic bombs, and genome transmuting devices in the hands of children and idiots. We must learn techniques that harness the future so it does not burn us, cripple us, or shoot us in the head.

## Animal Models

Animals are not very good talkers. Squirrels, for example, are practically unintelligible. They can communicate but they lack the nuances of a good stand-up comedian or a toastmaster after-dinner speaker. With apologies to our vegan friends, the only roast many animals are any good at is the one in which they may be featured as the main course. Baboons and dolphins may do tricks, jump through hoops for a smelt or herring, or smoke a cigar for a banana reward, but few of them ever get linguistically agile. So is an animal model of human speech production out of the question? Perhaps not. Incredible advances are being made in work with the learned vocal utterances of some species, including our fine-feathered friends.

### Birdsong and Us

Species-specific vocal production represents one of many strategies by which organisms communicate. Birds do it. Bees do it. Only a few (oscine passerines and humans) develop their vocal behavior through precisely orches-trated experience against the backdrop of time-sensitive sensory and motor experiences. One unique vocal learning exemplar is the zebra finch (*Taeniopygia guttata*) (Figure 11–1). Zebra finches are a species of passerine songbird that learns and produces a motif of stereotyped sequences of three to seven harmonically complex syllables. Analyses of both vocal development and experimental manipulation of adult motifs focus on vocal features that individuate birds. These vocal features include the sequential order and acoustic structure of birdsong syllables.

How similar is birdsong learning to human speech and language acquisition? Can destabilized birdsong inform us about recovery of speech and language in humans? When birds have an impairment of learned song motifs because of brain damage, how do they recover it? Do they lose the individual notes or syllables? Do they lose the order or the syntax of notes in the song? Is their destabilized singing characterized by imprecise movements in attempts to produce notes? How long

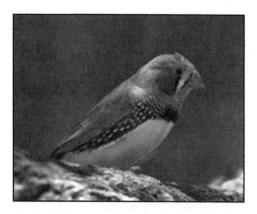

**FIGURE 11–1.** A zebra finch, a fine utterer of learned vocal sequences, is shown.

does it take a bird to recover his song to its pre-surgical state? Does destabilized birdsong relate to neurologically destabilized speech and language in humans? Would birds be a viable animal model for manipulations or interventions that could alter the quantity and quality of recovery? What are the limitations of a birdsong–human language analogy?

These questions have piqued our curiosity about similarities and differences between the tuneful noises that birds generate and the communicative audible patterns of sound that humans produce. A group of us at Florida State University and the University of Pittsburgh have been pondering these issues for several years (LaPointe, Johnson, McNeil, & Pratt, 2012; LaPointe, Johnson, Thompson, McNeil, & Pratt, 2009). Our initial findings are more than mildly interesting and cautiously encouraging. Perhaps an animal model of dissolution and recovery of birdsong would allow us to explore a variety of intrinsic (neural) and extrinsic (social and facilitative) manipulations that might inform us about correlates in human communication recovery after brain damage.

## Birds and Humans

Speech has long been thought of as a uniquely defining characteristic of humans; yet songbirds, like humans, communicate using learned signals (song, speech) that are acquired from their parents by a process of vocal imitation. Both song and speech begin as amorphous vocalizations (subsong, babble) that are gradually transformed into an individualized version of the parent's speech, including dialects (Ziegler & Marler, 2008).

Species-specific vocal production represents one of many strategies by which organisms communicate. Only a few organisms (oscine passerines and humans) develop their vocal behavior through experience against the backdrop of time-sensitive sensory and motor experiences (Goldstein, King, & West, 2003). Human speech and birdsong have numerous rather striking parallels.

Both humans and songbirds learn their complex vocalizations early in life, exhibiting a powerful dependence on hearing the adults they will imitate, as well as themselves as they practice, and a fading of this dependence as they develop and become more proficient and practiced in their emissions (Kuhl, 2003). As pointed out by Berwick Okanoya, Beckers, and Bolhuis (2011), unlike our primate relatives, many species of bird share with humans this significant capacity for vocal learning, a crucial factor in speech acquisition. Striking and perhaps unexpected behavioral, neural, and genetic similarities exist between auditory–vocal learning in birds and human infants. Only relatively recently have the linguistic parallels between birdsong and spoken human language begun to be investigated. Although both birdsong and human language are hierarchically organized according to particular syntactic constraints, birdsong structure is best characterized as "phonological syntax," resembling aspects of human sound structure (Berwick et al., 2011).

Some of our early analysis of destabilized birdsong and the subsequent path to recovery of these rather intricate combinations of learned vocal utterances suggest some room for optimism about the future use of birdsong as an animal model for both intrinsic and extrinsic manipulations that might influence patterns of both destabilization and recovery (LaPointe et al., 2012). Birdsong is not human speech and language. Significant differences exist, particularly in the area of lexical–semantic richness. The complexity of human language is unparalleled among biological communication systems, and there are no completely suitable animal models. Recognizing these limitations is crucial, and we do not want to overstate the case or the aptness of human speech and language to that of songbird learned vocalizations; however, songbirds are considered by many researchers to be the best animal model as they are unique among non-humans in their combination of vocal sophistication and experimental accessibility (Proposal, 2005).

Scientists now realize that the cortex and basal ganglia dominate the songbird's brain. The zebra finch's learning to produce songs is anything but instinctual and involves complex interactions between the cortex and other brain regions, and research laboratories, such as that at Florida State University, are bringing sophisticated clarification to what is known about the birdsong brain in dissolution and recovery of its song. A consortium of leading scientists has outlined well the biological and biomedical rationales for the pursuit of research on birdsong (Proposal, 2005).

Our research has suggested that not only is destabilized birdsong defective in motoric aspects, but also loses aspects of syntax (order of syllables or notes), and surprisingly, some elements of lexical-semantic behavior (the pro-duction of neologistic syllables or notes that have never before been uttered in the bird's repertoire). These aspects of destabilized birdsong (and subsequent recovery of presurgical vocal utterances in a matter of days or weeks) leads us to be optimistic about further intrinsic or extrinsic manipulations that might hasten recovery (Presence of a community of tutors during recovery? Cellular implantation?).

Birds are our friends. We should feed them, care for them, nurture them, and perhaps they will assist us in unlocking some of the secrets of learned and lost vocal utterances.

## Heavy Duty Magnets and Drugs, More Drugs

The machines and cameras will help us as well and will raise new and unusual bioethical and legal questions. These cautions, mentioned first above, must be part of futuristic and technological deliberations. The days of human–machine interface and fusion are no longer the fodder of science fiction but instead will force us to confront tricky and deep-seated ethical issues (LaPointe, 2012). Surely, there will be increased use of brain imaging techniques for both diagnostic and prognostic purposes and surveillance as well. With the age of the rise of the drones that allow us to survey and observe any place on the planet with pinpoint resolution, we are on the threshold of internal observation that matches that precision. Soon the nano-drones will be in our bloodstream, with orders to search and repair, rather than search and destroy.

New drugs, too, are on the horizon, and we can only hope that the commercial and bottom-line economics that now steer the ethics of pharmaceutical research and drug availability will be tempered with some seasoning of altruism that will guide widespread use for human benefit. New and better-targeted psychoactive and psychomotor drugs to treat neurologic diseases, such as Parkinson disease as well as other degenerative movement disorders, are in clinical trials constantly. The other plagues to human well-being, such as Alzheimer disease, depression, and anxiety and related conditions, are being battled with greater insights into these disorders through advances in neurogenetics and neurochemistry. "Lucy in the sky with diamonds" is now in the research laboratory working on cures for many of our ills.

The future may hold widespread use of "protective" drugs to prevent neurodegeneration. This means that the horrible degenerative movement disorders with subsequent devastating effects on motor speech production and communication may well be slowed, stopped in their tracks, or even repaired. The future of these disorders may be characterized if not with eradication, then at least with significant lessening of their gruesome effects. We can only work. We can only hope.

## References

Bad Predictions. (2013). Top 87 bad predictions about the future. Retrieved January 29, 2013 from http://www.2spare.com/item_50221.aspx/

Berwick, R. C., Okanoya, K., Beckers, G. J. L., & Bolhuis, J. J. (2011). Songs to syntax: The linguistics of birdsong. *Trends in Cognitive Sciences, 15*, 113–121.

Doige, N. (2007). *The brain that changes itself.* New York, NY: Penguin Books.

Goldstein, M. H., King, A. P., & West, M. J. (2003). Social interaction shapes babbling: Testing parallels between birdsong and speech. *Proceedings of the National Academy of Sciences, 100*(17), 9645–9646.

National Institute of Neurological Disorders and Stroke (NINDS). (2013). Future of neuroscience. Retrieved January 29, 2013 from http://www.ninds.nih.gov/about_ninds/plans/strategic_plan/A%20Blue%20Sky%20Vision%20for%20the%20Future%20of%20Neuroscience.htm/

Institute for the Study of Disability and Bioethics. (2013). About the Institute. Retrieved February 6, 2013 from https://www.regent.edu/acad/schedu/isdb/about.cfm/

Kuhl, P. K. (2003). Human speech and birdsong: Communication and the social brain. *Proceedings of the National Academy of Sciences, 100*(17), 9645–9646.

LaPointe, L. L. (2012). *Brain-based communication disorders: Pearls from 51 years of dredging oysters.* Invited lecture by American Speech-Language-Hearing Association Special Interest Group 2, Neurophysiology and Neurogenic Speech and Language Disorders. Annual convention of American Speech-Language-Hearing Association, Atlanta, November 2012.

LaPointe, L. L., Johnson, F., McNeil, M. R., & Pratt, S. (2012). Birdsong and human speech and language: What the zebra finch uses, loses, and regains. In R. Goldfarb (Ed.), *Speech and language pathology: Translational speech-language pathology and audiology.* San Diego, CA: Plural.

LaPointe, L. L., Johnson, F., Thompson, J., McNeil, M. R., Pratt, S. (2009). *How can destabilized birdsong inform us about language impairment in aphasia?* Paper presented to the Academy of Aphasia, Turku, Finland, October, 2009.

Proposal (2005). Proposal to sequence the zebra finch genome. Retrieved September 23, 2011 from http://www.genome .gov/Pages/Research/Sequencing/Seq Proposals/ZebraFinchSeq2.pdf/

TED.com. (2013). TED talk: Anthony Atala, Printing a human organ. Retrieved January 29, 2013 from http://www.ted .com/talks/anthony_atala_printing_a_ human_kidney.html/

Ziegler, P., & Marler, P. (2008). *Neuroscience of birdsong*. Boston, MA: Cambridge University Press.

# Glossary

**Ablation:** Surgical destruction or removal of tissue, an organ, or a precise region of a particular structure. Ablation may involve surgical cutting (excision); chemical destruction, such as injection of phenol; or the use of high-frequency electrical current or radio waves.

**Accelerometer:** A device used to measure the rate of change in velocity over a specific period of time. Measures the rate or "speed" of the tremor cycle.

**Acetylcholine (ACh):** A neurotransmitter present at junctions of nerve and muscle cells and various sites of the central nervous system, including the cerebral cortex and the basal ganglia. Primary functions of acetylcholine include regulating the delivery of messages from neurons to skeletal muscle fibers, smooth (involuntary) muscle fibers, and effector organs, as well as between nerve cells in the brain and spinal cord.

**Action tremor:** A tremor that occurs during the performance of voluntary movements. Such tremors include postural, isometric, kinetic, and intention tremors.

**Agonist:** A muscle whose contraction executes an intended movement.

**Akathisia:** A neurologic condition of motor restlessness, manifested by a sensation of muscular quivering, an urge to constantly move about, and an inability to sit still.

**Akinesia:** Absence of movement or loss of the ability to move, such as temporary or prolonged paralysis or "freezing in place."

**Akinetic:** Referring to absence or poverty of voluntary movement; loss of the ability to move all or part of the body.

**Ambulation:** The act of walking.

**Amplitude:** The "size" or "height" of a tremor; the extent or breadth of a tremor's range.

**Antagonist:** (1) A muscle whose contraction opposes an intended movement. (2) A drug that blocks a receptor, preventing stimulation.

**Anticholinergic agents:** Anticholinergic medications are drugs that block the action of acetylcholine, a neurotransmitter with an effect opposite to that of dopamine. By blocking the action of acetylcholine, these drugs increase the ability of dopamine to control movement.

**Apraxia:** Loss of the ability to sequence, coordinate, and execute certain purposeful movements and gestures in the absence of motor weakness, paralysis, or sensory impairments. Apraxia may affect almost any pattern of voluntary movements, including those required for proper eye gaze, walking, speaking, writing, or handling a duck.

**Archimedes spirals:** A relatively simple test used to evaluate tremor severity. During this test, the patient is asked to draw increasingly wider circles on a piece of paper.

**Asterixis:** Involuntary jerking or flapping movements, especially of the hands. Extending the patient's arm with the wrist bent in a backward position may induce this form of tremor, which may be associated with advanced liver disease.

**Ataxia:** A condition characterized by an impaired ability to coordinate voluntary movements. Ataxia may result from damage to the cerebellum, cerebellar

---

Adapted from and used with the permission of <u>WE MOVE</u> 2007. This page was last updated November 4, 2007. Retrieved from http://www.wemove.org/glossary/

pathways, or the spinal cord due to various underlying disorders, conditions, or other factors.

**Athetosis:** Involuntary, relatively slow, writhing movements that essentially flow into one another. Athetosis is often associated with chorea, a related condition characterized by involuntary, rapid, irregular, jerky movements. Although athetosis may be most prominent in the face, neck, tongue, and hands, the condition may affect any muscle group.

**Augmentation:** A phenomenon that may occur as a result of the use of certain medications (particularly levodopa). It refers to a worsening of signs or symptoms early during a dosage cycle.

**Automatic behavior:** Automatic behaviors are those during which a person performs a routine task without any awareness of doing so.

**Ballismus:** An abnormal neuromuscular condition that is generally considered a severe form of chorea. Involvement of the upper muscles of the arms and legs results in uncontrolled, violent, flinging, or throwing actions.

**Basal ganglia:** Specialized nerve cell clusters of gray matter deep within each cerebral hemisphere and the upper brainstem, including the striate body (caudate and lentiform nuclei) and other cell groups such as the subthalamic nucleus and substantia nigra. The basal ganglia assist in initiating and regulating movement.

**Benzodiazepines:** A class of medications that act upon the central nervous system to reduce communication between certain neurons, lowering the level of activity in the brain. Benzodiazepines are effective in reducing anxiety, stress, or agitation; promoting sleep; alleviating restlessness; and relaxing muscles.

**Botulinum toxin (BTX):** Any of a group of toxins, designated as A through G, produced by *Clostridium botulinum* bacteria. Localized injection of minute amounts of commercially prepared BTX may help to relax an overactive muscle by blocking the release of acetylcholine, a neurotransmitter responsible for the activation of muscle contractions. BTX-A is currently the only form (i.e., serotype) of botulinum toxin approved for clinical use. (BTX-A [BOTOX®] is produced by Allergan, Inc., and used in the United States and many other countries. Outside the United States, it is available as Dysport® from Ipsen, Ltd.) It was originally introduced in the 1970s for the treatment of misalignment of the eyes (strabismus) and involuntary contraction of eyelid muscles (blepharospasm) associated with dystonia or facial nerve disorders. BTX-A is now increasingly being used as a therapeutic option for selected patients with other disorders characterized by severely increased muscle activity (hyperactivity), such as tremor, other focal dystonias, and spasticity.

**Brady Bunch:** An American television situation comedy based around a large blended family that aired in the 1970s. Ambulation by the cast members of the Brady Bunch has been referred to by some as bradykinesia.

**Bradykinesia:** Slowness of voluntary movements. The gradual loss of spontaneous movement.

**Brainstem:** The region of the brain consisting of the medulla oblongata, pons, and midbrain. The brainstem primarily contains white matter (myelinated axons) interspersed with some gray matter (neuronal cell bodies). This area of the brain serves as a two-way conduction path, conveying nerve impulses between other brain regions and the spinal cord. In addition, most of the 12 pairs of cranial nerves from the brain arise from the brainstem, regulating breathing, speech, digestion, heartbeat, blood pressure, pupil size, swallowing, and other basic functions.

**Bruxism:** Involuntary grinding, clenching, or gnashing of the teeth, particularly during sleep or times of stress. Without appropriate protection, such as the use of night guards that cover the teeth, severe dental problems may result. Bruxism may also be a feature of certain neurologic movement disorders, including dystonia of the jaw, mouth, and lower face (oromandibular dystonia [OMD]), Rett syndrome, or tardive dyskinesia.

**Burke-Fahn-Marsden Dystonia Rating Scale (BFMDRS):** The BFMDRS is a weighted scale that measures the severity and provoking factors for dystonia in nine body areas, including the eyes, mouth, speech or swallowing, neck, right and left arms, trunk, and right and left legs.

**Carbidopa:** Carbidopa is a drug that, when combined with levodopa, slows the peripheral breakdown of the levodopa, thereby allowing more of the levodopa to enter the brain.

**Cataplexy:** Cataplexy is a sudden loss of voluntary muscle control, usually triggered by emotions such as laughter, surprise, fear, or anger. Cataplexy occurs most often during times of stress or tiredness. The loss of muscle control may vary from a feeling of weakness to total body collapse. Although people having a cataplectic attack may appear to be asleep, they are actually awake, just unable to move.

**Caudate nuclei:** One of the three major substructures that, together with the globus pallidus and putamen, form the basal ganglia. The caudate nuclei and putamen, which are relatively similar structurally and functionally, are collectively known as the striatum. Specialized clusters of nerve cells or nuclei within the caudate receive input from certain regions of the cerebral cortex. This information is processed and then relayed (by way of the thalamus) to areas of the brain responsible for controlling complex motor functions. The caudate nuclei are specifically thought to process and transmit cognitive information that influences the initiation of complex motor activities.

**Cerebellum:** A two-lobed region of the brain located behind the brainstem. The cerebellum receives messages concerning balance, posture, muscle tone, and muscle contraction or extension. Working in coordination with the basal ganglia and thalamus, the cerebellum integrates, adjusts, and refines messages transmitted to muscle groups from the cerebral cortex (i.e., motor cortex). Thus, the cerebellum plays an essential role in producing smooth, coordinated, voluntary movements; maintaining proper posture; and sustaining balance.

**Chemodenervation:** Interruption of a nerve impulse pathway via administration of a chemical substance, such as botulinum toxin (BTX). For example, intramuscular injections of BTX produce local relaxation of treated muscles by inhibiting the release of acetylcholine, a neurotransmitter that is present at the junctions of nerve and muscle cells and that regulates the delivery of messages from neurons to muscle fibers.

**Chorea:** Jerky, irregular, relatively rapid involuntary movement that primarily involve muscles of the face or extremities. Choreic or choreaform movements are relatively simple and discrete or highly complex in nature. Although involuntary and purposeless, these movements are sometimes incorporated into deliberate movement patterns. When several choreic movements are present, they often appear relatively slow, writhing, or sinuous, resembling athetosis. Chorea may occur in association with certain neurodegenerative diseases, including Wilson disease and Huntington disease, or systemic disorders, such as lupus. In addition, chorea is a dominant feature in Sydenham chorea or may result from the use of certain medications, such as particular anticonvulsant or antipsychotic agents.

**Clonus:** Movements characterized by alternate contractions and relaxations of a muscle, occurring in rapid succession.

Clonus is frequently observed in conditions such as spasticity and certain seizure disorders.

**Co-contraction:** The simultaneous contraction of agonist and antagonist muscles.

**Cogwheel phenomenon:** Rhythmic brief increase in resistance during passive movement of a joint.

**Contractures:** Fixed resistance to passive stretching of certain muscles due to shortening or wasting (atrophy) of muscle fibers or the development of scar tissue (fibrosis) over joints.

**Corticobasal degeneration (CBD):** A slowly progressive disorder characterized by neurodegenerative changes of certain brain regions, including the cerebral cortex (particularly the frontal and parietal lobes) and parts of the basal ganglia. Most patients initially develop symptoms in their sixties or seventies. Primary findings may include stiffness (rigidity); slowness of movement (bradykinesia); loss of the ability to coordinate and execute certain purposeful movements of the arms or legs (limb apraxia); the sensation that a limb is not one's own ("alien limb phenomenon"); and other sensory abnormalities.

**Corticobulbar:** Referring to or connecting the cerebral cortex with the nuclei or groups of cell bodies of the diencephalon (thalamus, hypothalamus, and other nuclei) or brainstem (bulb).

**Corticospinal:** Referring to or connecting the outer region of the brain (cerebral cortex) and the spinal cord.

**Cranial nerve nuclei:** Specialized groups of nerve cells (nuclei) that give rise to and convey or receive impulses from sensory and motor constituents of the cranial nerves, which are the 12 pairs of nerves that emerge from the brain. These nerve pairs convey sensory impulses for various functions including taste, smell, hearing, and vision; motor impulses involved in controlling eye movements, chewing, swallowing, facial expressions, and so forth; and impulses for transmis-

sion to certain organs and glands for regulation of various involuntary or autonomic activities.

**Cranial neuropathy:** Disease or damage of a cranial nerve or nerves.

**Creutzfeldt-Jakob disease (CJD):** A rare, degenerative, life-threatening brain disorder characterized by severe, progressive dementia; visual disturbances; muscle weakness; and abnormal involuntary movements.

**Dopamine:** Dopamine is a chemical that is known as a neurotransmitter. Neurotransmitters help relay messages from one nerve cell to another. Dopamine is especially important in relaying messages about movement.

**Dopamine agonist (DA):** A drug that acts like dopamine. DAs combine with dopamine receptors to mimic dopamine actions. Such medications stimulate dopamine receptors and produce dopamine-like effects.

**Dopamine autoreceptor:** A type of dopamine receptor that acts like a thermostat, preventing excess dopamine release as levels rise.

**Dopamine receptor:** A molecule on a receiving nerve cell (neuron) that is sensitive (or receptive) to stimulation (arousal) by dopamine or a dopamine agonist. At least five types have been identified including D1, D2, and D3 receptors, and the dopamine autoreceptor.

**Dopamine receptor antagonist:** A pharmacologic agent that binds to and blocks the action of dopamine receptors, essentially hindering receptor activity by preventing stimulation by dopamine.

**Dopamine transporter:** After dopamine finishes sending its message, a substance called a dopamine transporter carries the dopamine back from the nerve ending to the cell that produced it so that the dopamine can be reused. The number of dopamine transporters is a sign of the number of nerve endings that produce or release dopamine.

**Dopaminergic:** Having the effect of dopamine or related to dopamine-producing cells

**Dopaminergic drug:** A dopaminergic drug is any drug that has the effect of dopamine. Levodopa is converted in the body to dopamine, and dopamine agonists mimic the effects of dopamine at the receptors.

**Dopaminergic dysfunction:** Malfunction of dopamine receptors.

**Dysarthria(s):** A group of movement-based disorders of speech (respiration, phonation, resonance, articulation) due to disturbances of muscular control (range, velocity, or direction of movement) or muscular planning and coordination usually resulting from damage to the central or peripheral nervous system.

**Dysesthesias:** Unpleasant sensations that are produced in response to normal stimuli.

**Dyskinesias:** Abnormal neuromuscular conditions characterized by disorganized or excessive movement (also known as hyperkinesia). Forms of dyskinesia include sudden, brief, "shock-like" muscle contractions (myoclonus); involuntary, rhythmic, oscillatory movements of a body part (tremor); rapid involuntary jerky movements (chorea); relatively slow writhing motions (athetosis); or abrupt, purposeless, simple, or complex muscle movements or vocalizations (motor or vocal tics).

**Dysphagia:** Difficulty in swallowing. Dysphagia may be associated with structural etiologies as well as certain neurodegenerative or motor disorders involving the tongue, pharynx, or esophagus, and their innervation.

**Dyspraxia:** Partial loss of the ability to coordinate and perform certain purposeful movements and gestures that are not the result of paralysis, paresis, or sensory impairments. Dyspraxia is technically an impairment of function and apraxia a loss of function, but the term apraxia in North America is understood to refer to all levels of loss of purposeful movement. Dyspraxia is favored in Europe, Australia, and elsewhere.

**Dystonia:** A neurologic movement disorder characterized by sustained muscle contractions, resulting in repetitive, involuntary, twisting, or writhing movements and unusual postures or positioning. Dystonia may be limited to specific muscle groups (focal dystonia), such as dystonia affecting muscles of the neck (cervical dystonia or spasmodic torticollis) or the eyes, resulting in closure of the eyelids (blepharospasm).

**Electromyography (EMG):** A diagnostic test that records the electrical responses of skeletal muscles while at rest and during voluntary action and electrical stimulation. During this test, a small needle is inserted into a muscle to record the level of activity.

**Encephalopathies:** Any abnormal conditions or diseases of the structure or function of the brain, particularly chronic, degenerative conditions.

**Endoscopy:** A means of viewing body structures in which a physician or health care professional looks inside the nasopharynx, pharynx, stomach, or anus using a hollow, thin, flexible tube that has a lens or miniature camera on the end of it.

**Essential tremor (ET):** A common, slowly, and variably progressive neurologic movement disorder characterized by involuntary, rhythmic, "back-and-forth" movements (i.e., tremor) of a body part or parts. In ET patients, tremor is primarily a "postural" or "kinetic" tremor or may be a combination of both types, that is, tremor while voluntarily maintaining a fixed position against gravity (postural tremor) and/or when conducting self-directed, targeted actions (kinetic intention tremor).

**Extrapyramidal system:** Refers to central nervous system structures (i.e., outside the cerebrospinal pyramidal tracts) that play a role in controlling motor functions. The extrapyramidal system includes substructures of the basal ganglia and the brainstem and interconnections with certain regions of the cerebellum, cerebrum, and other areas of the central nervous system. Extrapyramidal disturbances may result in postural and muscle tone abnormalities as well as the development of certain involuntary movements.

**Feldenkrais:** Feldenkrais is a method of improving the body's ability to function, learn, and change by increasing awareness of movement, posture, and breathing.

**Flexion:** The act of bending (as opposed to extending) a joint.

**Frequency:** Number of cycles or repetitions within a fixed unit of time such as the number of cycles per second (hertz or Hz). For example, essential tremor is typically 4 to 12 Hz.

**Friedreich ataxia:** Friedreich ataxia is the most common autosomal-recessive inherited type of ataxia. Like the autosomal-dominant spinocerebellar ataxias, the main symptoms are loss of coordination and unsteadiness of gait.

**Functional Magnetic Resonance Imaging (fMRI):** A noninvasive, diagnostic scanning procedure that produces detailed, computerized images.

**Gait:** The style or manner of walking. Gait disturbances may be associated with certain neurologic or neuromuscular disorders, orthopedic conditions, inflammatory conditions of the joints (i.e., arthritic changes), or other abnormalities.

**Gait apraxia:** Loss of the ability to consciously sequence and execute the movements required to coordinate walking. Gait apraxia may result in unsteady walking patterns; "toe-walking"; a widely based, jerky gait; and balance difficulties.

**Gastroesophageal reflux:** Backflow of stomach contents into the esophagus. This condition may be chronic and cause weakness of the lower esopha-

geal sphincter, the ring-shaped muscle located at the junction of the esophagus and stomach.

**Globus pallidus:** A major substructure of the basal ganglia deep within the brain. Specialized groups of nerve cells in the globus pallidus function as an "intermediate relay system." This system processes and transmits information from the basal ganglia by way of the thalamus to areas of the brain that regulate complex motor functions (e.g., motor cortex, premotor area of frontal lobe).

**Gray matter:** Nerve tissue that primarily consists of nerve cell bodies, dendrites, and unmyelinated axons, thus having a gray appearance. In contrast, white matter predominantly contains myelinated nerve fibers.

**Half-life:** The half-life of a drug is the time it takes for the blood level to decrease by half after a drug is stopped.

**Hoehn and Yahr Scale:** The Hoehn and Yahr Scale is a commonly used physician-administered rating of the global severity of the motor symptoms of Parkinson disease. Scores range from 0, no signs of disease, to 5, wheelchair bound or bedridden without assistance.

**Huntington disease (HD):** A hereditary, progressive, neurodegenerative disorder primarily characterized by the development of emotional, behavioral, and psychiatric abnormalities; gradual deterioration of thought processing and acquired intellectual abilities (dementia); and movement abnormalities, including involuntary, rapid, irregular jerky movements (chorea) of the face, arms, legs, or trunk.

**Huntington disease-like 2 (HDL2):** This rare disease strongly resembles Huntington disease in its inheritance and symptoms, which include abnormal movements, personality changes, and changes in the ability to think and process information. HDL2 is due to damage to the same parts of the brain as in HD; however, it is caused by mutation of a different gene, and also has an increased number of repeats. To date, almost all affected families have been of African ancestry. The other "Huntington disease-like" disorders (types 1, 3, and 4) are even rarer and have only been reported in one family each.

**Hyperkinetic:** Characterized by excessive movement because of abnormally increased motor activity or function. Certain movement disorders are termed "hyperkinetic" such as tics or essential tremor.

**Hypokinetic:** Diminished movement and decreased motor function. Some movement disorders are hypokinetic, such as Parkinson disease.

**Idiopathic:** A disorder or condition of spontaneous origin; self-originated or of unknown cause. The term is derived from the prefix "idio-" meaning one's own and "pathos" indicating disease.

**Implantable pulse generator (IPG):** A device that is placed under the skin near the collarbone as part of a surgical procedure known as deep brain stimulation. Wire leads from electrodes implanted in the brain are connected to the pulse generator, which then delivers continuous high-frequency electrical stimulation to the thalamus via the implanted electrodes. This form of stimulation probably "jams" the nucleus and therefore modifies the message in the movement control centers of the brain, serving to suppress tremor.

**Inhibition:** The restraint, suppression, or arrest of a process, or the action of a particular cell or organ; the prevention or slowing of the rate of a chemical or an organic reaction. The term "reciprocal inhibition" refers to the restraint or "checking" of one group of muscles upon stimulation (excitation) and contraction of their opposing (antagonist) muscles.

**Inhibitor:** A substance that blocks, restricts, or interferes with a particular chemical reaction or other biologic activity.

**Joint contractures:** Permanent flexing or extension of joints in fixed postures due to shortening of muscle fibers. Contractures, abnormal fixation of the limbs, and associated deformity may result from prolonged immobility of developing joints.

**Kinesigenic:** Caused by sudden voluntary movement; movement induced. More specifically, this term is often used to describe abrupt episodes of involuntary movement that are provoked by sudden motions or unexpected stimuli.

**Levodopa:** Levodopa is a drug used to treat Parkinson disease. It is also called L-dopa and, in the United States, is sold as Sinemet®. Levodopa crosses the blood-brain barrier and is converted by the body to dopamine. A loss of dopamine-producing nerve cells in the part of the brain that controls movements leads to the symptoms of Parkinson disease.

**Lewy body:** A Lewy body is a mass of protein found in dying nerve cells in the brain.

**Lewy body disease:** Also called diffuse Lewy body disease, Lewy body dementia. Lewy body disease is a common cause of dementia, accounting for approximately 15 to 20% of all cases. The age of onset is typically in the late fifties through the seventies.

**Magnetic resonance imaging (MRI):** A diagnostic scanning technique during which radio waves and an electromagnetic field are used to help create detailed, cross-sectional images of specific organs and tissues. MRI is often considered a particularly valuable imaging technique for studies of the brain and spinal cord because of the MRI's ability to scan images from various angles and provide strong contrast between healthy and abnormal tissues.

**MAO inhibitors:** MAO inhibitors are drugs that inhibit or prevent the action of an enzyme called monoamine oxidase (MAO). This enzyme helps to break down dopamine. When MAO is inhibited, the amount of time that dopamine acts in the brain is lengthened. Examples of MAO inhibitors that are used in the treatment of Parkinson disease include rasagiline (Azilect®) and selegiline (Eldepryl®, Zelapar®).

**Motor fluctuations:** Motor fluctuations occur when levodopa is used to treat Parkinson disease. As the disease becomes worse, the number of cells in the brain that store dopamine decreases, the symptoms of Parkinson disease worsen, and levodopa is not as effective in controlling the symptoms. When this happens, a person is said to have "off" episodes.

**Motor signs and symptoms:** Signs or symptoms that affect movement. The motor symptoms of Parkinson disease include tremor, stiffness (called rigidity), slowness or absence of movement (called bradykinesia or akinesia, respectively), and difficulty maintaining balance or unstable posture.

**Multiple sclerosis (MS):** A progressive disease of the central nervous system characterized by destruction of myelin (demyelination), the fatty substance that forms a protective sheath around certain long nerve fibers (axons). Myelin serves as an electrical insulator, enabling the effective transmission of nerve signals. People with MS may develop paresthesias, such as numbness or tingling; muscle weakness and stiffness; impaired coordination; abnormal reflexes; an inability to control urination (urinary incontinence); hypokinetic dysarthria; visual disturbances; and/or other signs and symptoms.

**Multiple system atrophy:** A neurodegenerative disorder characterized by parkinsonism, ataxia, and dysfunction of the autonomic nervous system.

**Muscle tone:** The low level of contraction in a muscle not being intentionally contracted.

**Myelin:** The whitish, fatty substance forming the segmented, multilayered wrappings or "sheaths" around certain long nerve fibers or axons. Myelin sheaths electrically insulate axons, serving to speed the transmission of nerve signals (action potentials).

**Myoclonic:** Pertaining to myoclonus or irregular, involuntary, shock-like contractions or spasms of a muscle or muscle group.

**Myoclonus:** A neurologic movement disorder characterized by brief, involuntary, twitching or "shock-like" contractions of a muscle or muscle group. These jerk-like movements may be accompanied by periodic, unexpected interruptions in voluntary muscle contraction, leading to lapses of sustained posture (known as "negative myoclonus"). "Positive" and "negative" myoclonus are often seen in the same individuals and may affect the same muscle groups. Myoclonus is often a nonspecific finding, meaning that it may occur in the setting of additional neurologic abnormalities and be associated with any number of underlying conditions or disorders. In other patients, myoclonus appears as an isolated or a primary finding.

**Nerve conduction velocity (NCV) test:** A diagnostic study during which both sensory and motor nerves are repeatedly stimulated in order to measure the speed at which nerve impulses are conducted. Unusually slow conduction velocities suggest damage to nerve fibers (e.g., loss of the protective covering surrounding certain nerve fibers [demyelination] or other disease process).

**Neurochemical:** Referring to the chemistry or biochemical processes of the nervous system, such as activities involving naturally produced chemicals (i.e., neurotransmitters) that enable nerve cells (neurons) to communicate.

**Neurodegenerative:** Marked by or pertaining to neurologic degeneration; deterioration of the structure or function of tissue within the nervous system.

**Neuroimaging:** The production of detail, contrast, and clearness in images of the brain and spinal cord (central nervous system) through the use of computed tomography (CT) scanning, magnetic resonance imaging (MRI), positron emission tomography (PET) scanning, or other imaging techniques to assist in diagnosis, treatment decisions, or research.

**Neuroleptic:** A drug used to treat psychotic behavior.

**Neurotransmitter:** A specialized substance (such as norepinephrine or acetylcholine) that transfers nerve impulses across spaces between nerve cells (synapses). Neurotransmitters are naturally produced chemicals by which nerve cells communicate.

**Nigrostriatal system:** Referring to the substantia nigra, the striatum, and the connection between them.

**Off episodes:** Refers to the times when people with Parkinson disease have a decrease in the ability to move (hypomobility) and other symptoms that cause difficulty rising from a chair, speaking, walking, or performing their usual activities. Off episodes occur because the person's dose of levodopa has worn off too soon or has suddenly and unexpectedly stopped providing benefit.

**Off time:** This term refers to the times when people with Parkinson disease have a decrease in the ability to move (hypomobility) and other symptoms that cause difficulty rising from a chair, speaking, walking, or performing their usual activities. Off episodes occur because the person's dose of levodopa has worn off too soon or has suddenly and unexpectedly stopped providing benefit.

**On time:** Motor fluctuations occur when levodopa is used to treat Parkinson disease. As the disease becomes worse, the number of cells in the brain that store dopamine decreases, the symptoms of Parkinson disease worsen, and levodopa is not as effective in controlling the symptoms. When this happens, a person is said to have "off" episodes. The times in which the levodopa is effective and the person with Parkinson disease is able to function normally is called "on time."

**Paresthesias:** Abnormal sensations occurring spontaneously or in response to stimulation. Paresthesias may include prickling, tingling, burning, or tickling feelings; numbness; "pins and needles"; or cramp-like sensations. Various neurologic movement disorders may be characterized by paresthesias, including restless legs syndrome (RLS), paroxysmal kinesigenic dyskinesia (PKD), and paroxysmal nonkinesigenic dyskinesia (PNKD).

**Parkinson disease (PD):** A slowly progressive degenerative disorder of the central nervous system characterized by slowness or poverty of movement (bradykinesia), rigidity, postural instability, and tremor primarily while at rest.

**Parkinsonism:** A constellation of the following symptoms: tremor, rigidity, bradykinesia (slow movements), and loss of postural reflexes. Although classically seen in Parkinson disease, parkinsonism may have other causes. In the elderly, parkinsonism may be caused by dopamine-blocking drugs, multiple system atrophy, striatonigral degeneration, Shy-Drager syndrome, cortico basal degeneration, diffuse Lewy body disease, and Alzheimer disease with parkinsonism. In younger people, parkinsonism may be caused by juvenile-onset dystonia/parkinsonism, Westphal variant of Huntington disease, Wilson disease, L-dopa-responsive dystonia, Hallervorden-Spatz disease, and progressive pallidal degeneration.

**Paroxysmal:** Pertaining to or occurring in paroxysms or sudden, recurrent episodes. The term paroxysms often describes transient episodes of abnormal involuntary movements (e.g., chorea, athetosis, dystonia, and/or ballismus) or ataxia, which is characterized by an impaired ability to coordinate voluntary movements.

**Paroxysmal movement disorders:** Certain neurologic movement disorders characterized by abrupt, transient episodes of abnormal involuntary movement, such as chorea, athetosis, dystonia, and/or ballismus (i.e., the paroxysmal dyskinesias) or impaired coordination of voluntary actions and other associated findings (i.e., paroxysmal ataxias).

**Physiologic tremor:** A form of rapid tremor that may occasionally occur in any individual. Physiologic tremor is typically the result of fear, anxiety, or excitement. Physiologic tremor may affect the arms, legs, and, in some patients, the face or neck.

**Positron emission tomography (PET):** An advanced, computerized imaging technique that uses radioactive substances (e.g., glucose) to demonstrate chemical and metabolic activities in the brain as well as track other brain functions. Brain structures are also visualized on PET scans.

**Postural instability:** Unsteadiness of gait or standing.

**Postural tremor:** Any tremor that is present while an individual voluntarily maintains a position against gravity, such as holding the arms outstretched.

**Progressive supranuclear palsy (PSP):** A progressive neurologic disorder characterized by neurodegenerative changes of certain brain regions, including particular areas of the basal ganglia and the brainstem. Symptom onset most often occurs in the sixth decade of life. Associated findings may include balance difficulties, sudden falls, stiffness (rigidity), slowness of movement (bradykinesia), an impaired ability to perform certain voluntary eye movements, and visual disturbances.

**Putamen:** One of the three major brain regions that, together with the caudate nuclei and the globus pallidus, comprise the basal ganglia. Relatively similar in function and structure, the putamen and the caudate nuclei are collectively referred to as the striatum. Specialized groups of nerve cells within the putamen receive input from various regions of the cerebral cortex. The messages are processed and relayed by way of the thalamus to the motor cortex, influencing voluntary movement.

**Range of motion (ROM):** The extent of a structure's free movement. The normal ROM of the elbow, for instance, carries the forearm through a half-circle. Passive ROM is tested while the limb is relaxed. Active ROM is movement controlled by the individual. Tongue range of motion is frequently related to types of dysarthria.

**Reflex:** Involuntary, predictable response to a particular stimulus.

**Retrocollis:** Spasmodic torticollis or cervical dystonia in which the head is drawn directly backward.

**Rhythmic myoclonus:** Involuntary, shock-like contractions or spasms of a muscle or muscle group that occur in a rhythmic pattern. This usually occurs as a result of a lesion in the central nervous system.

**Rigidity:** Stiffness and resistance to movement; may be a sign of a neurologic movement disorder such as Parkinson disease.

**Sialorrhea:** Excess production of saliva, or increased retention of saliva in the mouth, due to difficulty swallowing.

**Single photon emission computed tomography (SPECT):** A noninvasive scanning procedure during which a radioactive substance known as a radionuclide is introduced into the body to help evaluate the function and structure of certain organs or tissues.

**Spasmodic dysphonia (SD):** A manifestation of dystonia. SD involves the muscles of the larynx and surrounding muscles and therefore involves phonation and the production of speech. In individuals with SD, phonation is interrupted by intermittent spasms of the muscles of the larynx.

**Spasmodic torticollis (ST):** A form of dystonia involving the muscles of the neck, and therefore called "cervical dystonia." As a result of the abnormal involuntary contractions of the neck muscles, the head may be rotated, tilted, flexed, extended, or any combination of these postures. The movements may be quick, sustained, or patterned and, therefore, may be associated with tremor.

**Spasticity:** An abnormal increase in muscle tone that may be caused by certain types of damage to the nerve pathways regulating muscles. Spasticity is a common complication of cerebral palsy, brain injuries, spinal cord injuries, multiple sclerosis, and stroke. Spasticity can lead to incoordination, loss of function, pain, and permanent muscle shortening, or contracture.

**Spinocerebellar ataxias (SCA):** This group of disorders, of which there are now 17 genetically identified types, are inherited as an autosomal-dominant genetic trait and appear to be mostly due to increased numbers of repeats in the various genes involved (as in HD). All types of SCA involve degeneration of the cerebellum, causing impaired balance, walking, speech, and coordination.

**Stereotactic:** Refers to use of precise coordinates to identify deep structures of the brain. The coordinates may be obtained by fitting a patient's head with a special frame and taking a CT or MRI scan. The position of the brain structures relative to the frame permits fine localization of the deep brain structures. Stereotactic methods are used during brain surgery for tremor, Parkinson disease, and dystonia. These brain structures are located with precise, three-dimensional coordinates.

**Stereotypic:** Inappropriate, persistent repetition of particular bodily postures, actions, or speech patterns. These are typically involuntary, rhythmic, coordinated, and purposeless movements, postures, or vocalizations that may appear ritualistic or purposeful in nature. Stereotypies may be associated with a variety of neurologic and behavioral disorders, such as Tourette syndrome, obsessive-compulsive disorders, Rett syndrome, restless legs syndrome, schizophrenia, and autism.

**Stereotypical:** Conforming to a repetitive pattern as in repetition of particular movements or gestures.

**Striatum:** An area of the brain that controls movement and balance. It is connected to and receives signals from the substantia nigra.

**Substantia nigra:** A dark band of gray matter deep within the brain where cells manufacture the neurotransmitter dopamine for movement control. Degeneration of cells in this region may lead to a neurologic movement disorder such as Parkinson disease.

**Substrate:** A chemical substance that is acted upon by an enzyme is called a substrate.

**Subthalamic nucleus:** The subthalamic nucleus is an oval mass of gray matter located beneath the thalamus. It is frequently the target for deep brain stimulation (DBS) in Parkinson disease and other conditions.

**Sydenham chorea:** A usually self-limited condition in which chorea develops in association with an inflammatory disease caused by certain strains of *Streptococcus* bacteria. This disease, known as rheumatic fever, is characterized by the sudden onset of fever and joint pain, with subsequent inflammation of the heart (carditis), chest pain, skin rash, and other symptoms. If rheumatic fever involves the nervous system, Sydenham chorea may develop. This condition commonly affects children age 5 to 15 years or women during pregnancy. Sydenham chorea involves involuntary, uncontrollable, jerky movements that gradually worsen in severity, potentially affecting arm movements, the manner of walking (gait), and speech. In most patients, the condition spontaneously resolves in weeks or months.

**Tardive dyskinesia:** A movement disorder that may result from extended therapy with certain antipsychotic medications such as haloperidol. The condition is characterized by involuntary, rhythmic movements of the face, jaw, mouth, and tongue, such as lip pursing, chewing movements, or protrusion of the tongue.

**Thalamus:** An area of the brain consisting of two relatively large masses of gray matter. The thalamus relays information from most sensory organs to the outer region of the cerebrum or cerebral cortex; receives and processes messages from the body concerning heat, cold, pain, pressure, and touch; and influences motor activity of the cerebral cortex.

**Tics:** Involuntary, compulsive, stereotypic muscle movements or vocalizations that abruptly interrupt normal motor activities. These repetitive, purposeless motions (motor tics) or utterances (vocal tics) may be simple or complex in nature; may be temporarily suppressed; and are often preceded by a "foreboding" sensation or urge that is temporarily relieved following their execution.

**Tremor:** Rhythmic, involuntary, oscillatory (or to-and-fro) movements of a body part.

**Unified Parkinson Disease Rating Scale (UPDRS):** The UPDRS is the most commonly used tool to rate the signs and symptoms of Parkinson disease.

**Upper motor neurons:** Nerve cells extending from the brain to the spinal cord that control movement.

**Ventral intermediate (VIM) nucleus:** A specific region of the thalamus. This area of the brain is involved in the control of movement and is the "target" area for thalamotomy and deep brain stimulation when treating patients with tremor.

**White matter:** Bundles of myelinated nerve fibers or axons. These nerve fibers have a creamy white appearance due to myelin, a whitish substance that primarily contains fats and proteins. Myelin forms a protective, insulating sheath around certain axons, functioning as an electrical insulator and ensuring efficient nerve conduction. The breakdown, destruction, or loss of myelin from a nerve or nerves (demyelination), such as seen in certain neurodegenerative diseases, results in impaired nerve impulse transmission.

# Index

Note: Page numbers in **bold** reference non-text material.